Persistent and Slow Virus Infections

Monographs in Virology

Vol. 3

Editor: J.L. MELNICK, Houston

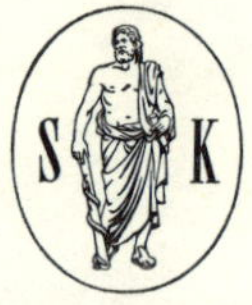

S. Karger · Basel · München · Paris · London · New York · Sydney

Persistent and Slow Virus Infections

JOHN HOTCHIN
Division of Laboratories and Research,
New York State Department of Health, Albany, N. Y.

With 26 figures and 11 tables

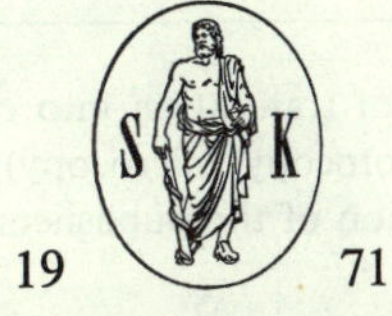

1971

S. Karger · Basel · München · Paris · London · New York · Sydney

Monographs in Virology

Vol. 1: HAMRE, D. (Chicago, Ill.): Rhinoviruses.
VIII + 88 p., 5 fig., 34 tab., 1968. sFr. 20.50

Vol. 2: KIT, S. and DUBBS, D.R. (Houston, Tex.): Enzyme Induction by Viruses.
X + 114 p., 7 fig., 11 tab., 1969. sFr. 27.–

S. Karger · Basel · München · Paris · London · New York · Sydney
Arnold-Böcklin-Strasse 25, CH–4000 Basel 11 (Switzerland)

Preface

This monograph by JOHN HOTCHIN represents an up-to-date review concerning presistent and slow virus infections. Included is a comprehensive bibliography of approximately 1200 references. The viruses capable of persisting within the infected host for long periods of time, sometimes for the life of the host, are heterogeneous in many respects, but there are important points of similarity. Their importance in a wide range of human and animal diseases is increasingly becoming recognized. It is not too much to conjecture that they may play a role in still other chronic degenerative diseases whose etiology is as yet unknown. Most appropriately the current status and future prospects of this fascinating and significant field are discussed in this volume by one of its pioneers, whose investigations, particularly in lymphocytic choriomeningitis, have contributed much toward moving the field forward and opening up new areas for its study.

As announced previously, suitable manuscripts in active areas of virus research for this series are welcomed by the editor. However, investigators who wish to submit material for a monograph are requested to make prior arrangements with the editor.

JOSEPH L. MELNICK

Acknowledgements

The author wishes to gratefully acknowledge the help he received from many friends during the complex and sometimes frustrating task of compiling and digesting the data for this monograph. Among others these include MARY CLARK, LOIS BENSON, DAGMAR MICHALOVA, ELIZABETH SEYMOUR, EDWARD SIKORA, WILLIAM KINCH, PEGGY and JENNIFER HOTCHIN. Drs. HUGH WEBB and CHARLES PFAU kindly read the LCM section, and specialized bibliographies were graciously supplied by Drs. M. C. CLARKE, R. L. CHANDLER, CARLETON GAJDUSEK, MARGRET GUDNADÓTTIR, WILLIAM HADLOW, JAMES B. HANSHAW, DONALD HARTER, J. H. LARSEN, I. H. PATTISON, RICHARD KIMBERLIN, NEVILLE STANLEY and HALLDOR THORMAR.

Contents

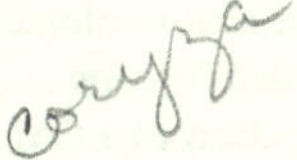

To ERIC TRAUB who started the whole thing

Introduction

It has become increasingly clear that the persistent viruses constitute an important, numerous and variegated group, which is responsible for a wide range of human and animal diseases. At the present time it is impossible to judge the limit of pathological effects of these viruses, which appear to involve the entire field of medicine. The close relationship between persistent virus infection and slow virus disease is self-evident. The spectrum of action of these agents suggests that no realm of biology is free from their impact. Although theoretically many cancer viruses qualify as persistent, they are excluded from this review, which will be confined to animal agents which are not usually regarded as tumorigenic and which can be readily isolated over a period of months from the infected host.

Arenaviruses

Lymphocytic Choriomeningitis

Lymphocytic choriomeningitis (LCM) virus has several claims as the primary model system of persistent virus infection. TRAUB's [1935a, b, 1936a, b, c] early studies of LCM constituted the first description of a persistent animal virus and stimulated BURNET and FENNER [1949] to suggest the concept of immunological tolerance as an explanation for the behavior of LCM virus in mice. This virus was last comprehensively reviewed by FARMER and JANEWAY in 1942, although VOLKERT and LARSEN [1965c] recently reviewed the question of tolerance to it and SCHEID [1957] has reviewed its neurological aspects. The findings of the many workers who have studied the pathogenesis of LCM appear to this writer to form the basis of a working concept of the mechanism of persistent infection which is used in this monograph as a basis of comparison for other persistent virus infections. The group is defined as those infections in which free virus is readily found, (without recourse to technics such as tissue culture or administration of immunosuppressive agents), for a period of months, in some or all tissues of the host.

Properties of LCM Virus

History

The discovery of LCM was made by ARMSTRONG and LILLIE [1934] on November 2, 1933, [KREIS, 1937] during investigation of the 1933 St. Louis encephalitis (SLE) epidemic, as a monkey isolate derived from a fatal human case. The agent behaved like SLE virus for five monkey passages, and since the final monkey had been immunized against SLE, it seems likely that the LCM originated from one of the monkeys and did not in fact arise from the human case. This possibility is supported by the isolation of LCM virus from tissue culture of an infected monkey by COUGHLIN and WHITNEY [1957]. In 1935 TRAUB [1935a, 1935b] isolated LCM virus from mice which had become sick only after intracerebral (IC) inoculation with sterile broth, and also from the blood of the animal caretaker who looked after the LCM-infected mice. Thus, very early in its history LCM demonstrated its now notorious propensity for inducing airborne laboratory infection. The virus was reported by ARMSTRONG and LILLIE [1934] and by TRAUB [1935b] to cause latent infection in mice.

BURNET and FENNER [1949] first drew attention to the possibility that LCM induced immunological tolerance in the host during intrauterine infection acquired from the mother. This concept was based on TRAUB's extensive work [1935a, b, 1936a, b, c, 1937, 1938a, b, 1939; TRAUB and SCHAFER, 1939] on the pathogenesis of this virus disease in mice.

Nomenclature and Classification

TRAUB pointed out [1936c] that the name lymphocytic choriomeningitis does not describe the disease naturally occurring in mice, since choriomeningitis is rare in such animals and naturally infected mice usually show no symptoms at all. The name applies mainly to the results of IC inoculation of mice and the meningitic complication of the human disease. The name *Armlillia erebea* was proposed [MERCHANT, 1961] for LCM but does not appear to have been used. The virus called pseudo-lymphocytic choriomeningitis [MACCALLUM *et al.*, 1939] appears to have been a strain of ectromelia [MACCALLUM *et al.*, 1957]. LCM virus has been experimentally transmitted by various bloodsucking insects [VIGOVSKII and GUTSEVICH, 1962] including the Rocky Mountain wood tick (*Dermacentor andersoni, Stiles*) [SHAUGHNESSY and MILZER, 1939], mosquitoes (*Aedes aegypti*) [COGGLESHELL, 1939], bedbugs *(Cimex lectularius)* [MILZER, 1942], fleas [FEDOROV and IGOLKIN, 1959] and trichinella spiralis nematodes [SYVERTON *et al.*, 1947] and grows in insect tissue cultures [REHÁČEK, 1965]. LCM can be regarded as an arthropodborne virus, and it has been suggested [SHAUGHNESSY and MILZER, 1939] that other blood sucking arthropods such as culicine mosquitoes, stable flies and body lice may transmit LCM from rodent to rodent and possibly to man. LCM pathogenesis reveals some resemblance to the mouse hepatitis virus group [GLEDHILL and SEAMER, 1960; SEAMER *et al.*, 1961]. However, LCM is capable of growing in many species of animals, fertile eggs, and tissue cultures in which mouse hepatitis virus will not grow. Both of these agents show a common, unexplained potentiation by coincident infection with the harmless murine blood parasite *Eperythrozoon coccoides* [GLEDHILL and SEAMER, 1960; GLEDHILL *et al.*, 1960; SEAMER *et al.*, 1961]. Recent work (see 'Physical and chemical properties') indicates that LCM is a lipoprotein-enveloped RNA virus with some similarities to the myxovirus group. The finding of multiple discrete electron-dense bodies within the virion gives a unique appearance, and the identical appearance of the Machupo-Tacaribe group [MURPHY *et al.*, 1969] and Lassa virus [BUCKLEY and CASALS, 1970; FRAME *et al.*, 1970; LEIFER *et al.*, 1970] suggests that LCM and these agents constitute a distinct new group. CASALS (personal communication) has found tentative evidence of some reciprocal complement-fixation (CF) cross reaction between Lassa, LCM and some Tacaribe strains. It has been proposed, on the basis of these and other findings, that this group be called the arenaviruses [ROWE *et al.*, 1970].

Strain Differences

TRAUB [1936a] showed that different strains of mice varied in the degree to which they became persistently infected with virus and that different strains of virus varied in pathogenicity. Similar results have been well established since then by other workers for both host [HOTCHIN and WEIGAND, 1961a; HOTCHIN and BENSON, 1963; ROGER and ROGER, 1963a, b, 1964a; HOTCHIN and COLLINS, 1964; VOLKERT and LARSEN, 1964; OLDSTONE and DIXON, 1968a, 1969] and virus [TRAUB, 1938a, 1960a; SCHWARTZMAN, 1946; HOTCHIN and WEIGAND, 1961a; HOTCHIN *et al.*, 1962; HOTCHIN and BENSON, 1963]. Strains of virus which have been passaged to develop viscerotropic properties readily induce tolerance, whereas those which have been passed in the brain, and are regarded as neurotropic, tend not to induce tolerance, but to kill newborn mice [HOTCHIN *et al.*, 1962]. Lethal strains were referred to as aggressive, and non-lethal as docile. Most wild strains of LCM virus are the docile or tolerance-inducing type. In spite of the occurrence of strains of LCM of different pathogenicity, no serologically distinct variants have been described, and all strains share common CF and neutralizing antigens [WILSNACK and ROWE, 1964; LEHMANN-GRUBE, 1964a, b; BENDA *et al.*, 1965]. One strain designated 'MP' virus [MOLOMUT *et al.*, 1965] has been shown to react in CF [MOLOMUT and PADNOS, 1965], mouse cross-protection, neutralization and footpad (FP) tests in the same way as LCM virus[1] and therefore it appears to be a strain of LCM. On the oth-

---

[1] J. HOTCHIN, unpublished results.

er hand, PADNOS *et al.* [1968] also reported that the MP strain produced a hemagglutinin for sheep red blood cells (SRBC) in serum and organs of infected mice [MOLOMUT and PADNOS, 1965; PADNOS *et al.*, 1968]. However, it was admitted by the authors that the mouse sera contained natural antibody to SRBC, and that the MP strain of LCM merely increased this existing SRBC hemagglutinin. The hemagglutinin was absent from the sera of tolerant mice. The hemagglutinating ability of the MP virus is therefore not comparable to other viral hemagglutinins, but appears to be related to an adjuvant-like property of the virus to enhance non-specific immunity. In all other respects, this strain behaves like LCM virus, and control mice used at the time of the original isolation were positive for LCM by CF test, suggesting that they carried LCM [MOLOMUT *et al.*, 1965; PADNOS *et al.*, 1968]. The biological, biochemical and biophysical properties of three LCM virus strains were compared by CAMYRE and PFAU [1968]. It was found that, although clearly belonging to the same group, the strains differed in terms of their stability to different physical agents. No difference could be detected between the virus from tolerant and acutely infected mice in terms of sedimentation, RNase susceptibility or neutralization [VOLKERT *et al.*, 1964].

Physical and Chemical Properties

The size of LCM virus was first determined by SCOTT and ELFORD [1939] to be 37 to 55 nm by centrifugation studies, while ultrafiltration gave a particle size of 40–60 nm. The virus can be separated from a soluble antigen by centrifugation [SMADEL *et al.*, 1939a]. PFAU [1965a] found it to be unstable in density gradients of RbCl or CsCl, but surviving virus was found in two bands at densities of 1.15 and 1.24. Morphological studies by DALTON *et al.* [1968] suggested that LCM virus was a pleomorphic agent with a variable size range from 50 to greater than 200 nm. While it usually appeared to be spherical, it was often cup-shaped. All the particles were found to contain 1 to 8 or more electron dense granules which were removed by ribonuclease. The virus particles were formed by budding from the plasma membrane and appeared to have spikes. These findings have been confirmed by ABELSON *et al.* [1969], who used peroxidase-labeled anti-virus sera to locate the virions by light and electron microscopy, and by KAJIMA [1970] (fig. 1). Electron microscopy of the MP strain was reported by PADNOS *et al.* [1968] to show spherical particles 80 nm in diameter, having a double limiting membrane with a corona of attached particles 10 nm in diameter.

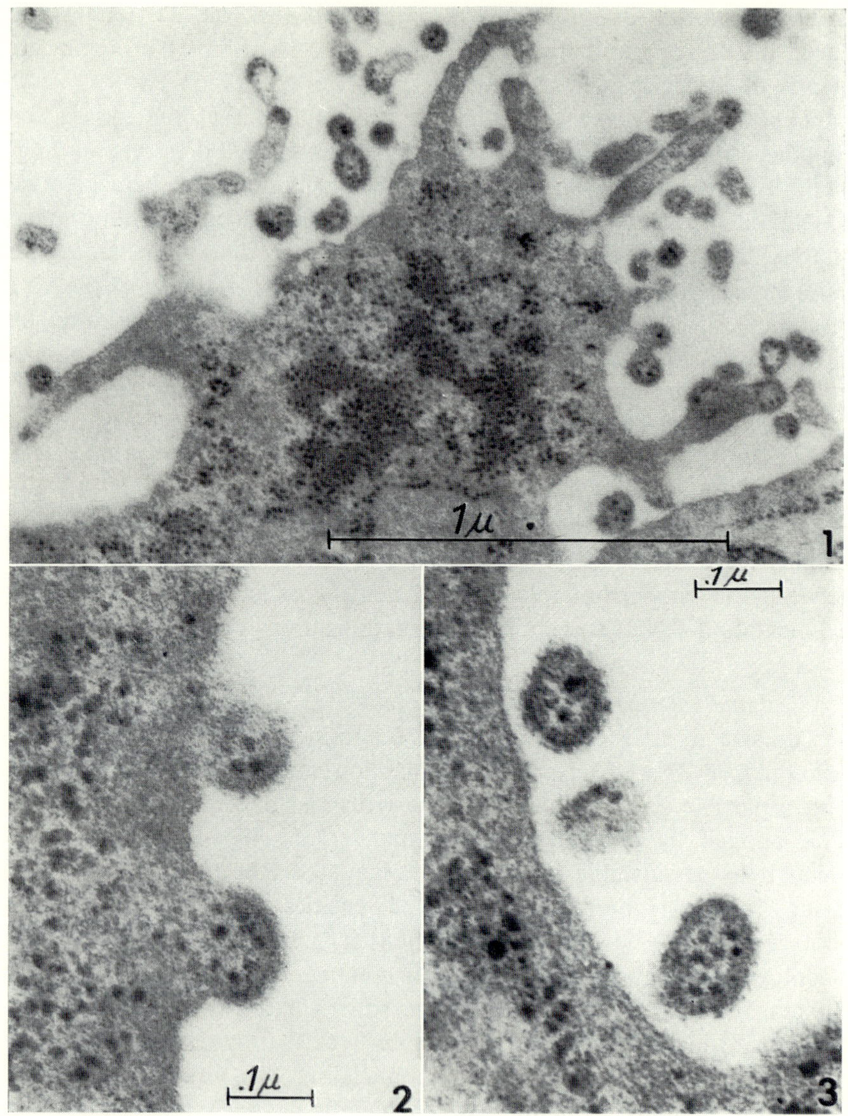

Fig. 1. Electron micrographs showing thin sections of Earle's strain L-929 cells infected with LCM strain CA1371. Virus particles can be seen budding from the cell surface, and electron dense bodies (20 nm) can be seen inside both cells and mature virus particles. Reproduced by permission of Dr. MASAHIRO KAJIMA. Figure 1.1 ×53,000. Figures 1.2 and 1.3 ×150,000.

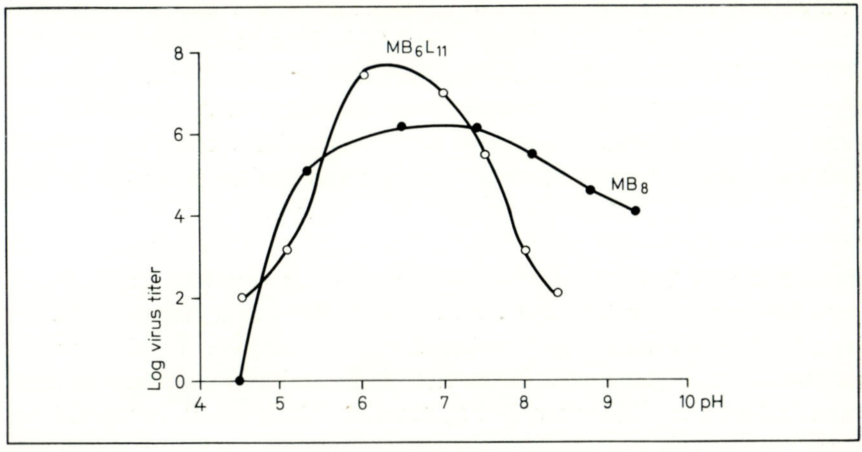

Fig. 2. Titer of LCM virus relative to pH after addition of citrate or borate buffer. pH measurements were made after mixing.

LCM virus is inactivated by soaps, detergents, ether [STOCK *et al.*, 1943; ANDREWES and HORSTMANN, 1949], merthiolate [ROGERS, 1951], pH 3 [PADNOS *et al.*, 1968] and divalent cations [PFAU and CAMYRE, 1968]. Although some conflicting evidence exists [MOLOMUT *et al.*, 1965], 0.05 to 0.005 M Tris buffer has a stabilizing effect, provided the solution contains large amounts of protein [PFAU, 1966]. Resuspension of virus pellets in 8.5% sucrose after centrifuging was found to increase the recovery [PFAU, 1965b]. Stabilization by haemaccel was also reported [LEHMANN-GRUBE, 1968]. The virus can be precipitated with methanol and eluted in phosphate buffered saline (PBS) with a fifty-fold concentration [PEDERSEN, 1966]. However, this virus is by ordinary standards very unstable to most purification procedures [PFAU and CAMYRE, 1967; LEHMANN-GRUBE, 1968]. At 37° C in tissue culture fluid the half-life was found[2] to be approximately 5 h, and at 56° C a 20% liver suspension in PBS showed an inactivation curve equivalent to a half-life of 2.1 min[2]; pH stability[3] is shown in figure 2.

In tissue culture the growth of LCM was not limited by halodeoxyuridines [BARLOW and KELLER, 1964a, 1965; BARLOW *et al.*, 1965a, b; PFAU *et al.*, 1965; FURUSAWA *et al.*, 1964], which are traditional inhibitors

[2] J. HOTCHIN, unpublished results.
[3] J. HOTCHIN and E. SIKORA, unpublished results.

of the synthesis of DNA-containing viruses. However, it was found by PFAU and CAMYRE [1968] to be inhibited by 2-(α-hydroxybenzyl)-benzimidazole (HBB) which was believed to selectively inhibit only the picornaviruses. However, unlike the HBB-sensitive picornaviruses, LCM virus multiplication was not inhibited by guanidine HCl. *In vitro* studies also showed that the antiviral agent 1, 3-bis (2-chloroethyl) 1-nitrosourea (BCNU) is active against LCM [SIDWELL *et al.*, 1966]. Some inhibition of LCM replication occurs with the addition of actinomycin D and 6-azauridine; the implications of this for the possible role of DNA template function during LCM replication have been discussed by BUCK and PFAU [1969]. Infected cells stain orange with acridine orange, in a pattern which is similar to the distribution of antigen visualized by indirect immunofluorescence microscopy [BARLOW *et al.*, 1965b]. The general conclusion of these studies was that LCM is an RNA virus. The NY 621 strain was reported [FURUSAWA *et al.*, 1967] to be susceptible to inhibition by a plant extract 'Propionin' when tested in mice but not when adapted in KB cell tissue culture. However, the tissue culture strain is not LCM virus but appears to belong to the picornavirus group [PFAU and CAMYRE, 1968].

Contamination of Viruses with LCM

LCM virus has been repeatedly found as a contaminant of other systems, starting with the initial isolate of the virus by ARMSTRONG and LILLIE [1934] as a contaminant of SLE virus. Other instances include LCM virus contamination of canine distemper [DALLDORF and DOUGLASS, 1938; DALLDORF, 1939a], mycoplasma [FINDLAY *et al.*, 1938] which it potentiates sufficiently to cause murine 'rolling disease', rabies virus [CASALS-ARIET and WEBSTER, 1940; WIKTOR *et al.*, 1965, 1966], murine poliovirus [WENNER, 1948], lymphosarcoma [DEBRUYN, 1949], Ehrlich carcinoma [MOLOMUT *et al.*, 1965; PADNOS *et al.*, 1968], leukemia [STEWART and HAAS, 1956], guinea pig leukemia [JUNGEBLUT and KODZA, 1963] and Toxoplasma gondii [VERMEIL, 1956].

Tissue Culture

LCM virus has been found to grow in most of the tissue culture systems tested including minced mouse [HOTCHIN and CINITS, 1958; ACKERMANN, 1960; BENSON *et al.*, 1960; BENDA and ČINÁTL, 1962; MOLOMUT and PADNOS, 1965], chick embryo [MACCALLUM and FINDLAY, 1940; HOTCHIN, 1958; HOTCHIN and CINITS, 1958; BENSON and HOTCHIN, 1960; DEIBEL *et al.*, 1964; WIKTOR *et al.*, 1966], mouse macrophages

[SEAMER, 1965a], L cells [BENSON, 1960a; BENDA and ČINÁTL, 1962; HOTCHIN, 1962a; PEDERSEN and VOLKERT, 1966], 3T3 cells [ABELSON *et al.*, 1969], monkey kidney [BENDA and ČINÁTL, 1962; HOTCHIN, 1962a; LEWIS *et al.*, 1965] and heart [HOTCHIN, 1962a], BHK-21 [BARLOW and KELLER, 1964b], RE, MK-2, primary human amnion [PARIKH, 1961], WI-26 [WIKTOR *et al.*, 1966], CMH, human embryo, Hep-2, Chang liver [BENDA and ČINÁTL, 1962] and guinea pig embryo [HOTCHIN and CINITS, 1958]. It also grows in cultures of tick tissue [REHÁČEK, 1965]. Failure was reported in only a few cell types, e.g. Novikoff rat hepatoma cells [HOTCHIN, 1957] and hamster kidney cells [WILSNACK and ROWE, 1964]. Cytopathic effects have been reported in mouse embryo [ACKERMANN, 1960], chick embryo [BENSON, 1959; BENSON and HOTCHIN, 1960; DEIBEL *et al.*, 1964], primary human amnion [PARIKH, 1961], Detroit-6 cells [STULBERG *et al.*, 1956], L cells [BENSON, 1960a; BENSON *et al.*, 1960; LEHMANN-GRUBE, 1967], mouse lymphosarcoma [MOLOMUT and PADNOS, 1965], and KB cells [EAGLE *et al.*, 1956; HOTCHIN, 1958; HOTCHIN and CINITS, 1958] and were absent in the rest; conflicting reports on CPE are given for L cells [BENDA and ČINÁTL, 1962; HOTCHIN, 1962a; WAGNER and SNYDER, 1962; PEDERSEN and VOLKERT, 1966].

In the presence of 2×10^{-7} M fluorodeoxyuridine (FUDR), LCM virus was found to cause a CPE in L cells with cell destruction reaching a maximum 3 to 4 days after infection [PFAU *et al.*, 1965] but the effect was not suitable for use in a plaque assay (PFAU, personal communication). Control cells showed no effect when treated with LCM, or with FUDR separately.

Using the indirect fluorescent antibody (FAB) method with hyperimmune rabbit or guinea pig sera, BENDA *et al.* [1965] noted that LCM antigen first appeared after 9 h in some LCM-infected strain L cells; it was distributed within the cytoplasm, sometimes attached to one side of the nuclear membrane, and coincided with the logarithmic phase of virus multiplication as detected by titration. These observations were confirmed by WIKTOR *et al.* [1966], who detected LCM antigen 12 h after infection of human diploid cells; staining was most intense 48 h after infection, thereafter fading and disappearing completely 5 days after infection, although at this time the yield of virus in mice or tissue culture was quite high. Large cytoplasmic ribosomal aggregates were observed by ABELSON *et al.* [1969] within LCM-infected mouse 3T3 cells; by means of peroxidase-labeled anti-LCM serum, virus-specific antigens were shown to be associated with these structures.

In a study of cellular tolerance to LCM *in vitro*, TRAUB [1961a] found that lymph node cells from mice with persistent tolerant infection (PTI) exhibited a continuous level of LCM titer for 6 or more weeks, whereas LCM-infected lymph node cells from nontolerant mice showed a fluctuation in virus titer during the same period. After prolonged cultivation, nontolerant cells tended to acquire the character of tolerant cells. TRAUB and KESTING [1963a] noticed that after subcutaneous (SC) inoculation of mice with LCM virus there was a period around day 7 and 8 when trypsinized cells grew very poorly *in vitro*, and also showed a marked tendency to clump when washed with PBS. Before and after this period, normal cell growth occurred in spite of the fact that the cultures were infected with LCM virus. MIMS and SUBRAHMANYAN [1966] observed that LCM tolerantly infected mouse macrophages could not be infected *in vitro* in spite of the fact that nearly all of the cells did not contain antigen demonstrable by FAB test.

Titration Methods

Since LCM virus has proved somewhat difficult to titrate in animals (see HDIP section) or in tissue culture, several workers have attempted to overcome these difficulties. A detailed study of the different host responses during mouse titration of LCM was made by HOTCHIN and BENSON [1963] who concluded that inoculation of the FP was the most sensitive route for virus assay. An LCM titration method was devised by LEHMANN-GRUBE and HESSE [1967] by detecting CF antigen released from infected L cell cultures. However, the method was 9 times less sensitive than standard mouse titration. Tissue culture assay combined with direct immunofluorescence has also been described [OLDSTONE and DIXON, 1968b].

A plaque assay for LCM was first reported in 1959 [BENSON, 1959; BENSON and HOTCHIN, 1960] using mixed chick embryo cell monolayers; it gave a plating efficiency of 0.23 mouse LD_{50}. Since plaques only appeared on the 12th day of incubation, it proved difficult to maintain the monolayers for this length of time. Plaques also were shown to develop in L cells within 4 to 6 days [BENSON, 1960a] but the plating efficiency was only 0.003. CHASTEL [1965] confirmed the ability of several strains of LCM to produce plaques on chick embryo tissue. Plaques appeared after 4 to 6 days and reached a diameter of 2 to 3 mm by 7 or 8 days. LCM virus strains were identified by plaque inhibition with hyperimmune rabbit serum. WAINWRIGHT and MIMS [1967] utilized hemadsorption interference in a plaque assay, whereby challenge with Sendai virus and hemadsorption revealed LCM plaques as clear areas. The method was one-tenth as sensitive as mouse IC titration. Another LCM plaque assay system was devised by SEDWICK and WIKTOR [1967] using BHK21/13S cells in agarose suspension; plaques appeared after only 4 days incubation. At the present time none of these methods has proven entirely satisfactory.

Autointerference

ROWE [1954] noticed that viscerotropic LCM virus conferred protection against a more virulent neurotropic strain. The effect was not obtained with heat-killed virus. TRAUB and KESTING [1963b] suggested that the immunity of mice to LCM was due in part to the interference phenomenon, particularly in the early stages of infection. TRAUB [1960b] observed that non-lethal viscerotropic LCM virus or congenital infection [TRAUB, 1959] could protect mice against challenge with a neurotropic strain; he concluded that cells which were persistently infected with a mild strain could not be reinfected with the more virulent strain. The frequent presence of nuclear LCM antigen, which was often the only antigen demonstrable in the cells of LCM tolerant mice, suggested to MIMS and SUBRAHMANYAN [1966] the possibility that virus was replicating in the cell nuclei, and raised the question of its ability to limit the infective process by autointerference. A similar conclusion was made by WILSNACK and ROWE [1964]. Intracerebrally injected LCM virus did not grow (as judged by immunofluorescence) in Kupffer cells or ependymal cells of LCM-PTI mice, in spite of the fact that most of those cells contained no demonstrable antigen. Controls showed that Kupffer cells support virus growth in uninfected mice; the effect was not interferon mediated [MIMS and SUBRAHMANYAN, 1966]. BENSON *et al.* [1960; BENSON, 1961] showed that a persistent infection could be obtained with LCM-infected L cells after a brief period of partial CPE. Fluid from the persistently infected cultures protected uninfected cultures from CPE following virus challenge. The result was confirmed by LEHMANN-GRUBE [1967], who concluded that interferon was not involved. It is clear that in cells persistently infected with LCM, both *in vitro* or *in vivo,* virus growth is partially inhibited or regulated in many of the cells by an unknown process which does not apparently involve interferon. The same appears to hold true for acute LCM virus disease, where interferon does not appear to play a role [TRAUB, 1961b; WAGNER and SNYDER, 1962;

Volkert *et al.*, 1964; Mims and Subrahmanyan, 1966; Lehmann-Grube, 1967] since all experiments failed which were designed to demonstrate the presence of interferon in LCM-infected animals or tissue cultures. Tests of the interfering capacity of liver versus brain virus showed[4] that the degree of interference was associated with active virus and did not appear to depend upon a soluble factor or inactive virus particles.

Interference with Other Viruses

LCM has been shown to interfere *in vivo* with several viruses including Western equine encephalomyelitis (WEE) [Hotchin and Cinits, 1958], Eastern equine encephalomyelitis (EEE) [Traub, 1961a; Wagner and Snyder, 1962], poliovirus [Dalldorf and Douglass, 1938], MM [Rhodes and Chapman, 1949, 1950], polyoma [Hotchin, 1962a], leukemia [Nadel and Haas, 1955, 1956; Jungeblut and Kodza, 1963; Barski and Youn, 1964] and vesicular stomatitis virus (VSV) [Traub and Kesting, 1963b]. *In vitro* interference by LCM was reported for VSV [Wagner and Snyder, 1962] and WEE [Hotchin and Cinits, 1958]. No *in vitro* interference could be produced by LCM against CPE due to poliovirus, WEE [Hotchin and Cinits, 1958] or EEE [Traub and Kesting, 1963b]. Rabies virus multiplication was reported [Ko-

Table I. The effects of Coxsackie viruses A-14 and B-1 on the % mortality of mice after IC inoculation with LCM virus

IC[1] LCM day 0	P[2] A-14 day	% mortality
+	6	40
+	7	8
–	0	100
–	7	100
	SC[3] B-1 day	
+	2	100
+	6	31
–	0	100
–	6	100

[1] IP = Intraperitoneal. [2] IC = Intracerebral. [3] SC = Subcutaneous.

[4] J. Hotchin and E. Sikora, unpublished results.

PROWSKI *et al.*, 1966] to be enhanced by the simultaneous infection of tissue cultures with LCM virus. An interference-like effect was described between LCM virus and *Rickettsia prowazeki* [REISS-GUTFREUND, 1962]. An apparent interference between LCM and coxsackieviruses A-14 and B-1 was demonstrated by HOTCHIN and SIKORA[5]. 0.02 ml of a 10^{-3} dilution of LCM MB_6L_{11} was inoculated IC into 16 mice/group followed by intraperitoneal (IP) injection of 0.2 ml coxsackievirus-infected monkey kidney tissue culture (MKTC) as shown in table I. However since the effect only developed after 6 or 7 days, it is possible that it was not mediated by interference, but involved an increased immune responsiveness or maturity by the LCM-infected mice via an adjuvant effect, since these coxsackieviruses normally cause high mortality only in immunologically immature mice.

Acute Disease

Harmlessness of LCM

There are numerous indications that LCM is capable of behaving as a harmless agent as well as a lethal one. LCM produces inapparent disease in chicks [ALICE and McNUTT, 1945], dogs [DALLDORF, 1943], and in adult rabbits [SMADEL and WALL, 1942] (although retardation of growth is caused in newborn rabbits [SMADEL and WALL, 1940]), newborn [VOLKERT and LARSEN, 1965c] and adult Syrian hamsters [SMADEL and WALL, 1942], and sometimes the mouse [HAAS, 1954]. It grows without forming lesions on the chorioallantoic membrane of embryonated hen eggs [BENGTSON, 1936; PRICK, 1946] and causes minimal lesions in the embryo [LILLIE, 1936a] which develops into a normal chick.

In 1958 it was proposed by HOTCHIN and CINITS that LCM is only harmful to the mouse if the latter responds to it immunologically as a foreign antigen. This concept was later developed [HOTCHIN, 1958; COLLINS *et al.*, 1961; HOTCHIN and WEIGAND, 1961a, b; WEIGAND and HOTCHIN, 1961; HOTCHIN *et al.*, 1962] to a hypothesis of LCM as a basically harmless agent capable of inducing a homograft response which causes sickness and death in mice. MIMS [1966] and MIMS and SUBRAHMANYAN [1966] noted an absence of pathological changes which was almost complete for the first ten months of age after congenital infection of mice with LCM. MIMS emphasized that this demonstrated the normal

---

[5] J. HOTCHIN and E. SIKORA, unpublished results.

functioning of cells heavily infected with LCM, particularly in the cerebellar neurons and retinal cells, all of which contained large amounts of antigen.

Clinical Manifestations

LCM susceptible species include the mouse, rat, guinea pig, and rhesus and macaque monkeys, all of which develop central nervous system (CNS) disease. Acute LCM disease of mice begins 5–7 days after IC or IP inoculation and includes a hunched posture, ruffled fur, blepharitis and facial edema, and is typically culminated at 6–8 days by convulsions and death. In a convulsion the mouse exhibits rigid, extended hind limbs, which remain extended briefly after recovery of the forelimbs, in non-fatal cases. The convulsions may be induced by twirling the sick mouse by the tail. Intranasal (IN) or subcutaneous (SC) inoculation produces temporary illness in mice, followed by solid immunity. All inoculation routes cause weight loss in mice, which can be used [HOTCHIN and BENSON, 1961] as an end point method for detecting and titrating strains of low pathogenicity. Clinical and pathological details of acute and chronic LCM have been summarized by MAURER [1964] and by FARMER and JANEWAY [1942]. The detailed pathological histology of murine LCM will not be included in this review; it has been excellently summarized by LILLIE and ARMSTRONG [1945] and consists essentially of lymphocytic infiltration of virtually the entire animal. Lesions are most severe in the liver and kidneys and vary somewhat in severity with different strains. Neurological findings are relatively mild even with neurotropic strains and consist of meningitic infiltration and sometimes mild encephalitis. LCM virus can infect guinea pigs through the normal, apparently intact skin [SHAUGHNESSY and ZICHIS, 1940]; guinea pigs and monkeys are particularly sensitive to LCM infection by inhalation[6] [DANEŠ *et al.*, 1963; BENDA *et al.*, 1964].

Man

LCM virus causes a disease in man [ADAIR *et al.*, 1953], first described by ARMSTRONG and DICKENS [1935], ranging in severity from inapparent infection to a rare fatal systemic response. The virus has also been regarded as harmless to man and has been injected into human volunteers [KREIS, 1937; LÉPINE *et al.*, 1937; RASMUSSEN, 1946; BLANC,

---

[6] J. HOTCHIN, unpublished results.

1952], and the MP strain has been used therapeutically as an oncolytic agent (WEBB, personal communication). The disease [ARMSTRONG, 1940–1941] is usually manifested as a mild influenza-like illness sometimes with meningitis [HOWARD, 1940], rarely with encephalitis [TREUSCH *et al.*, 1943; SHVAREV and REMEZOV, 1959], myocarditis [THIEDE, 1962], parotitis, orchitis [LEWIS and UTZ, 1961; BLATTNER, 1962], pneumonia [COLMORE, 1952] and very rarely as a fatal systemic disease [MACHELLA *et al.*, 1939; HOWARD, 1940; SILICOTT and NEUBUERGER, 1940; ARMSTRONG, 1942; SMADEL *et al.*, 1942; SCHEID *et al.*, 1956]. Cases with chronic sequelae have been reported which involved fatigue, headache, impairment of memory, mental depression, personality changes [GUNTHER, 1930; VIETS and WATTS, 1934; SKOGLAND and BAKER, 1939; BAKER, 1947; CHANG *et al.*, 1954] and more rarely meningoencephalitis [SKOGLAND and BAKER, 1939] or paralysis [FINDLAY *et al.*, 1936; MACCALLUM and FINDLAY, 1939]. Complement-fixing [KÜPPER *et al.*, 1964] but not neutralizing [HEYL, 1948] antibody to LCM has been found in man during surveys where no human disease was reported [SCHEID *et al.*, 1964], but where there was association with persistent murine infection. A case of LCM in a newborn human infant was reported [KOMROWER *et al.*, 1955] which was believed to have been acquired *in utero* from the mother. Domestic [ARMSTRONG and SWEET, 1939; SMITHARD and MACRAE, 1951; DALLDORF *et al.*, 1946] and laboratory infections of man from infected animals are very easily contracted[7] [LÉPINE and SAUTTER, 1938; ARMSTRONG, 1942; MILZER and LEVINSON, 1942; HAYES and HARTMAN, 1943; SCHEID *et al.*, 1956; LEHMANN-GRUBE *et al.*, 1959; Amer. Assoc. Lab. Anim. Sci., 1966; BAUM *et al.*, 1966; ARMSTRONG *et al.*, 1969], though human to human infection does not appear to be common, in spite of the presence of virus in the nasal secretions of patients with LCM [SMADEL, 1942].

Pathogenesis

Animals which develop signs of LCM disease show infiltration of the viscera with lymphocytes especially in the liver, suprarenals, kidneys, lungs and meninges [FINDLAY and STERN, 1936; LILLIE, 1936; FARMER and JANEWAY, 1942]. High titers of virus are found in all organs [ARMSTRONG *et al*, 1936]. LCM virus in the blood was found by SHWARTZMAN [1943, 1944] to be in close association with erythrocytes. NIKOLITSCH

---

[7] J. HOTCHIN, unpublished results.

[1959] used LCM virus to demonstrate that viremia was a prerequisite for CNS invasion. Recent studies have confirmed and extended the early findings on the pathogenesis and spread of this virus within the tissues of the mouse. REMEZOV and TOPLENINOVA [1961] showed that the FAB method could be used to detect LCM antigen in infected cells and WILSNACK and ROWE [1964] followed its development in infected mice by the indirect technic. They concluded that LCM infection in the brain is almost completely restricted to meninges, choroid plexus, and ependyma with little or no multiplication of the virus in brain parenchyma. Evidence of antigen formation began 24 h after IC inoculation and was extensive by the second day. After viscerotropic virus inoculation, antigen appeared in the lung, bronchial epithelium, alveolar cells and occasional macrophages. The liver was the most consistently infected organ, as judged by immunofluorescence, and was the best sentinal organ for the detection of LCM in the mouse. Antigen was evident in hepatic cells 72 h after IP inoculation of viscerotropic virus. Ten percent of erythrocytes contained specific fluorescent staining granules, but antigen could not be seen in lymphocytes, except for rare examples in congenitally infected mice.

The indirect FAB technic was also employed by BENDA et al. [1965] who showed that antigen appeared in brain tissue 2 days after infection and then increased in amount for 6–7 days, by which time deaths had begun to occur among the animals. In the brain, viral antigen was found to occur only in the choroid plexus, ependymal lining, and leptomeninges, and occasionally in foci around vessels and capillaries. No specific fluorescence was present in perivascular infiltrates in the brain tissue itself. Fluorescence was localized exclusively to the cytoplasm of the cells; it also occurred in some macrophages. Similar studies have been made by MIMS [1966] and MIMS and SUBRAHMANYAN [1966] and by BROWN [1968] (see section on 'Tolerance induction in the perinatal period'). LCM antigen was visualized in peripheral leucocytes of infected mice by BARATAWIDJAJA et al. [1965] using the direct FAB technic. Positive cells were present from the 7th day onwards.

The pathogenicity of LCM is greatly enhanced by coincident infection of mice with *Eperythrozoon coccoides* [GLEDHILL and SEAMER, 1960; GLEDHILL et al., 1960; SEAMER et al., 1961]. The nature of this interaction and its mechanism is not understood, but SEAMER and GLEDHILL [1965] showed that IP inoculation of *E. coccoides* could enhance the liver titer of LCM by a factor of 10^4.

The major histological changes in mice after IC or IP inoculation with LCM virus were confirmed to be lymphocytic infiltration of the viscera [Rowe *et al.*, 1963] and meningoencephalitis and hepatitis on the 5th day, with a peak in severity on the 7th day [Collins *et al.*, 1961]. When mice were pretreated 24 h before virus inoculation with 500 r of total body X-irradiation, none of the normal LCM lesions were present, and the mice showed the same, essentially normal, histological picture found in the control mice receiving X-irradiation alone. Histological lesions in the brain and liver were entirely absent in spite of virus multiplication which occurred at the normal rate in these organs (see section on 'X-irradiation'). It was concluded [Collins *et al.*, 1961] that the X-ray-induced protection from clinical and histological evidence of LCM disease occurred as a result of the inhibition of the host leucocyte response. Acute LCM disease was therefore seen [Hotchin, 1962a; Hotchin *et al.*, 1958] as a manifestation of a homograft rejection of the virus-infected tissue by the host. Volkert [1963, 1964] commented on this theory, with the view that an immunological response to LCM virus should cause a clinical illness, but his experiments on adoptive immunization did not support the theory. However, he admitted that some batches of transplantation cells had a harmful effect on the virus carriers, with illness and death of the recipients 3 weeks after transplantation. Histological examination showed no inflammatory reactions, but did show extensive liver necrosis and a marked reduction of the lymphoid tissue in the spleen.

Traub and Kesting [1963a] agreed with the homograft rejection concept of Hotchin's theory of LCM pathogenesis, and believed that an immunological response was developed against a non-viral antigen arising in the body in the course of the disease. He found an anticomplementary effect of spleen extracts from mice during the acute disease, and also observed the spontaneous clumping of trypsinized and washed lymph node cells in such animals. Traub interpreted these phenomena as indications of an antigen-antibody reaction in the pathogenic mechanism. Volkert *et al.* [1964] agreed that the immunological responsiveness conferred by grafts of lymphoid cells to tolerant mice had many similarities to immune reactions against skin and tumor grafts, and that the two phenomena might therefore be caused by the same immune mechanism. East *et al.* [1964] concluded that the laboratory findings supported Hotchin's concept that the pathogenic effect of LCM virus in adult mice results from the immune reaction of the host to the virus, rather than from the direct cytopathic effect of the virus upon the host cells. For further discussion on the pathogenesis of acute and tolerant LCM infection see 'Pathogenic mechanisms'.

Subcutaneous Sensitization, Followed by Intracerebral Inoculation of Mice with LCM (The SC/IC Effect)

Several workers have investigated SC sensitization of mice to LCM followed at different time intervals by IC challenge. These experiments appear to have originated from Traub's description [1936b, 1938a] of an 'accelerated reaction' to IC challenge by mice which retained only 'partial immunity'. From the 3rd to the 5th day after the test injection, these animals showed malaise, loss of appetite and weight, and ruffled fur and tremors, but no convulsions of the hind extremities when lifted by the tail. The brains of mice killed during the accelerated reaction revealed marked meningoencephalitis comparable to controls with acute LCM. Traub concluded that the accelerated reaction represented an allergic state of the mice with waning immunity. He noted that no mice with partial immunity were viremic, although virus could be detected in the organs of some. The observation was confirmed by Lyon [1940], Haas [1954] and Rowe [1954]. Burnet and Fenner [1949] concluded that this effect was due to a sensitivity reaction. Haas [1954] and Hotchin [1958] showed that IC inoculation of sterile material 2–6 days after SC or IP LCM inoculation induced the meningitic form of the disease with convulsions. An accelerated response to IC challenge was found by Haas [1954] and Rowe [1954] to occur at the start of the immune response 3 or more days after SC or IP inoculation. After 3 days, the accellerating effect was found by Haas to give way to a sparing influence. Lyon [1940] also observed that mice became progressively more immune to LCM IC challenge, beginning on the 5th day after SC inoculation with the virus. The SC/IC phenomenon was reinvestigated by Seamer et al. [1963] and by Seamer and Hotchin [1960] who showed that SC virus inoculation sensitized the mice in such a way that subsequent IC inoculation within a few days caused early death; the time of death after IC challenge had been set by the time of SC inoculation. After the 4th day, IC challenge caused decreasing mortality and progressively later times of death, indicating that at day 4 the mice passed from a state of hypersensitivity into a state of immunity, with increasing resistence to challenge. These observations confirmed the impression that death from LCM was due to the effects of an immune response. Titrations of the brain virus of SC/IC inoculated mice at different intervals after infection showed that when the SC/IC interval was within 4 days, brain virus titers rose to the same height (approximately 10^8 ID_{50}/g) as without SC sensitization. However, when the SC/IC interval was greater than 4 days, titers only rose to approximately 10^6 and then declined [SEAMER *et al.*, 1963].

Endotoxin Sensitivity

Mice inoculated with LCM virus have been found to develop extreme sensitivity to *Escherichia coli* endotoxin during the incubation period following inoculation [BARLOW and FAIRLEY, 1962; HOTCHIN, 1962a]. By the sixth day, following a large dose (6×10^5 LD_{50}) of LCM virus, sensitivity to fatal endotoxin shock increased 3,000-fold. Smaller inocula produced the effect about one day later. Under these conditions, the fatal endotoxin shock presented the same clinical signs as IC LCM virus inoculation including typical convulsions. The mechanism of the interaction between endotoxin and LCM virus infection appears to be similar to that described by SUTER and KIRSANOW [1961] following endotoxin injection of mice infected with mycobacteria, and the endotoxin shock syndrome is the same [SUTER, 1962]. It is noteworthy that increased sensitivity to endotoxin occurs during infection of mice with mouse hepatitis virus and *E. Coccoides* [GLEDHILL and NIVEN, 1957; GLEDHILL, 1958]. STETSON [1959] suggested that the common feature shared by these reactions is the mechanism of delayed hypersensitivity. In addition to endotoxin, the radiomimetic nitrogen mustard derivative chlorambucil (Leukeran) has been shown by BARLOW [1964] to precipitate a similar endotoxin shock during the incubation period after LCM virus inoculation of mice.

Skin and Foot Pad Reactions to LCM

SHAUGHNESSY and ZICHIS [1939, 1940] concluded that LCM virus can infect guinea pigs through the normal, apparently intact skin. A papular skin reaction following inunction of LCM virus was reported in rhesus monkeys [DALLDORF, 1939b]. Similar lesions were frequently noted in the late stages of LCM infection in these monkeys; histological examination of the lesions showed edema of the epithelium. Human volunteers [BLANC, 1952] and rabbits [ROGER, 1962] inoculated intradermally (ID) with LCM virus also exhibited a local skin reaction.

Inoculation of mice with LCM virus into the FP was found by HOTCHIN [1962b] and ROGER and HOTCHIN [1961] to cause an unusual response in which animals sustained a mild immunizing infection. On the eighth day after injection, the inoculated FP became swollen followed by gross edema of the leg, lasting approximately one week, after which there was full recovery. The FP effect was shown to require live LCM virus. The response was not neutralized by anti-vaccinia nor anti-ectromelia serum but was neutralized by anti-LCM serum; it was obtained with many different strains of LCM virus. Histological study revealed a severe obliterative lesion of the local lymph node during and after the FP response. The FP response to LCM virus was confirmed by ROGER [1963b], ROGER and ROGER [1964a, b, c, d] and TRAUB [1963] who found it to be more sensitive than the IP route for the demonstration of neutralizing antibody in organ extracts. A similar effect occurred in guinea pigs [ROGER, 1963a]. The FP route was found to be the most sensitive one for detecting strains of LCM virus [HOTCHIN and BENSON, 1963]. It was shown by BENSON [1962a] that whole body irradiation of mice prior to inoculation prevented the FP response but local irradiation of the FP of the hind leg failed to prevent FP response in the same leg. The results conformed with the concept that the FP reaction is a local manifestation of the general immunological response of the host to the virus infection.

Immune Responses to LCM

As early as 1938 TRAUB suggested that there might be two different types of immunity to LCM in the mouse according to whether the infection was acquired before birth or as an adult [1938a]. More recently WEIGAND and HOTCHIN [1961] proposed that these two types be called 'tolerant' and 'active' immunity. Immunity is used to denote [Brit. Med. Dictionary, 1961] the state of resistance of an animal to a particular disease (not to infection by an agent) and does not necessarily imply the presence of humoral or cellular immune response. In tolerant immunity the mice are fully resistant to challenge with all strains and carry high titers of virus throughout their tissues. There is neither cellular nor humoral immune response and no virus suppression. In active immunity the animals are resistant to challenge but little or no virus is detectable in their tissues; humoral and cellular immune responses occur and virus is rapidly suppressed. Since virus challenge causes no symptoms in these two conditions, they are indistinguishable without recourse to tests for virus or antibody. LARSEN [1968] pointed out that the disappearance of virus, and subsequent reappearance after long intervals of time, in anti-lymphocyte serum (ALS)-treated mice, could be explained by two separate immune reactions which may run synchronously or independently, showing dissociated immune functions. One was responsible for elimination of viremia, and the other was a humoral immune response in which only CF antibodies were found. These two types of active immunity will be considered separately.

Humoral Immune Response

Comparison of titers of LCM immune sera by TRAUB [1963], SMADEL and WALL [1940, 1942], SMADEL *et al.* [1940], COHEN *et al.* [1966], WILSNACK and ROWE [1964] and BENDA *et al.* [1965] showed that the CF, neutralizing and FAB were independent. These are discussed separately.

Complement-fixing Antibody

Soluble CF antigen, widely distributed in tissues of infected guinea pigs, mice [GRĚSIKOVÁ and CASALS, 1963], monkeys [SMADEL *et al.*, 1939a] and chick embryos [WHITNEY *et al.*, 1953] is separable by centrifugation from the virus which fixes complement poorly [SMADEL *et al.*, 1939b]. It was stable at $+4°$ C [SMADEL and WALL, 1941] and apparently of protein nature and gave a specific CF [HOWITT, 1937b] and precipitin reaction with immune serum [SMADEL and WALL, 1940]. BARLOW and MUSTICO [1964, 1965] found at least three serologically distinct antigens from infected mouse and guinea pig tissue and separated the CF antigen by gel filtration. The antigens were stable for 1 h at $60°$ C, high salt concentration and a pH range between 3 and 9. CF antibody to this antigen appears early in the disease of man and experimental animals [HOWITT, 1937a; SMADEL *et al.*, 1939a; TRAUB and SCHÄFER, 1939b; JOCHHEIM *et al.*, 1957; TRAUB, 1960a, 1963] and its appearance has been adapted as a quantitative diagnostic tool for LCM [EGGERS, 1958]. Tissue culture antigen gives the most sensitive diagnostic test [SCHELL *et al.*, 1966]. LARSEN [1969a] has shown that CF antibody appears one week after vaccination of mice with live LCM virus and that this antibody is of the 7S (IgG) type.

Neutralizing Antibody

Neutralizing antibody has been found by many workers [TRAUB, 1936b, 1960a; SMADEL and WALL, 1940; HAAS, 1954; ROWE, 1954;

WEIGAND and HOTCHIN, 1961; VOLKERT *et al.*, 1964] to be consistently absent from the sera of LCM immune mice although it was readily found in other animal species [MILZER and LEVINSON, 1949 ; HAAS, 1954; ROWE, 1954; LEHMANN-GRUBE *et al.*, 1959; VOLKERT *et al.*, 1964] including man [WOOLEY *et al.*, 1937, 1939]. Non-specific heat labile [POL-LIKOFF and SIGEL, 1952] accessory neutralizing factors have also been described [ACKERMANN *et al.*, 1962] in human sera. Neutralizing anti-body was tested by BENDA [1964] for ability to protect guinea pigs against LCM virus challenge after IN administration but only minimal protection occurred. The inability to find LCM-neutralizing antibody in immune mice led some workers [ROGER and ROGER, 1965] to conclude that LCM virus could not be inactivated by antibody at all. By using special test procedures mainly dependent upon suppression of symptoms in the test animal, ROWE [1954] was able to detect low levels of neutral-izing and protective antibody in LCM immune mice. TRAUB [1960d] con-firmed this (using prolonged incubation for 24 h at 37° C) but found that the results were weak and irregular. Only 5 to 250 infectious doses of virus were neutralized in a virus preparation which originally contained 10^8 infectious doses, and the results were at the borderline of signifi-cance. Using a more sensitive method HOTCHIN *et al.* [1969] found LCM to be similar to other viruses in respect to neutralization suscepti-bility. The method utilized salt-free albumin solution as diluent, based on observations by BARLOW and WEILAND [1959] and inoculation of the animals in the FP. A mouse which had recovered from LCM 20 months previously was found to possess high titer (1/625) neutralizing antibody in the serum. From this and other similar results, it was concluded that mice are fully capable of making high titer neutralizing antibody to LCM but only after a delay of 10–12 months. While the improved tech-nical method offers considerably greater sensitivity, the main factor in the discovery of murine LCM-neutralizing antibody lay in the unusually large time interval required for significant antibody to appear. The pos-sible relationship of this to the mechanism of LCM persistence is dis-cussed in the section on pathogenic mechanisms.

Fluorescent Antibody

The immunofluorescent technic has been applied to LCM-infected tissue by the direct and indirect methods; the antibody which reacts in this test with LCM antigen is referred to as FAB. BENDA *et al.* [1965] found the FAB technic to be insensitive for detecting LCM antibody,

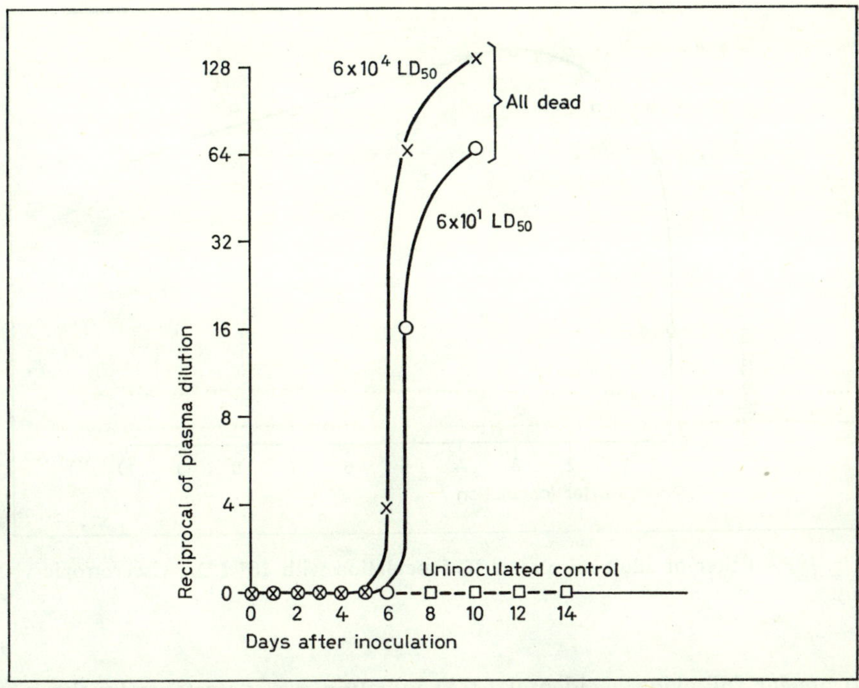

Fig. 3. Development of fluorescent antibody in adult mice inoculated IC with LCM M/B$_8$ virus. Two different virus doses were used, 6×10^4 or 6×10^1 LD$_{50}$.

but BENSON and HOTCHIN [1969] developed a quantitative method which showed that adult mice produced high levels of detectable FAB, beginning on the 6th day after inoculation and rising rapidly to titers of 1/64 to 1/128 before death by day 10 (fig. 3). The FAB was found to be a separate entity from both CF and neutralizing antibody [BENDA *et al.*, 1965; COHEN *et al.*, 1966]. Similar results were obtained using high doses of a viscerotropic LCM strain (M/B$_6$L$_{11}$); in this case mice did not die, but survived with the high dose immune paralysis (HDIP) effect, exhibiting high titers of FAB for many months (fig. 4) with concomitant high virus titer, which only gradually declined. The FAB did not protect against death nor neutralize blood virus at all. FAB has also been found by BENSON and HOTCHIN [1969] in mice with persistent tolerant LCM virus infection (see section on 'Neonatal infection').

In man, the appearance of FAB was studied as a diagnostic test by TRIANDAPHILLI *et al.* [1964] and COHEN *et al.* [1966]. The first antibody

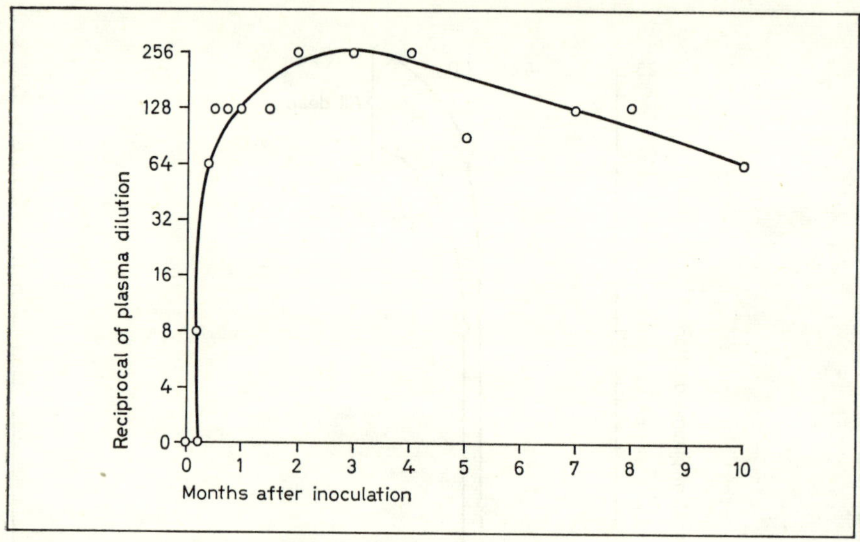

Fig. 4. FAB titer of adult mice after IC inoculation with 10^6 LD_{50} viscerotropic virus.

to appear following accidental LCM infection was detectable by the indirect FAB test, using LCM-infected tissue culture cells; in some cases a significant titer appeared between 1 and 6 days after the onset of meningeal symptoms, declining slowly after several months. In contrast, CF antibody usually appeared considerably later, between 8 days and 2 months after infection; neutralizing antibody was last to show a significant rise, usually after 2 months.

Cellular Immunity

TRAUB's [1936b] early studies led him to believe that neither humoral antibody nor leucocytes were involved in the immunity of mice to LCM virus, which he thought [1937] was closely linked with a special property of the tissues, since circulating antibodies appeared to play only a secondary part in immunity to this virus. ROWE [1954] and HAAS [1954] showed that in LCM-immune mice, challenged weeks or months after IC inoculation, the peak brain virus titer was lower than in non-immunized mice, and quickly dropped. In spite of the lack of significant neutralizing antibody titer, these mice were able to eliminate challenge virus rapidly. A search for neutralizing factors in lymph node extracts by Traub [1963] was negative, but very slight neutralizing capacity was shown by extracts of spleen tissue from LCM-immune mice. Attempts were made by Benson [1960b] to demonstrate a cytotoxic effect of anti-LCM sera or immune spleen cells upon LCM-infected cell monolayers; virus could be suppressed in Maitland cultures by antiserum but not by spleen cells. No visible effect was obtained using antibody, with or without complement, on LCM-infected monkey kidney or L cells[8], although in a comparable system cytotoxicity of suitable anti-sera could be demonstrated with influenza virus-infected cells [Weiland and Hotchin, 1959]. However, destruction of LCM-infected mouse testis monolayers was noted by Benson [1962b] 7 days after exposure to LCM-immune mouse spleen cells, in the absence of comparable effect by normal spleen cells (table II). The effect was accompanied by a less well-marked but definite destruction of normal cells exposed to the immune lymphocytes, presumably due to infection of the normal cells by virus in the immune spleen. In repeat experiments the severity of the effect was variable. More recently Lundstedt [1969] has described similar experiments in which LCM-infected L cells were destroyed by LCM-immune splenocytes. Only half of Lundstedt's experiments showed a positive result and non-LCM-specific destructive effects also occurred in the normal tissue controls exposed to LCM-sensitized lymphocytes. Similar results have been obtained by Oldstone et al. [1969]. Considerable additional evidence concerning the role of cellular immunity in the pathogenesis of LCM virus infection has accrued from in vivo studies using agents known to affect the system (see section on 'Tolerance induction in the adult animal by immune suppressive agents').

Table II. The cytotoxic effect of lymphocytes on LCM infected tissue cultures

Mouse lymphocyte suspension	Mouse testis culture	Total CPE[1]
Normal	Normal	2
LCM immune	Normal	7
Normal	LCM infected	1
LCM immune	LCM infected	9

[1] Based on coded 'blind' scoring on a scale of 0–4 plus CPE.

[8] J. Hotchin and L. Benson, unpublished results.

Immunization

No satisfactory human LCM vaccine has been prepared and animal vaccination attempts have been relatively unsuccessful. MILZER and LEVINSON [1946, 1949] were unable to immunize mice or monkeys with LCM-infected guinea pig spleen suspensions inactivated by heat or formalin. However, these workers claimed to have successfully immunized mice with an ultraviolet light inactivated LCM virus vaccine. Virus inactivated by oleate or ether was ineffective as a mouse vaccine [STOCK *et al.*, 1943]. TRAUB [1937, 1938b] showed that injections of formolized LCM-infected tissue only immunized guinea pigs when homologous tissue was used and there was no parallel between immunizing power and virus content prior to formolization. Similar results were obtained by SMADEL and WALL [1940] who showed that soluble antigen was an ineffective immunizing agent, and for virus particles to be effective considerable purity was necessary. Slight protection of guinea pigs against IN challenge with small doses of LCM virus was obtained by BENDA and ČINÁTL [1964] by SC injection of formolized LCM-infected monkey kidney tissue culture fluid. HOTCHIN and SIKORA[9] found that heat or 1% formalin-inactivated mouse liver suspension given by SC, IC, or FP inoculation did not protect mice against IC challenge with live LCM virus.

Persistent Tolerant Infection (PTI)

The congenital transmission of LCM in mice was apparently responsible for the persistent nature of this virus to be noticed [ARMSTRONG and LILLIE, 1934; TRAUB, 1935b, 1936b] very early after its discovery. Evidence exists for less prolonged persistence in guinea pigs [TRAUB, 1936b], Syrian hamsters [SMADEL and WALL, 1942; VOLKERT and LARSEN, 1965a], chicks[10] [TOBIN, 1954], rats and rabbits[10] [BLANC and BRUNEAU, 1951]. Some cases of LCM in man have shown minimal signs of persistence [SCHNEIDER, 1931; GRUN, 1932; DOLESCHALL and PAUL, 1936; BARKER and FORD, 1937; GLATZEL, 1938; MACCALLUM and FINDLAY, 1939; VOGT, 1939; HOWARD, 1940; LEICHENGER *et al.*, 1940; TREUSCH *et al.*, 1943; BAKER, 1947; CHANG *et al.*, 1954].

The term PTI was coined by HOTCHIN and WEIGAND [1961a] to refer specifically to virus infections which exhibited long-term persistence of

---

[9] J. HOTCHIN and E. SIKORA, unpublished results.
[10] J. HOTCHIN, unpublished results.

the agent in the absence of significant virus-suppressive immunological response. This form of persistence is thereby distinguished from latency in which immunologic tolerance plays no part, but in which the virus is present at very low titer, frequently in 'masked' form due to failure of the host to completely eradicate the agent. In this situation, a strong suppressive immune response is detectable. HOTCHIN pointed out [1967] that PTI can be readily distinguished from latent infections since the two types have quite different characteristics. Some of these are summarized in table III.

LCM can exist in a latent form in mice which have not suppressed all the virus; this situation is very common in actively immune animals. The term 'carrier state' as used by TRAUB [1936c], PFAU [1965a] and MIMS [1966] to denote long-continued virus carriage does not clearly exclude latent infection and appears to be a less precise term than 'persistent infection', though the adjective is convenient. TRAUB [1938a] restricted the use of 'carrier mice' to describe those animals with demonstrable virus in the blood. However, he also stated that in some cases virus was excreted in the urine when it could not be found in the blood of carrier mice; such animals seem to be more properly regarded as having latent infection. The results of experiments on congenital and neonatal LCM-PTI infection in mice will be discussed separately.

Tolerance Induction in the Perinatal Period

Congenital Persistent Tolerant Infection

In 1935, TRAUB [1936c] began to publish his observations on a colony of mice which had become naturally infected with LCM; this pro-

Table III. Comparison of latent and persistent tolerant infections

Factor	Latency	Persistent tolerant infection
Virus titer	Low	High
Antibody	Present	Absent
Virus	Masked	Unmasked (free)
X-ray, UVL[1], etc.	Activated	No effect
Immunosuppressive agents	Activated	No effect

[1] Ultraviolet light.

vided knowledge of the ability of LCM to cause persistent infection and congenital transmission. Although 50% of the mice in the colony were infected, morbidity was less than 20% since the majority of the infected stock mice showed no definite symptoms, and infection could only be determined by inoculation of blood into susceptible animals or IC challenge with known LCM virus. Some or all of the young mice were runted at 2 to 6 weeks but about 40% of these recovered completely [TRAUB, 1936a]. They showed slow and stiff movements, somnolence, ruffled fur and sometimes diarrhea. Pathological change was scanty, consisting of collections of round cells in the vicinity of blood vessels in the liver, and patchy reticuloendothelial hyperplasia. Mature mice infected by contact showed circulation of virus for about 3 weeks at the most; the younger the mice were at infection, the longer they carried virus in the blood [TRAUB, 1938a]. Mice infected *in utero* retained virus so that even in old age blood titers had only fallen to about half the neonatal level. In an infected colony, the proportion of PTI mice increased with time, and after two years even immune mice, with no circulating virus, sometimes had detectable virus in certain organs [ROWE, 1954; VOLKERT and LARSEN, 1964]. At 4 years the virus persisted at high titer in all animals, without causing disease [TRAUB, 1939] and was transmitted to the offspring by the intrauterine route through the female; infection of the ovum was believed [TRAUB, 1960c] to be the initiation of congenital infection. This became the only mode of transmission, in contrast to the earlier situation when some mice were born virus-free and became infected by contact shortly after birth.

Many of TRAUB's early observations on the congenital transfer of LCM virus were confirmed and amplified by HAAS [1941], who showed that virus transmission only occurred via the infected mother. He emphasized a basic difference in response to infection between mice infected *in utero* and after maturity, and made many fruitless attempts to induce suppression of LCM infection acquired *in utero* [HAAS, 1954], e. g. by repeated IC LCM virus inoculation or injection of SLE or influenza PR-8 vaccine, cortisone or insulin. TRAUB [1960b] reinvestigated the nature of the transmission mechanism responsible for congenital infection of mice with LCM virus, and confirmed the transovarial transmission route for congenital infection of the entire litter. Infection by a male at impregnation, or infection during pregnancy, only infected a proportion of the embryos. SEAMER [1965b] reported that mice congenitally infected with LCM virus showed a lower birth rate, growth rate, and smaller litter size, with higher mortality during the first year of life than normal control animals. In congenitally LCM-infected females there was a considerable amount of infectious virus in the ovaries and uterus [TRAUB, 1960b]. TRAUB concluded that the role of spermatozoa in the infection of normal females was probably not important, although HAAS [1941] demonstrated LCM virus to be present in the sperm of male virus carriers. Mice which had been infected *in utero* with LCM virus failed to produce CF and neutralizing antibodies, either immediately or when hyperimmunized later in life [TRAUB, 1960a, b]. Congenital LCM infection has been studied in the gnotobiotic state [POLLARD *et al.*, 1968a, b], although in this study since no virus-free control mice were available the findings were complicated by the possible presence of additional agents such as leukemia virus. The LCM-infected gnotobiotic mice were shown to have increased levels of gamma globulin which were 2.7% at 2 months rising to 49.7% in 8-month-old mice. A histological study of congenitally LCM-infected mice by MIMS [1966] using the FAB method to detect LCM antigen, showed that almost all cells were infected in early embryos and a very high proportion of cells of virtually all tissues were found to contain LCM antigen for at least 8 months after birth. Antigen was most often seen in the form of fine fluorescent particles which appeared to be in both the cytoplasm and nucleus. Fluorescence of cells tended to decrease as mice became older. Brain showed faint fluorescence, both in meninges and in brain parenchyma, particularly in Purkinje cells. Infected lymphoid cells were seen in the spleen, lymph nodes and thymus, particularly in the larger mononuclear cells. In these organs there were small cells which did not contain antigen. Infected monocytes and lymphocytes were seen in blood smears. Almost every cell in the ovaries was involved, and infected ova were clearly identified.

A similar immunofluorescent study by WILSNACK and ROWE [1964] showed congenitally infected animals to contain less antigen than those with acute infection, except for the kidney where the antigen content was greater.

Neonatal Persistent Tolerant Infection

After the intensive period of work on congenital LCM infection of mice for a few years after 1935 by TRAUB and HAAS there occurred an extensive period with very little research on mice carrying persistent LCM infection. In 1951 WHITNEY noticed that neonatal inoculation of mice with LCM virus did not produce disease when freshly isolated vi-

rus strains were used. She concluded that newborn mice were insusceptible to these strains and suffered only an inapparent infection which produced active immunity; no tests were made for persistence of the virus.
In 1958 HOTCHIN reopened the subject of persistent LCM infection by
demonstrating the increasing mortality of LCM in newborn mice with
respect to age at inoculation. He showed that the survivors exhibited a
persistent infection with high blood virus titers fulfilling all the require-
ments of acquired immunological tolerance to the virus and its products
[HOTCHIN and WEIGAND, 1959]. The term 'persistent tolerant infection'
(PTI) was therefore used to describe the condition [WEIGAND and
HOTCHIN, 1961; HOTCHIN, 1962a]. Very low mortality (approximately
10%) occurred in neonatal mice inoculated 24 h after birth, but by
about two weeks of age mortality increased to 100% (fig. 5). The persistent infection resulting from neonatal inoculation constitutes a reproducible state, comparable to congenital infection and lacking the uncer-
tainties inherent in using an infected colony. Most neonatally inoculated
animals showed few or no signs of disease but others were runted
[HOTCHIN and CINITS, 1958; HOTCHIN, 1961; TRAUB and KESTING,

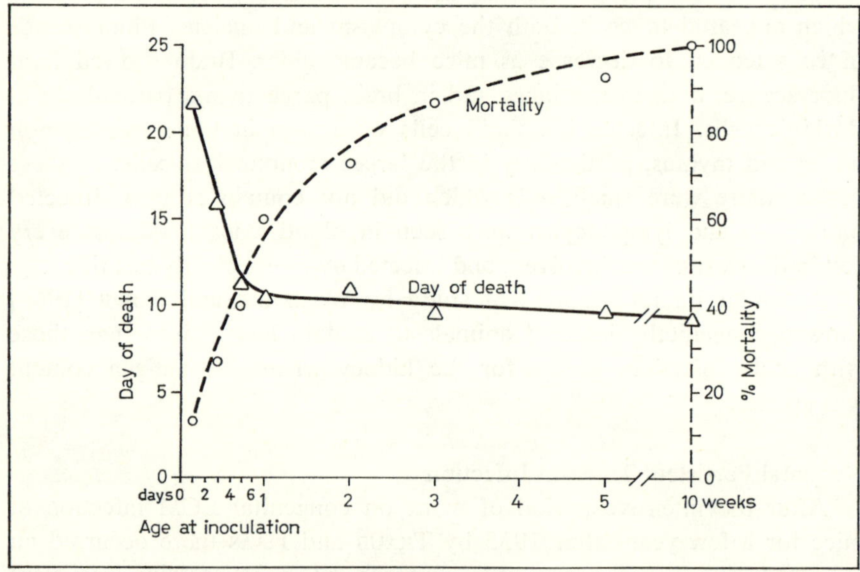

Fig. 5. The relationship between the age of mice at inoculation (IC with LCM virus)
and the mortality and time of death after inoculation.

1963b] and exhibited scant hair, a dainty bird-like behavior and unusual jumpiness. These animals either died quickly, or recovered and appeared normal. Mortality of the neonatally inoculated infants is caused in part by maternal morbidity which results from contact infection of the mother [HOTCHIN et al., 1970]. Mouse and virus strain variations influence the severity of reactions of newborn mice to LCM [HOTCHIN et al., 1962] and viscerotropic (or 'docile') virus strains and high virus doses were the most tolerogenic [HOTCHIN et al., 1962; LEHMANN-GRUBE, 1964b; VOLKERT and LARSEN, 1965a; LARSEN, 1969]. Litters born to female PTI mice were also PTI. Neonatal inoculation of newborn mice regularly caused transmission of the infection to mothers by contact [TRAUB and KESTING, 1963b; BENSON and HOTCHIN, 1969] causing inapparent infection and active immunity. No protective antibody appeared to be transmitted from immune mothers to infants [WEIGAND and HOTCHIN, 1961] and the latter reacted [TRAUB, 1960d] more severely to LCM infection than normal controls. However antibody detectable by the FAB technic is transferred from contact infected mothers to neonatally inoculated infants [BENSON and HOTCHIN, 1969]. Virus was present in the milk of PTI mothers (WEIGAND, personal communication) and invariably caused infection of normal mice suckled by this type of mother. Titers of virus in congenital PTI mice resembled those found in the brains of adult animals suffering from a lethal infection. For example 195 days after inoculation [WEIGAND and HOTCHIN, 1961] titers in brain and blood were approximately 10^6 and 10^4 LD_{50}/g or ml respectively, regardless of whether the mice were inoculated 2 h or up to 6 days after birth. PTI mice resisted repeated LCM virus challenge by various routes and the resulting immunity was referred to as tolerant [WEIGAND and HOTCHIN, 1961], since no antibody was involved. Both CF and neutralizing antibody were absent [TRAUB, 1960a; WEIGAND and HOTCHIN, 1961; VOLKERT et al., 1964; LARSEN, 1969a], but persistent low levels of FAB have been found by BENSON and HOTCHIN [1969]. The late onset of disease and glomerulonephritic changes in LCM-PTI mice described by HOTCHIN [1962a] (see section on 'LCM-induced glomerulonephritis'), suggested [HOTCHIN and COLLINS, 1964] that neonatal LCM tolerance was gradually waning, with development of cellular or humoral immunity. In this light, the finding of low titer FAB in these animals takes on greater significance. FAB appeared in the blood of neonatal PTI mice 10 days after inoculation, with peak titers at 14 to 20 days [BENSON and HOTCHIN, 1969] (fig. 6). The mothers of these mice developed high FAB

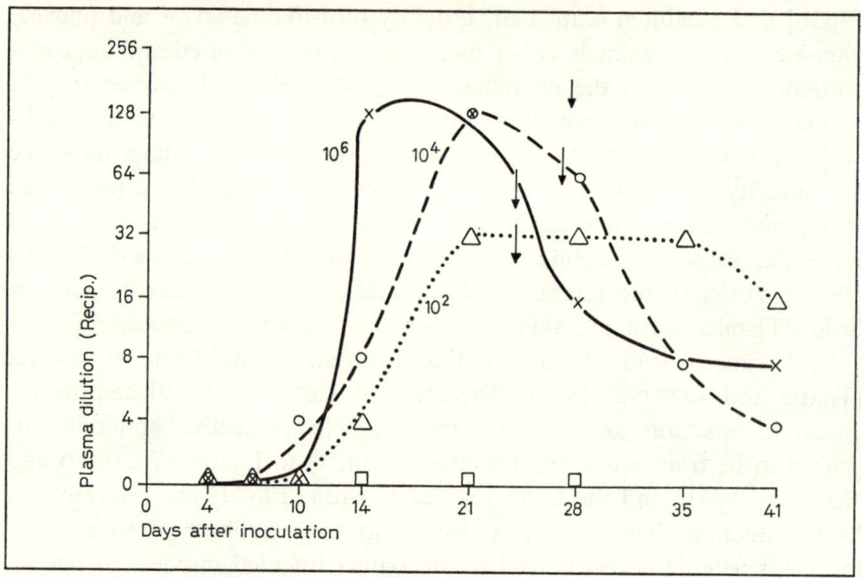

Fig. 6. Development of FAB in infant mice which were neonatally inoculated IC with LCM virus. Mice were weaned on day 24 or 27 ($\downarrow$ = mother removed). Three different virus doses were used: 10^6, 10^4 or 10^2 LD_{50}. Points show lowest plasma dilution producing fluorescent staining of LCM-infected BHK cells by indirect immunofluorescence.

titers (1/64 to 1/256) by 8 to 10 days after exposure to the infected infants. Mother exchanges between uninfected and LCM-infected litters showed that maternal FAB passed to normal offspring (fig. 7), and FAB was found in the milk at 12 days post-infection (BENSON, personal communication). Control, uninoculated infant mice with normal mothers consistently gave negative results (titers of <1/4). When a fresh uninfected mother was provided every 7 days to neonatally LCM-inoculated mice, no FAB was found in them for 63 days after infection. Thereafter a persistent low titer (1/8) was obtained. This late antibody could not have come from the mothers and therefore must have been made by the PTI mice themselves (fig. 8). There was some suggestion that the elimination of maternal antibody caused a higher titer of FAB in PTI mice in later months. Congenitally infected mice also showed FAB after the 3rd month. It is evident that antibody to LCM viral product is produced in LCM-PTI mice and that immunological tolerance to LCM antigens is not absolute.

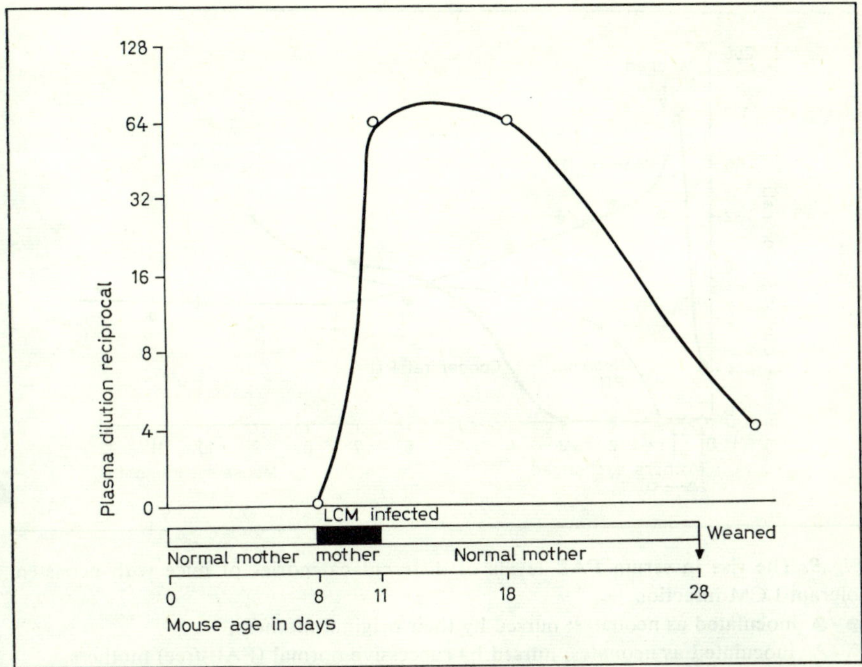

Fig. 7. The transfer of FAB from an LCM contact infected foster mother to uninoculated infant mice within a 3-day period. The foster mother had suckled LCM inoculated infants for 18 days previously and exhibited a high FAB titer (1/512) [BENSON and HOTCHIN, 1969]. Reproduced by permission of the editors of Nature.

A similar conclusion was inferred independently by VOLKERT [1962]. The findings are in keeping with the hypothesis [HOTCHIN, 1962a] that the gradually waning LCM tolerance is responsible for the late onset disease and glomerulonephritis of PTI mice.

The distribution of LCM antigen in neonatal PTI mice has been studied by WILSNACK and ROWE [1964] and BROWN [1968] utilizing the FAB technic which showed very generalized distribution of antigen, comparable to that found in congenitally LCM-infected mice by MIMS [1966]. BROWN [1968] showed a progressive development of fluorescence of cells distributed throughout virtually the entire mouse during the first five days after neonatal inoculation. Thereafter fluorescence remained at the same high level throughout the animal for as long as 20 months. On the first day post-infection, foci of antigen were limited to

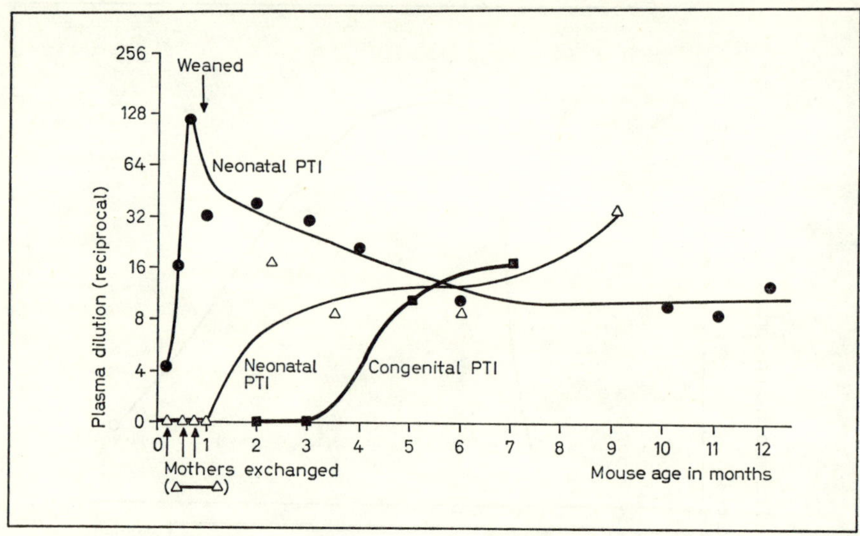

Fig. 8. The rise in serum FAB levels of different categories of mice with persistent tolerant LCM infection.
●–● inoculated as neonates; nursed by their original mothers;
△–△ inoculated as neonates; nursed by successive normal (FAB-free) mothers;
■–■ congenital LCM–PTI mice nursed by their original PTI mothers.

the vicinity of the IC injection site (table IV), choroid plexus, meninges, and rare clusters of fluorescent cells in the liver. The sequence of spread involved the liver at day 1, spleen and kidneys at day 2 and all other organs by day 3, including the entire remaining lymphoreticular system, thymus, lymph nodes, Peyer's patches, bone marrow and tissue macrophages. Antigen production was particularly intense in cells of the skin, gastrointestinal tract and kidneys. Similar findings were reported by WILSNACK and ROWE [1964] who observed much more antigen in the kidneys of PTI mice than in animals infected in adult life. Antigen was particularly plentiful in the proximal and distal convoluted tubules (both intracellular and free in the lumen), glomeruli, parietal layer of Bowman's capsule, uriniferous tubules, papillary ducts and connective tissue cells. In the glomerulus, antigen was coalesced into inclusion-like masses, while in the tubules it was evident as fine, granular cytoplasmic particles. The punctate distribution of LCM antigen visualized by the FAB technic has been shown by ABELSON *et al.* [1969] to correspond with aggregates of ribosomes in the infected cell. WILSNACK and ROWE

Table IV. Intensity of fluorescence in tissues of neonatal mice inoculated with lymphocytic choriomeningitis virus during the period of spreading infection [1]

	Time after inoculation				
	12 h	1 day	2 days	3 days	5 days
Site of inoculation	0	+	+ +	+ + + +	+ + + +
CNS	0	+	+ +	+ + +	+ + + +
Liver	0	+	+ +	+ + +	+ + + +
Spleen	0	0	+ +	+ + +	+ + + +
Kidneys	0	0	+	+ +	+ + + +
Blood	0	0	+	+ +	+ + +
Lymph nodes	0	0	0	+ +	+ + + +
Thymus	0	0	0	+ +	+ + + +
Other	0	0	0	+ +	+ + + +

[1] BROWN [1968].

[1964] found extreme variation between mice in amount and distribution of antigen. In some animals antigen was located primarily in the glomeruli while in others it was chiefly in the tubules. There were also big variations in the extent of involvement in different areas of the same kidney. The liver was found to be the most extensively involved organ and the pattern of parenchymal cell staining was indistinguishable from that in the acute infection, although different sections varied in the amount and distribution of antigen. The cells were situated in foci or cords with a distribution that was not lobular or confined to any particular area of a lobule. Antigen was sparse in bile ducts, connective tissue, Kupffer cells and arterial endothelium. Viral antigen was detected in the spleens of all mice examined, mainly localized in reticular and other connective tissue of the red pulp. Only rarely was antigen noted in lymphocytes of the Malpighian corpuscles. The capsule and trabeculae were invariably negative.

The most noteworthy difference between the results of antigen distribution studies in neonatal and congenital PTI mice appears to be the relative disappearance of antigen from the congenital group [WILSNACK and ROWE, 1964; MIMS, 1966] in older animals. While this phenomenon may be due to differences in the virus or mouse strains used, it nevertheless represents a profitable area for the study of the control mechanisms which regulate LCM replication in the tolerant animal.

LCM-induced Glomerulonephritis

Persistent infection of mice with LCM was at first thought to result in a completely harmless lifelong infection. However, HOTCHIN [1962a] reported that 10 to 14 months after neonatal inoculation with LCM virus, PTI mice gradually developed ruffled fur, blepharitis and hunched posture, resembling the early stages of acute LCM disease. This condition, tentatively termed 'late disease', did not progress to the convulsive stage but showed degenerative changes of the skin with marked hair loss and a generalized dilapidated appearance reminiscent of an adult runting syndrome. Mortality rose steeply after a 10-month incubation period (fig. 9) and the affected mice showed progressive weight loss. The premature aging and weight curves were similar to the results obtained in

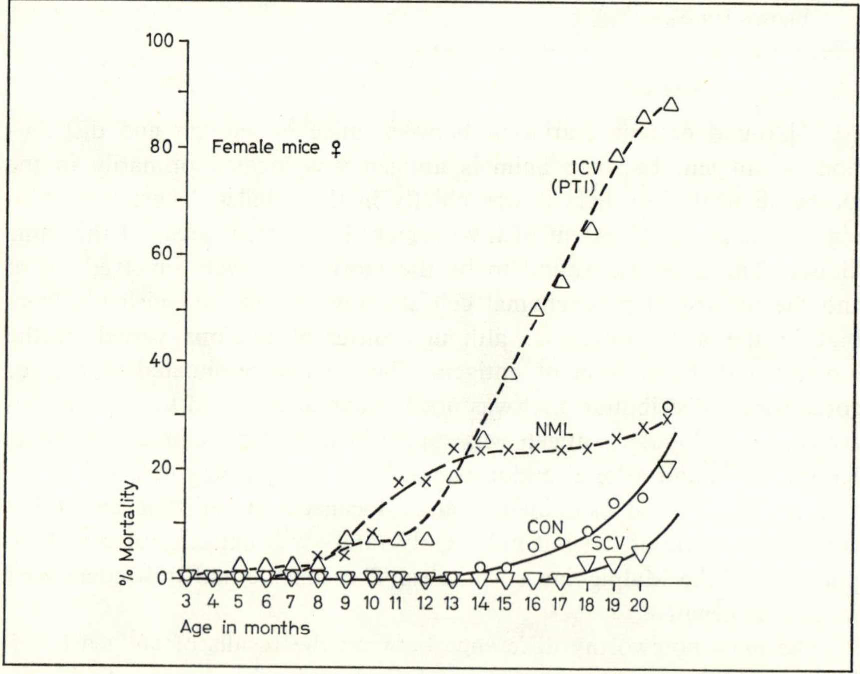

Fig. 9. The relation between cumulative mortality and time, in four groups of female mice. ICV = mice received LCM mouse liver IC at one day of age. NML = mice received normal mouse liver IC at one day of age. CON = mice received no inoculation. SCV = mice received LCM virus (same dose as ICV) at one month of age, by the SC route (this produces active immunity with suppression of virus). Reproduced by permission of Springer, New York/Berlin.

mice infected with the mammary-tumor-inciting virus [STORER, 1966]. All of the PTI mice finally succumbed to this condition. Virus titrations during their lifetime, with a few exceptions, showed very high levels in all animals examined. Representative titers of brain, liver and blood averaged 10^5, 10^6 and 10^5 LD_{50}/g or ml respectively. Histological investigation [COLLINS and HOTCHIN, 1963; HOTCHIN and COLLINS, 1964] showed splenic hyperplasia and pigment deposition, hepatitis with round cell infiltration, and pyelonephritis. Some kidney sections showed lesions typical of systemic lupus erythematosus [COLLINS and HOTCHIN, 1963]. The PTI mice remained well for approximately 7 to 10 months and then began to show 'late disease'. The disease was strain-dependent since 85% of Albany strain mice showed clinical late disease by 1 year of age compared to 46% of Swiss mice. Histological evidence of chronic glomerulonephritis was found in 34% of the Albany and 16% of the Swiss mice. This example of virus-induced glomerulonephritis was believed by HOTCHIN and COLLINS [1964] to be the result of an autoimmune process consequent upon a gradual waning of virus tolerance. This conclusion was strengthened by their finding deposits of antibody-containing material in the affected glomeruli which stained with fluorescent anti-mouse gamma globulin rabbit serum. The disease was proposed as an example of slow virus infection. The fluorescent staining of the glomerular deposits was confirmed by OLDSTONE and DIXON [1967]. The proposed mechanism would fit the observation of gradual lymphoid hypertrophy reported in LCM tolerant mice [TRAUB and KESTING, 1963a].

Accelerated LCM late disease could be produced in PTI mice by coelomic parabiosis with an LCM immune partner, using relatively inbred but not completely isologous mice [HOTCHIN, 1965]. In retrospect it appears that LCM late disease was possibly seen during the early studies by TRAUB [1938a], who noted that at the age of about 10 months, several mice which had congenital LCM infection began to show signs of old age, such as lack of liveliness, adiposis and ruffling of the fur. TRAUB and KESTING [1963a] later found a 40% increase in the weights of spleens of 6-month-old PTI mice compared to controls. These mice had virus titers of about $10^{6.5}$ ID_{50} in the spleen and lymph nodes over a 20-month period.

The occurrence of subacute glomerulonephritis similar to that described by HOTCHIN and COLLINS [1964] in the kidneys of neonatal LCM-PTI mice was confirmed by WILSNACK and ROWE [1964], POLLARD *et al.* [1968a, b], OLDSTONE and DIXON [1967, 1969], BROWN [1968] and

HIRSCH *et al.* [1968], but not in congenital LCM-PTI mice used by MIMS [1966], MIMS and SUBRAHMANYAN [1966], VOLKERT [1965], and VOLKERT *et al.* [1964]. These differences suggest that congenital infection is less likely to induce nephritis than neonatal inoculation and that the C_3H mouse strain is relatively insusceptible to glomerulonephritis. The nephritis was similar to that described by HELYER and HOWIE [1963] in NZB mice and may have a similar mechanism [MCGIVEN and HICKS, 1967]. It is also similar to the nephritis found in AKR [DMOCHOWSKI *et al.*, 1966] or Balb/C/DM/Tex [RECHER *et al.*, 1954] mice inoculated with Friend or Rauscher virus. The lesions are also similar to those found in Aleutian mink disease [HENSON *et al.*, 1967; KINDIG *et al.*, 1967] with the suggestion that a similar virus-induced circulating antigen/antibody complex is responsible. POLLARD *et al.* [1968a] reported high levels of IgM in gnotobiotic LCM-PTI mice with glomerulonephritis, and OLDSTONE and DIXON [1967] found the sera of their three-month-old mice to be antibody free, but reported the acid elution of low titer CF antibody from homogenates of nephritic kidneys. Using the same method HOTCHIN and BAKER[11] were unable to elute detectable CF antibody or FAB from the kidneys of PTI or HDIP mice, although they were able to demonstrate that both antibodies were stable during the elution procedure. Virus was inactivated by the procedure but antigen was unaffected. Very low levels of anticomplementary (AC) activity were found in the eluates from occasional mice in the series. It may be prudent to consider also the entire pathological picture of these LCM glomerulonephritic kidneys, which are clearly the site of a complex pathogenic process and contain excess soluble antigen and a large number of infiltrated round cells (fig. 10). Therefore, the specificity of the AC effect cannot be tested, and the origin of eluted antibody cannot be ascribed to the glomerular deposit rather than the cellular infiltrate. Normal kidney tissue is reported to have AC activity [HAMPERS *et al.*, 1967]. However, these findings at least conform with the concept that the glomerular deposit is formed from circulating antigen-antibody complexes. WILSNACK and ROWE [1964] reported that in contrast to the other tissues of congenital PTI mice, the kidney contained more fluorescent antigen than those of acutely sick mice. Antigen occurred in the glomeruli of some mice, but in others it was more obvious in the tubules.

BAKER and HOTCHIN [1967] found that kidneys of PTI mice were smaller than normal, particularly in male mice. Renal function tests showed that PTI mice without significant signs of disease nevertheless

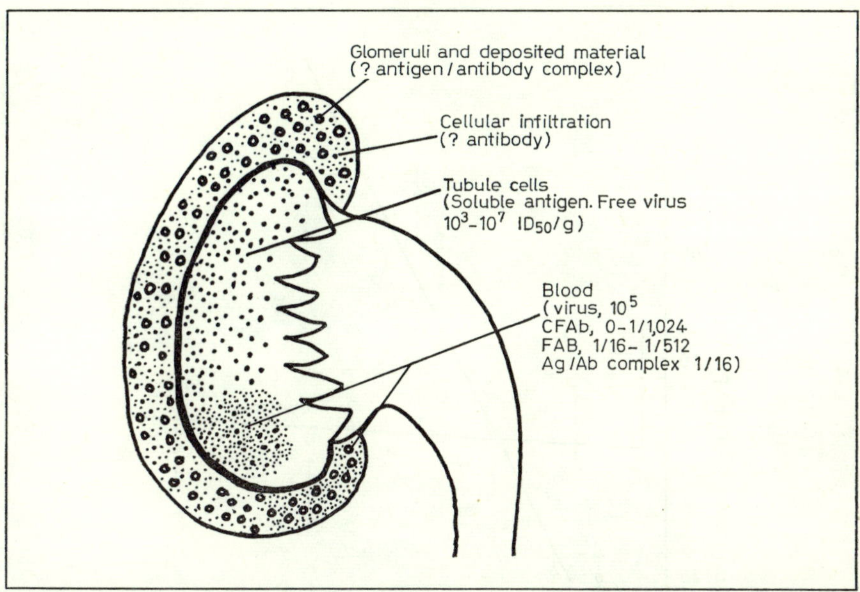

Fig. 10. Diagram showing the complex nature of the pathogenic process in nephritic kidneys of LCM-PTI mice.

had progressively impaired ability to clear urea from their blood[11] (fig. 11). The onset of kidney failure showed a parallel relationship to the incubation period and mortality curve of mice with late disease (fig. 9). Similar results were obtained with a separate group of mice utilizing creatinine clearance as a measure of kidney function. In the study by HIRSCH *et al.* [1968] using mice inoculated neonatally and treated with *RAMT*, and also in HDIP mice[12], circulating antigen-antibody complexes have been detected, suggesting that the renal lesions may be secondary to immunopathological mechanisms initiated by antigen-antibody complexes. These authors [HIRSCH *et al.*, 1968] proposed that the earlier onset of glomerulonephritis in *RAMT* serum-treated animals than in animals neonatally inoculated with virus, is attributable to the increased amount of circulating antibody present. They suggested that the presence and amount of circulating and nephritogenic antibody is dependent on various factors, such as timing of inoculation, strain of virus, or

[11] J. HOTCHIN and F. BAKER, unpublished results.
[12] J. HOTCHIN, unpublished results.

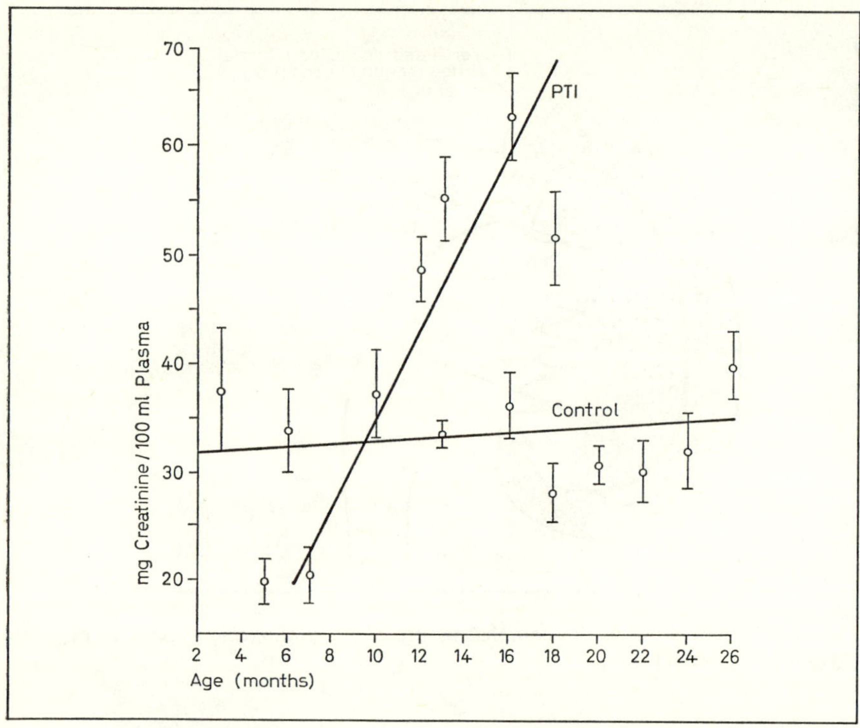

Fig. 11. Creatinine clearance values (± standard error) of non-infected control and PTI mice over 26 months. All PTI mice were dead after 18 months.

strain of mouse used. Before the antigen-antibody concept can be concluded to provide the entire explanation for the onset of glomerular disease after LCM inoculation in mice, it will be necessary to investigate whether the presence of antigen complexes induced by persistent viruses other than LCM, such as lactic dehydrogenase elevating virus (LDV), also produce renal damage.

Tolerance Breakage

Many attempts have been made to reverse or break the immunological tolerance of LCM-PTI mice. The approach seems to have been suggested by TRAUB's early observations on the totally different effect, in which IC injections of sterile fluids induced LCM disease in partially immune animals (see section on 'The SC/IC effect'). Failure to break tolerance occurred after repeated inoculation with homologous virus,

SLE virus and influenza virus by Haas [1954], after IC inoculation of broth by Traub [1963] and after IC inoculation with sterile fluids, cold stress, X-irradiation and superinfection with ectromelia or WEE viruses by Hotchin [1958] and Hotchin and Cinits [1958]. Superinfection with *E. coccoides* [Hotchin, 1965] induced temporary illness lasting about one week in PTI mice 2 to 7 months old, without causing appreciable change in virus titer. Hotchin [1962a] attempted to induce acute disease in PTI mice by the IV or IP inoculation of varying amounts of viable cell suspensions obtained from lymph nodes, spleen, thymus and bone marrow of LCM-immune inbred mice. Although illness was induced, no specific induction of LCM disease occurred in PTI animals during the 14-day period of observation. Similar attempts using coelomic parabiosis of immune and tolerant mouse pairs [Hotchin, 1965] caused 'late disease' in the virus-carrying animal. However, the effect depended also on minor degress of tissue incompatibility since it could not be reproduced in isologous mice. Volkert [1963, 1965] and Volkert and Larsen [1964] made a very thorough study of passive tolerance reversal by transplantation of isologous immune lymphoid cells to LCM-PTI mice and followed virus titer and antibody production. Marked reduction of virus titer in blood and spleen occurred, with production of high titer CF and neutralizing antibody. The effect began about 10 days after transplantation and virus titer fell by 10^4 during the next 5 weeks and remained just detectable in many mice. The rate at which virus was eliminated was roughly proportional to cell dose in the range of 12×10^6 to 200×10^6 cells and the effect was somewhat mouse strain dependent. With normal (non-immune) cells the effect took 9 weeks and was only 25% effective, but homologous (non-isologous) cells did not confer any immunity. The efficacy of virus clearing occurred in the descending order of spleen, lymph nodes, lungs, liver, brain and thymus to kidney, where relatively large amounts remained. A noticeable feature of this work was the exceptionally high titer of antibody which was 100 times higher in lymph node cell transplanted tolerant mice than that seen in hyperimmunized control animals, or in the donor mice that had provided the transplant (fig. 12) [Volkert *et al.*, 1964; Volkert and Larsen, 1965b]. The immunity could be secondarily conferred by lymphoid cells harvested from transplanted virus carriers [Volkert *et al.*, 1964]. No parallelism occurred [Larsen and Volkert, 1967] between antibody formation and virus suppression, which suggested that the two functions involved different systems of immunologically

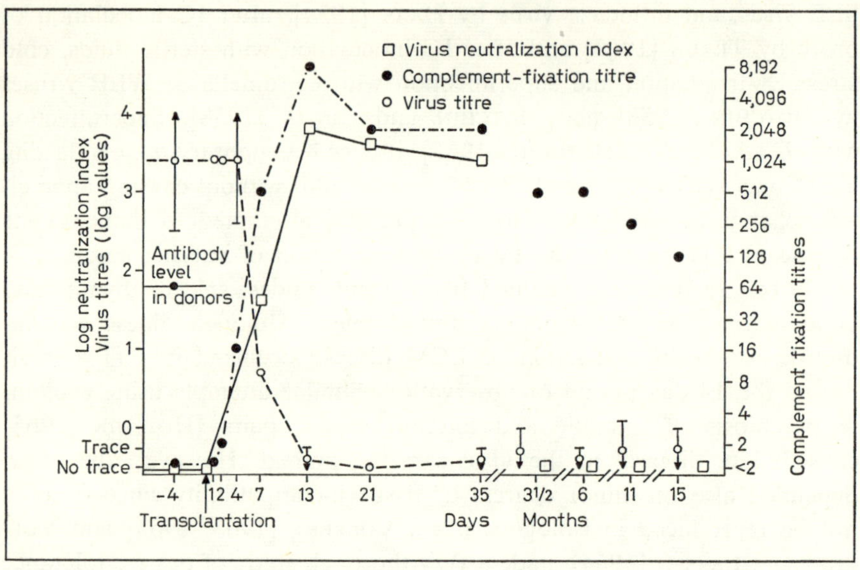

Fig. 12. Virus titers and antibody titers of the blood from LCM-PTI C₃H mice and after transplantation of 100×10⁶ lymphoid cells from immune donors [VOLKERT, LARSEN and PFAU, 1964]. Reproduced by permission of the author and editor.

reactive cells. Both CF and neutralizing antibody were claimed by VOLKERT *et al.* [1964] to be present in serum at the same time as infectious virus. High titered neutralizing antiserum given without cells to LCM-PTI mice caused only a temporary depression of virus titer, of approximately 2 logs [VOLKERT and LARSEN, 1965b]. The series of experiments by VOLKERT and LARSEN clearly established that passively acquired cellular immunity, but not humoral antibody, could abolish LCM tolerance and virtually eliminate the virus infection. The effect occurred slowly and for the most part without obvious disease [VOLKERT, 1965]. VOLKERT and LARSEN [1965b] proposed that if the level of viral antigen could be temporarily reduced to a critical level in LCM tolerant mice, the state of tolerance should be reversed, by allowing immunologically competent host cells to react to the virus and initiate virus suppression. However, a temporary reduction of tolerance caused by the administration of non-isologous immune lymphoid cells failed to support the concept, and tolerance returned to its previous level [VOLKERT and LARSEN, 1965b]. The negative result is reinforced by the fact that donated normal lymphoid cells do not all become tolerant on exposure to the high antigen concentrations in the recipient animal, since such transplants can slowly abolish tolerance [VOLKERT, 1963].

Tolerance Induction in the Adult by Immune Suppressive Agents
X-irradiation

ROWE [1956] found that pre-irradiation of mice with X-rays protected them from the acute disease, but left a persistent infection which lasted for several weeks. This effect was confirmed [HOTCHIN, 1958; HOTCHIN and CINITS, 1958; HOTCHIN and WEIGAND, 1959; REMEZOV, 1959]. When IC inoculation preceded X-irradiation, partial protection was achieved, which decreased as the interval between inoculation and irradiation increased. When LCM was given by IP inoculation a day or two before X-irradiation, an unexpected effect occurred whereby cerebral symptoms were induced by the irradiation and the mice died in convulsions [HOTCHIN and CINITS, 1958]. UPHOFF and HAAS [1960] used lethal X-irradiation, followed by protective bone marrow grafts, to show that resistance to subsequent LCM challenge was determined by the immune status of the host rather than that of the graft donor. Bone marrow tissue from LCM-immune donors did not confer immunity to LCM. The X-ray protection mechanism was studied in detail [BENSON *et al.*, 1959; SCHLEIFSTEIN and COLLINS, 1959; COLLINS *et al.*, 1961; HOTCHIN and WEIGAND, 1961b] and was found to coincide with severe depression of the total blood leucocyte count, to levels of approximately 1,000 cells/mm³. Virus multiplication was unaffected or slightly enhanced as a result of the prior X-irradiation. It was clear that the protective effect was not due to inhibition of virus multiplication, but was possibly a consequence of the depression of cellular immune response caused by the X-irradiation. Histological study showed that none of the normal LCM-induced lesions were present in the X-irradiated animals. The radiation therefore prevented the host response of lymphocytic infiltration and the associated tissue damage, which suggested that the cellular immune response caused the tissue lesions previously ascribed to the virus. Mice were protected against LCM challenge for about 10 days after irradiation [HOTCHIN and WEIGAND, 1959]. Comparable amelioration of clinical murine virus disease by X-irradiation has been reported and reviewed by WEBB and SMITH [1966] for other viruses, including SLE [GOLDBERG *et al.*, 1935] and Langat virus [WEBB *et al.*, 1968a, b]. These results strengthen the conclusion that the cellular immune response of the host is responsible for a significant portion of virus disease, and that possibilities exist for some therapeutic effect of immune suppressive agents, if the intrinsic destructive effect of the virus is not great.

Chemical Immune Suppressants

HAAS and STEWART [1956] noticed that an antifolic agent, amethopterin, and also an antipyrimidine, guanazolo, both prolonged or spared the lives of mice infected with normally lethal doses of LCM virus. The infection was not eradicated by the drugs and surviving mice had an inapparent persistent infection [HAAS et al., 1957a] with viremia and CF antibody formation. The authors suggested that amethopterin probably interfered with antibody development [LEVY and HAAS, 1958], thereby allowing the infection to persist. Two substrains of leukemia from which LCM virus was isolated could only be propagated in mice treated with either amethopterin or 8-azaguanine [STEWART et al., 1957; HAAS, 1960]. These chemicals appeared to contribute to the ability of LCM to persist in the tumor-bearing animal by inhibiting the immune response [POTTER and HAAS, 1959]; histological study by LERNER and HAAS [1958] showed that the normal lesions of LCM were almost completely suppressed by the drug. The amethopterin sparing effect was reversed by administration of citrovorum factor or folic acid [HAAS et al., 1957b]. Similar protection was afforded by myleran, chlorambucil [BARLOW, 1961], 1, 3-bis-(2-chloroethyl)-1-nitrosourea (BCNU) [SIDWELL et al., 1965], cortisone [HOTCHIN and CINITS, 1958], stress[13] [HOTCHIN, 1958], azaserine, 6-diazo-5-oxo-nor-1-leucine (DON) and 5-fluorouracil [LEVY and HAAS, 1958]. An extract of a higher plant *Sambucus sieboldiana* was reported [FURUSAWA et al., 1968] to be capable of reducing mortality of LCM virus infection in mice. This has not been confirmed, and the mechanism of the effect is unexplained. BARLOW and HOTCHIN [1960, 1962; HOTCHIN, 1962a] studied the time of administration of amethopterin relative to virus inoculation and found that a single injection of 8 mg/kg of the drug would completely prevent death if given at 100 h after IC inoculation (fig. 13). The single inoculation appeared to act upon the immune response at a critical time, converting it to a temporary tolerance. After drug inoculation, virus titer in brain and blood gradually decreased (fig. 14). Repeated virus challenge during this period had no effect upon virus level. The sparing effect of amethopterin upon LCM-infected mice was thought at this time

---

[13] E. SIKORA, L. BENSON, and J. HOTCHIN, unpublished results.

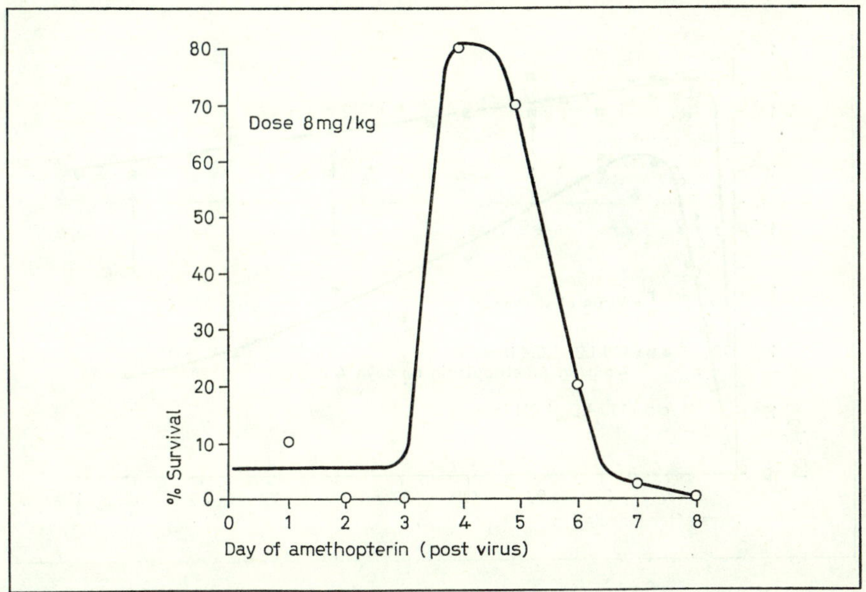

Fig. 13. The relationship between percent survival and day of administration of 8 mg/kg amethopterin, after IC inoculation of approximately 100 LD$_{50}$ LCM virus, in adult mice. This dose of drug had no visible effect upon uninoculated mice [HOTCHIN, 1962a]. Reproduced from Cold Spring Harbor Symposia, vol. 27, 1962.

[BARLOW and HOTCHIN, 1962] to be dependent upon its ability to block a generalized immune response to soluble antigen. Similar experiments were made with 1, 3-bis-(2-chloroethyl)-1-nitrosourea (BCNU) by SID-WELL *et al.* [1965] who concluded that the theory proposed by Hotchin that a tolerance-inducing mechanism was the probable explanation of the amethopterin protection. They felt that this theory is likely to hold for the BCNU effect which primarily suppressed the cellular immunity. The results with chemical immunosuppressants tended to confirm the concept that the host's immune mechanisms may be depressed at a critical time during the immune response to LCM antigens, causing the animal to exhibit tolerance rather than a lethal immunological reaction [HOTCHIN, 1962a].

SIKORA and HOTCHIN [1962] noticed that the administration of amethopterin daily from day 0 to day 6 post virus, converted a nonlethal infection after FP inoculation into a lethal infection and abolished the FP re-

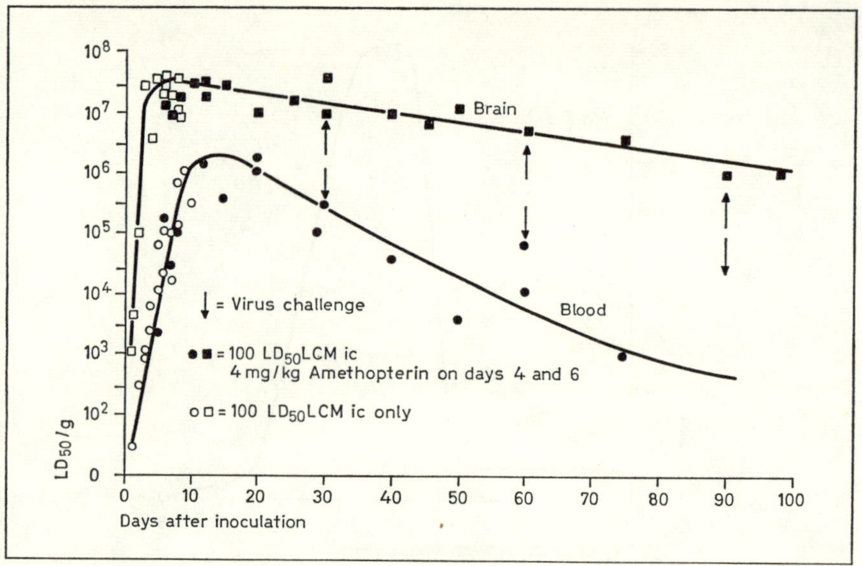

Fig. 14. Virus titer in brain and blood of mice with and without amethopterin treatment (4 mg/kg on days 4 and 6). The untreated mice died, but treated ones showed only slight temporary illness. Arrows show times of IC virus challenge. Reproduced from Cold Spring Harbor Symposia, vol. 27, 1962.

sponse. This may be equivalent to the observation[14] that in young animals FP inoculation of LCM causes a lethal infection with no FP response. Both of these situations may arise when the local lymph node response to LCM is inadequate to restrain the virus, either due to immaturity or amethopterin suppression. A similar conversion of the LCM-FP response to lethal generalized infection without FP swelling is caused by IV injection of Evans blue during the first 2 days post-inoculation of virus [CUTIE and SIKORA, 1964]. An extract of herbs reported [FURUSAWA and CUTTING, 1966; CUTTING *et al.*, 1965; FURUSAWA *et al.*, 1967] to have an ameliorative effect upon LCM infection in mice may owe its modest success to an immunosuppressive effect upon the mice. However, PFAU and CAMYRE [1968] have reported that the tissue culture adapted variant of this strain is not LCM virus but is a picornavirus.

Thymectomy

If acute LCM disease is due mainly to a cellular immune response

[14] J. HOTCHIN, unpublished results.

comparable to the homograft rejection mechanism, neonatal thymectomy should prevent the acute disease. ROWE *et al.* [1963] and SIKORA [1963] showed this prediction to be correct.

ROWE *et al.* [1963] noticed that mice with minor amounts of thymus tissue still remaining showed some cellular infiltration of the meninges, whereas those with complete thymectomy showed negative or minimal infiltration. Thymectomized animals showed less sickness and increased survival after IC or IP injection of LCM. The effect was obtained in mice of differing strains, with continuing virus multiplication in spite of the appearance of CF antibody. Thus, cellular virus-suppressive immunity was abolished by thymectomy, but humoral CF antibody production was left intact indicating a dissociation of the two types of immune response or 'split tolerance', in the thymectomized mouse. Thymectomy differed from other immunosuppressive measures since it did not induce marked lymphopenia in the NIH strain of mice that were used. Its effect was 52% reversed by inserting a 0.45 μ millipore filter chamber containing thymus tissue [LEVEY *et al.*, 1963; OLDSTONE and DIXON, 1968a] in the peritoneal cavity. Similar results following neonatal thymectomy and LCM inoculation were obtained by EAST *et al.* [1964], HOTCHIN and SIKORA [1964] and FÖLDES *et al.* [1964]. Chronic disease and persistent viremia of differing durations occurred in surviving mice, some of which showed wasting disease, retardation, dermatitis and spleen atrophy [FÖLDES *et al.*, 1964]. These experiments added valuable new evidence which confirmed the immune conflict concept of acute LCM disease, and provided additional evidence that the cellular response, and not the humoral one, caused virus elimination and acute disease.

Immune Suppressive Serum

When the technic of causing temporary extirpation of lymphocytes or thymocytes by injection of specific antiserum became available, several workers successfully applied it to the LCM system as a further test of the role of cellular immunity in this disease. GLEDHILL [1967] found that a regime of ALS injections given to mice after LCM inoculation protected against the lethal effect of the virus, although some mice became ill if fewer doses of serum were given. The blood of these animals still retained large amounts of virus one month after inoculation although they were free from disease. Similar results were obtained by LUNDSTEDT and VOLKERT [1967] who obtained ALS-induced inapparent persistent infection lasting for more than 12 months, with variable levels of CF antibody.

Normal rabbit serum caused similar but less marked effects, in which there was prolonged viremia and delayed antibody response to LCM virus. These facts seem to indicate that relatively little inhibition of the immune system of the host animal was sufficient to tip the scale in favor of tolerance. When ALS was given [VOLKERT and LUNDSTEDT, 1968] to mice which had suppressed LCM infection, viremia developed temporarily in all of the treated mice to very high titers without affecting antibody level. In a few mice, CF antibody increased at the same time as virus titer.

Rabbit anti-mouse thymocyte serum (RAMT) was given by HIRSCH and MURPHY [1967] and HIRSCH et al. [1967] at 3-day intervals to 3–4-week-old mice which were challenged 6 days later with LCM virus; no clinical signs developed while the mice were under treatment. There was no histological evidence of infection despite brain titers of 10^6–10^7 LD_{50}/g and blood titers of 10^3–10^5 LD_{50}/ml. When RAMT serum was discontinued, characteristic clinical and histological choriomeningitis with convulsions developed in 1–2 weeks. In mice under continuous serum treatment, brain titers diminished to 10^3 LD_{50} after 40 days and were undetectable by day 76. In these animals the RAMT appears to have exerted a therapeutic effect by prolonging the course of the infection and ameliorating the severity of the animal's defense mechanism in suppressing the virus. Shorter exposure of the animals to serum treatment caused a delay in onset of clinical and histological signs of infection; even one dose of serum given 6 days prior to virus inoculation was sufficient to prolong life significantly. Treated animals showed evidence of small lymphocyte depletion from thymus-dependent areas of the spleen and lymph nodes, with replacement of these cells by large mononuclear and plasma cells. There was also a moderate depletion of small thymocytes from the thymic cortex. Seven to fourteen days after discontinuation of serum therapy, repopulation of lymphoid organs and restoration of peripheral lymphocytes was complete. RAMT also extended [HIRSCH et al., 1968] the period after birth during which inoculation with LCM virus induced PTI instead of causing acute death. Although the lethal cellular immune response was depressed, humoral (CF) antibody production was normal and a state of split tolerance ensued. One-fifth of the RAMT treated virus-inoculated animals developed a severe wasting disorder between one and two months of age, with retarded growth, hunched posture, facial edema, alopecia, oily skin and a mincing gait; in later stages, joint stiffness and ataxia was seen. The condition was characterized histologically by reticular cell hyperplasia and generalized infiltration. The remaining animals developed severe glomerulonephritis at 3 months of age. The runting syndrome appears to be similar to that produced by neonatal thymectomy and virus inoculation at weaning [SZERI *et al.*, 1966] and by neonatal inoculation of LCM virus alone [HOTCHIN, 1962a]. These syndromes have in common [HIRSCH *et al.*, 1968] a poorly functioning cellular immune system, and the reticular cell hyperplasia and infiltration may play a part in the pathogenesis of the disease. There appears to be a direct correlation between reticuloendothelial hyperactivity and the degree of wasting [DEVRIES *et al.*, 1964; MILLER and HOWARD, 1964; SCHOOLEY *et al.*, 1965]. HIRSCH and MURPHY [1968] concluded that the circulating CF antibody caused the development within a few months of chronic glomerulonephritis, characterized by deposition of gamma globulin and viral antigen in glomerular tufts. They considered that their results confirmed the earlier conclusions [HOTCHIN, 1962a] that cellular immune phenomena are critically important in murine LCM-virus pathogenesis.

Mice exhibiting the graft versus host reaction (GVH) were used by KOLTAY *et al.* [1968] for challenge with LCM virus; more rapid weight loss and later deaths occurred in the grafted mice than in LCM-infected non-GVH controls. Animals that survived LCM, which had also received GVH treatment, had viremia for at least 37 days. The authors suggested that the development of active neurological symptoms and early mortality in LCM-infected mice are closely correlated to the availability of active lymphocytes. The rapid weight loss was believed to be comparable to the runting syndrome in thymectomized mice, which is aggravated by LCM infection [FÖLDES *et al.*, 1964]. Runting or wasting was regarded as a nonspecific syndrome which could be caused by a variety of factors, including viruses, in host animals with impaired immunological competence.

High Dose Immunological Paralysis with LCM Virus

HAAS [1954] observed that among adult mice which had received lethal IC or IP doses of LCM, a certain proportion remained well but were immune and a few showed chronic illness. HOTCHIN and BENSON [1963] reported that IC inoculation was frequently followed by fewer deaths when high doses of LCM virus were used than with lower doses. This effect was particularly marked when using viscerotropic LCM. Surviving mice, though immune to challenge, proved to be persistently infected and carried virus at high titer, in a state of immunological tolerance or paralysis. The effect was referred to as 'high dose immune paralysis' (HDIP).

These results were confirmed by LARSEN [1967, 1968] who found that the viremia decreased slowly from a high level during the first week, to a low level two to three months later. Titers of CF antibody were constant during this period, but in some mice CF titer fell after 8 months and viremia reappeared. LARSEN [1969b] obtained various levels of antibody and viremia by inoculating mice of different ages up to 9 days after birth.

High antibody titer, coexisting with high levels of viremia, was also described in HDIP mice by BENSON and HOTCHIN [1969]. The levels of FAB and viremia in mice following a high IC dose (10^4 ID_{50}) of viscerotropic LCM are shown in figures 15 and 16[15]. The mice exhibited high FAB titers for many months, with concomitant high virus titer which only gradually declined. This antibody did not protect against death nor neutralize blood virus, but significant levels of AC activity[16] were found in the blood which were presumed to be due to antigen/antibody complexes. It is clear that in the HDIP mouse there is a spontaneous state of split tolerance similar to that described by HIRSCH and MURPHY [1968] in ALS-treated LCM-infected mice, since humoral antibody production is normal but cellular immune response to LCM is impaired. Situations comparable to the HDIP state also occurred with variable frequency when inoculation was made shortly after birth [LARSEN, 1969b]. The inhibition of

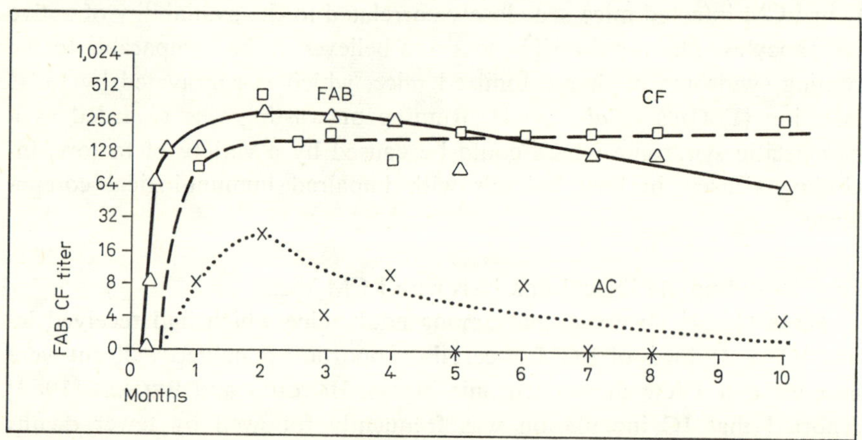

Fig. 15. Antibody titers and anticomplementary (AC) activity of plasma in HDIP mice.

[15] J. HOTCHIN, unpublished results.
[16] J. HOTCHIN and W. DECHER, unpublished results.

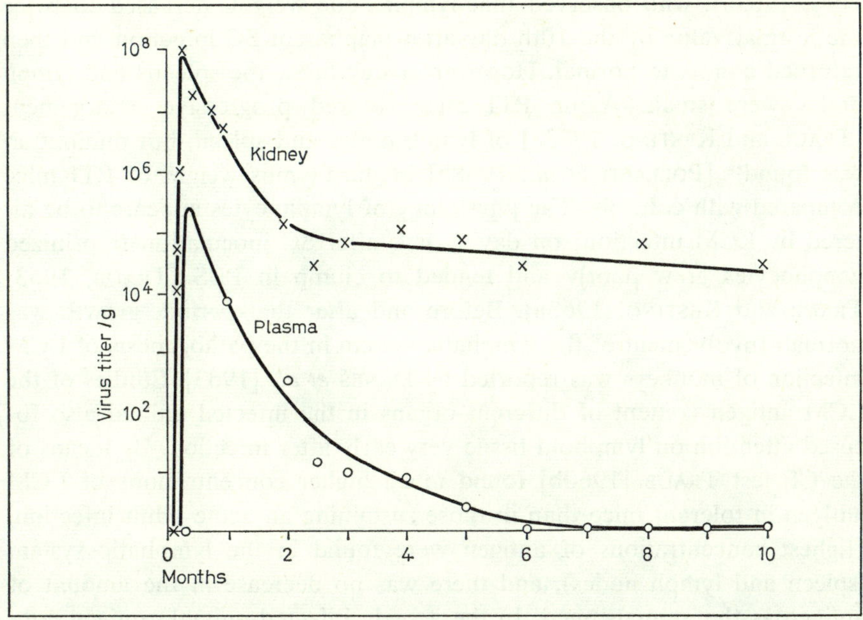

Fig. 16. Virus titer in kidney and plasma of HDIP mice.

cellular immunity is apparently related to the lysis of thymus-dependent lymphocytes described by HANAOKA *et al.* [1969]; these cells are normally responsible for LCM virus suppression. The paralysis of the host cellular immunity, however, is not complete, as shown by ability of the HDIP mouse to reject skin grafts from mice of a different strain[17]. Neither is the state permanent, since after 20 months HDIP mice were shown [HOTCHIN *et al.*, 1969] to have suppressed virus and to have developed high titer (1/625) neutralizing antibody. The differential inhibition of cellular, relative to humoral immune response, is similar to that produced by BOREL *et al.* [1966] by injection of proteins into newborn animals.

Lymphoreticular Lesions

Enlargement of lymph nodes and spleen in LCM-infected animals was noted in early reports of the disease [FARMER and JANEWAY, 1942] and confirmed by HAAS [1960] and TRAUB [TRAUB, 1960b; TRAUB and KES-

[17] J. HOTCHIN and S. SUZUKI, unpublished results.

TING, 1963a], who observed that lymph node weight increased to twice the normal value by the 10th day after inapparent SC infection and then returned almost to normal. However in sick mice, the spleens and lymph nodes were small. Aging PTI mice showed progressive enlargement [TRAUB and KESTING, 1963a] of lymph nodes and spleen, but diminution was found[18] [POLLARD et al., 1968b] in the thymus weight of PTI mice compared with controls. The physiology of lymphocytes appears to be altered by LCM infection; on day 7 or 8 after SC inoculation trypsinized lymphocytes grew poorly and tended to clump in PBS [TRAUB, 1963; TRAUB and KESTING, 1963a]. Before and after that period, growth was normal. Involvement of the lymphatic system in the pathogenesis of LCM infection of monkeys was reported by DANEŠ et al. [1963]. Studies of the LCM antigen content of different organs in the infected animal also focused attention on lymphoid tissue very early after infection. By means of the CF test TRAUB [1960b] found much higher concentrations of LCM antigen in tolerant mice than in those sustaining an acute adult infection. Highest concentrations of antigen were found in the lymphatic system (spleen and lymph nodes), and there was no decrease in the amount of antigen as the animals aged. In the acutely infected animal, antigen concentrations in lymph nodes and spleen were highest by the 3rd day of infection and then declined to zero by the 21st day. In other organs, such as the liver, peak titers occurred about the 7th day. Fluorescent antibody studies confirmed the rapid development of high concentrations of antigen in the spleens and lymph nodes [WILSNACK and ROWE, 1964; BROWN, 1968] of PTI mice but only rarely in the lymphocytes [WILSNACK and ROWE, 1964]. Conflicting evidence is reported [WILSNACK and ROWE, 1964; BARATAWIDJAJA et al., 1965; MIMS, 1966] on the fluorescence of lymphocytes in acute disease.

The histology of the lymphoreticular system during acute LCM infection of adult mice was studied by HANAOKA et al. [1969] who found specific lymphoid cell destruction by the third day after viscerotropic or neurotropic virus. The lesions were visible as pale areas of reticulum with a relative absence of small lymphocytes, beginning in the cortex of lymph nodes and in the white pulp of the spleen around the central artery. By the 7th day, destruction of small lymphocytes was prominent in the whole lymph node, with extensive cell debris and phagocytosis, and by the 10th day, small lymphocytes were almost entirely absent. The distribution of

---

[18] J. HOTCHIN and S. SUZUKI, unpublished results.

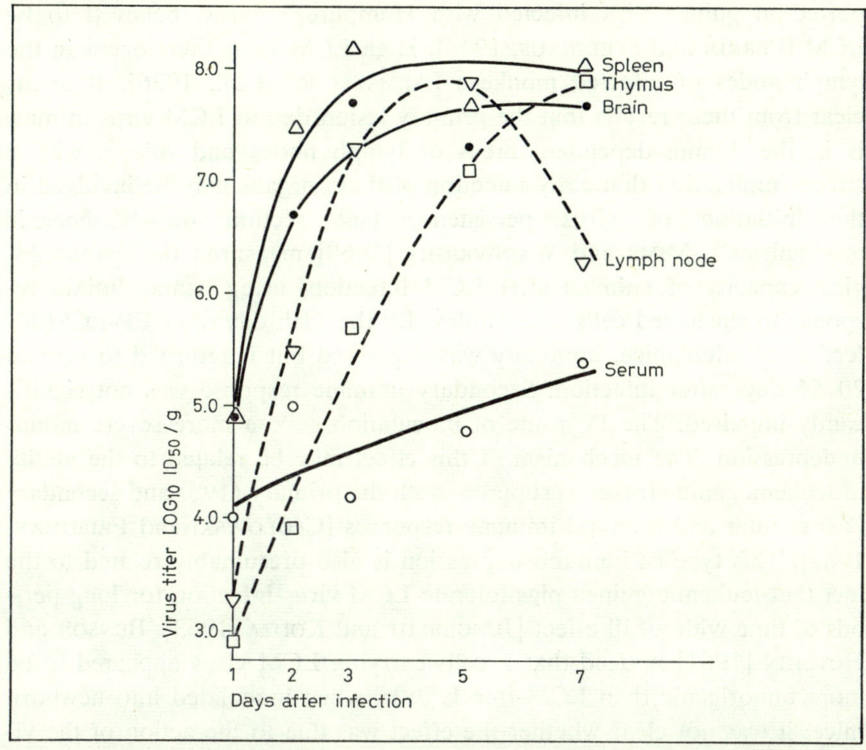

Fig. 17. Virus titer of lymphoreticular system, brain and serum, after infection with
10^3 MID$_{50}$ neurotropic LCM virus IC (SUZUKI and HOTCHIN, unpublished results).

the lesions corresponded to the areas believed to be occupied by thymus-
dependent lymphocytes (TDL). Cortical thymic lymphocytes were destroyed, beginning on the 5th day until by the 10th day thymic lymphocytes had almost completely disappeared from the cortex, causing a 4-fold
decrease in thymus weight. During this period virus titers in these organs
increased steeply (fig. 17). Similar lymphoreticular changes were reported
as early as 1945 for LCM by LILLIE and ARMSTRONG [1945], and more
recently for the MP strain of LCM [MOLOMUT *et al.*, 1964; MOLOMUT
and PADNOS, 1965; MOLOMUT *et al.*, 1965; PADNOS *et al.*, 1968] and for a
virus from DBA mice [LAW and DUNN, 1951] which appeared to be LCM
(DUNN, personal communication). Lymphoreticular damage has been reported to occur in guinea pigs with LCM [LILLIE and ARMSTRONG, 1944;
BENDA *et al.*, 1964] and severe lymphoid and thymic degeneration was re-

ported in guinea pigs infected with Humphrey's virus, believed to be LCM [PERRIN and STEINHAUS, 1944]. High LCM virus titers occur in the lymph nodes of infected monkeys [ARMSTRONG *et al.*, 1936]. It seems clear from these results that the primary lesion due to LCM virus in mice is in the thymus-dependent areas of lymph nodes and spleen, with a strong implication that early infection of these organs may be involved in the initiation of virus persistence (see section on 'Pathogenic mechanisms'). MIMS and WAINWRIGHT [1968] measured the immunological capacity of animals after LCM infection, using hemagglutinin response to sheep red cells as an index. By the 11th day after FP-LCM infection of adult mice, immunity was depressed but it returned to normal 20–56 days after infection. Secondary immune response was not significantly impaired. The IV route of inoculation gave a more severe immunodepression. The mechanism of this effect may be related to the ability of leukemogenic viruses to suppress both the primary (19S) and secondary (7S) cellular and humoral immune responses [CEGLOWSKI and FRIEDMAN, 1967]. This type of immunosuppression is also presumably related to the fact that leukemic guinea pigs tolerate LCM virus infection for long periods of time without ill effect [JUNGEBLUT and KODZA, 1963]. BENSON and HOTCHIN [1961] noticed that L cells carrying LCM virus appeared to be more tumorigenic than LCM-free L cells, when inoculated into newborn mice; it was not clear whether the effect was due to the action of the virus upon the L cells, or conceivably via its immunosuppressive effect upon the host. SUZUKI and HOTCHIN[19] tried to detect a depression of homograft rejection capability induced by LCM virus, but found no significant change in rejection of homologous grafts following or during LCM infection. HOLTERMANN and MAJDE [1969b] found that isografts from PTI donors were uniformly rejected in 14 days by normal recipients but concurrent autografts on these recipients were frequently also rejected. While the infected isograft rejection could be explained on the basis of rejection of LCM-induced new transplantation antigens, the autograft rejection is harder to understand and suggests heightened rather than diminished homograft rejection consequent upon the infection. However, it is likely that the autograft becomes infected during the generalized LCM infection of the recipient from the isograft, and that it is particularly susceptible to the generalized rejection of virus-infected tissue which results from the cellular immune response of the host.

[19] S. SUZUKI and J. HOTCHIN, unpublished results.

The Interaction of LCM with Leukemia

A remarkable number of examples has been reported in which LCM has been found to contaminate leukemias [HUMPHREYS *et al.*, 1956; TAYLOR and MACDOWELL, 1949; LAW and DUNN, 1951; NADEL and HAAS, 1955, 1956; STEWART and HAAS, 1956; HAAS, 1960; TRAUB, 1962; JUNGEBLUT and KODZA, 1963; MOLOMUT and PADNOS, 1965]. In several instances, the presence of LCM has appeared to moderate the severity of the leukemia to a significant degree. LCM virus was found by HOTCHIN [1962a] to induce resistance to tumor induction by polyoma virus, when the LCM was given to newborn mice a few hours after birth, and polyoma virus was administered one day later. However, LCM infection of L cells did not prevent them from inducing tumors in newborn mice [BENSON and HOTCHIN, 1961] but on the contrary appeared to increase the incidence of tumors. BARSKI and YOUN [1964] showed a similar interference of the leukemogenic effect of Rauscher virus when LCM virus was given 1 or 2 days previously. TAYLOR and MACDOWELL [1949] isolated an unidentified viral contaminant of a mouse leukemia which exerted an ameliorative effect upon the leukemia and caused signs of disease in mice very similar to those produced by LCM. LAW and DUNN [1951] isolated a virus believed to be LCM (DUNN, personal communication) which had an ameliorative effect upon murine leukemia. Experimental infection of guinea pigs with LCM significantly increased the survival and decreased the spleen size of animals bearing the transplantable leukemia L2B/N [NADEL and HAAS, 1956] and L2C [NADEL and HAAS, 1955; JUNGEBLUT and KODZA, 1963]. The effectiveness was limited to injection of virus 2 days before to 7 days after transplantation of the leukemia [NADEL and HAAS, 1956]. Previous immunization of the guinea pigs with LCM virus prevented the effect, and killed virus offered no protection. Other viruses were tested, including SLE, influenza and yellow fever, but these did not have a similar or additive effect. In contrast, LCM infection did not significantly increase the survival of mice with leukemia L1210, showing the effect to be very specific with respect to cell type. STEWART and HAAS [1956] recovered and identified LCM virus in 2 sublines of leukemia, including L1210. Presumably this explained the previously mentioned failure of LCM to affect this leukemia since it already carried LCM. HUMPHREYS *et al.* [1956] reported a similar contaminant in the same leukemia strain. Administration [BARSKI and YOUN, 1964] of Armstrong strain LCM 48 h before giving Rauscher leukemia virus cut down the number of enlarged spleens (measured 30 days later) from 91% to 45%. It was concluded that LCM virus interfered with Rauscher leukemia virus and caused a lower incidence and later onset of leukemia. In newborn mice the leukemia shielding effect of LCM infection persisted longer [YOUN and BARSKI, 1966]. MOLOMUT and PADNOS [1965] and MOLOMUT *et al.* [1964] found that treatment with the MP strain of LCM caused remission of transplantable lymphoid leukemia in some mice which were still grossly normal 60 days later. A similar effect occurred in mice with Ehrlich ascites carcinoma after IP inoculation with the virus, which induced lymphocytopenia in mice, kittens, dogs, rats and swine. This virus has been used cautiously as a therapeutic agent by WEBB *et al.* [1968c] in a few human cases of neoplastic disease including Hodgkin's disease. There was some evidence that the Hodgkin's disease tissue had suffered disintegration as a result of the virus therapy. Some of the leukemias [STEWART and HAAS, 1956] which gave rise to LCM virus also yielded cell-free extracts with high tumor-inciting properties, suggesting that LCM might have been related to the tumor-inciting substance. However, the studies by STEWART *et al.* [1957] indicated that LCM was not in fact a tumor agent. TRAUB and KESTING [1963a] suggested that LCM pathogenesis included features which were similar to leukemogenesis, and TRAUB [1941, 1962] concluded that LCM virus caused lymphomatosis in a persistently infected mouse strain. However, this data can also be interpreted to indicate that the tumorigenic agent is either another carried virus or a host genetic factor rather than LCM virus. It may be relevant that LCM virus induces the formation in infected cells of large aggregates of ribosomes [ABELSON *et al.*, 1969] resembling the aberrant cytoplasmic structures seen in chicken cells infected with avian tumor viruses [HEINE *et al.*, 1968].

The LCM-leukemia interaction appears to justify further investigation, both from the point of view of a possible therapeutic approach, and also to gain insight into leukemogenesis. RUBIN *et al.* [1962] considered the acute LCM disease model as a possible explanation of avian leukosis but rejected a cellular immune mechanism, although they concluded [RUBIN *et al.*, 1961] that the persistently infected hosts were immunologically tolerant to the virus. However, there remain some suggestive pointers; it is clear that LCM-specific cellular immune response is inhibited in the LCM tolerant animal. The nature of the virus-induced cellular lesion responsible for this inhibition is obscure, but appears to involve failure of antigen recognition rather than failure of cellular proliferation or homograft rejection mechanisms. If a virus-induced lesion allowed a proliferative response of immunologically defective cells to occur, a state indistinguishable from leukemia would be produced.

Pathogenic Mechanisms of LCM Infection

As a result of his studies on the pathogenesis of LCM in mice, ROWE [1954] suggested that the acute cerebral symptoms might be due to the effect of the meningeal infiltrate itself, either through pressure effects or some substance present in the infiltrate. A similar concept led HOTCHIN [1958] to propose that LCM virus is only harmful to mice if they respond to it immunologically as a foreign antigen, since the virus is capable of initiating immunological tolerance [HOTCHIN, 1959] in this host. He suggested that this pathogenic mechanism is probably similar to that of human serum hepatitis and infectious equine anemia [HOTCHIN, 1958]. A comparison of the properties of LCM virus inoculated into mice either neonatally or after 1 week of age revealed the properties shown in table V.

As a result of experiments on LCM inoculation at different time intervals after birth, HOTCHIN [1962a] concluded that both the lethal disease and the PTI state depend upon the induction of a new cellular antigen by the virus. This antigen was seen as either initiating and maintaining an immunological conflict (in the adult animal) directed towards elimination of the pathogen, or, in the case of the newborn animal, initiating immunol-

Table V. Properties of mice infected with LCM [1]

Infected neonatally (PTI)	Infected after 1 week of age
1. Carry virus indefinitely	1. If not lethal, virus is usually quickly suppressed
2. Minimal AB formed	2. Rapid CF and FAB formed + very late NAB
3. No cytopathogenicity *in vitro* Little inflammation *in vivo*	3. No cytopathogenicity *in vitro* Violent inflammatory response *in vivo*
4. Same titer of virus as in sick older mice	4. Same titer of virus as in disease-free infected mice
5. Acute disease cannot be induced in these mice	5. Disease can be largely eliminated by immunosuppressives

[1] Modified from HOTCHIN and CINITS [1958].

ogical tolerance, thereby allowing the otherwise harmless virus to maintain a persistent symptom-free infection. This hypothesis would explain acute LCM disease as the result of an immunological conflict in which the sick animal attempted to reject the virus-infected tissue via the homograft response [BILLINGHAM *et al.*, 1956]. The fact that acute LCM disease and its associated histopathology is completely prevented by immunosuppressive measures (including X-irradiation, cortisone, thymectomy, chemical immunosuppressants and anti-lymphoreticular cell sera), provides solid verification for the immune disease concept. The basic events underlying LCM pathogenesis have therefore been regarded as the result of a choice between dual alternative pathways of the host immune response, depending on whether this is positive (active immunity with virus suppression) or negative (immunological tolerance or paralysis) to LCM [HOTCHIN, 1962a]. These alternative routes are summarized diagrammatically in figure 18. The positive response has two parts, cellular and humoral. It appears from the foregoing sections that the two parts can be separated as 'split tolerance' in the HDIP state and in the tolerance induced by ALS or RAMT treatment, in both of which cellular immunity is impotent but high titers of humoral antibody are found (CF antibody and FAB but not neutralizing antibody). The occurrence of persistent infection during these states makes it clear that these two humoral responses do not affect virus

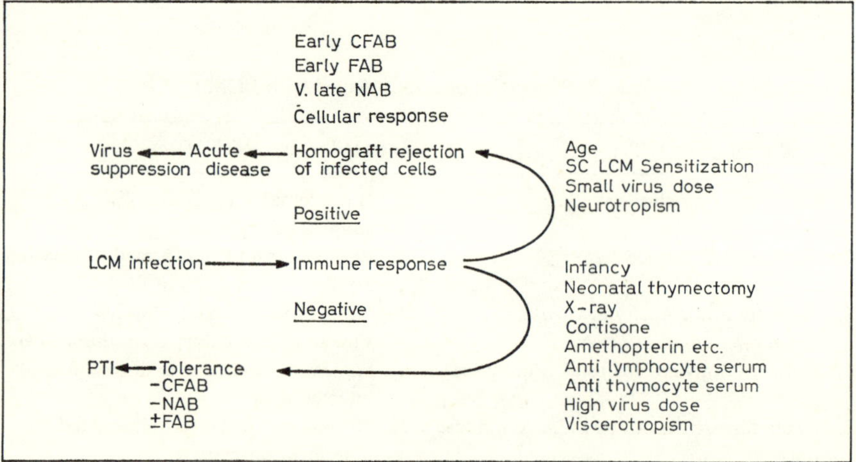

Fig. 18. Alternative pathways of host immune response in LCM pathogenesis and the major factors influencing the direction of the response.

titer, and that virus suppression only occurs as a result of a cellular immune response. TRAUB [1960b, 1963] concluded that Hotchin's theory, postulating an immunological reaction as the cause of disease in murine LCM, could explain much of the pathogenic mechanism, including the accelerated reaction of reinoculated mice with waning immunity, and also the state of PTI in the absence of an immune response. LEHMANN-GRUBE [1964b] emphasized the concept of BURNET and FENNER [1949] that LCM virus is integrated into the animal's own antigenic make-up when present during a period of immunological unresponsiveness, being recognized as 'self', i. e., non-antigenic thereafter. In this view, he agreed with the Hotchin theory that the virus itself is quite harmless for the mouse, whose fate is determined solely by an interaction between the virus as antigen and the host's immune mechanisms. The observation that mice do make significant titers of neutralizing antibody to LCM virus many months after they have suppressed LCM infection [HOTCHIN *et al.*, 1969] is in keeping with the slow or persistent aspect of infection with this virus, and it also accords with the view that the process of recovery from the disease is not mediated by neutralizing antibody but by cellular immunity. ROWE *et al.* [1963] considered that the classical delayed hypersensitivity phenomenon was not necessarily the sole mechanism involved because of the observation of HOTCHIN [1962a] that mice may die of typical convulsions as early as 30 h after virus inoculation if challenged by IV endotoxin. They suggested that there is an early change in vascular reactivity to nonspecific stimuli, such as that seen in the Shwartzman phenomenon. It was also felt that, since antibody was present in thymectomized mice which survived, the simple humoral antigen-antibody reaction was unlikely to be the mechanism of disease production. The protection of thymectomy closely resembles that produced by X-irradiation and folic acid deficiency, in that virus multiplication was not inhibited but lymphocytic infiltration was prevented or ameliorated.

These facts strongly support the contention [HOTCHIN, 1962a] that viral tolerance is not an all-or-none phenomenon, but is more akin to a spectrum of immune responses, ranging from complete tolerance (possibly found in some LCM-PTI strains of congenitally infected mice) to the acute lethal infection of the adult mouse. This viewpoint appears to be shared by VOLKERT and LARSEN [1965c]. The different spectral colors in this analogy would correspond for example to neonatal PTI [HOTCHIN and WEIGAND, 1961a], split tolerance following ALS or RAMT serum [HIRSCH and MURPHY, 1967], the HDIP state [HOTCHIN and BENSON,

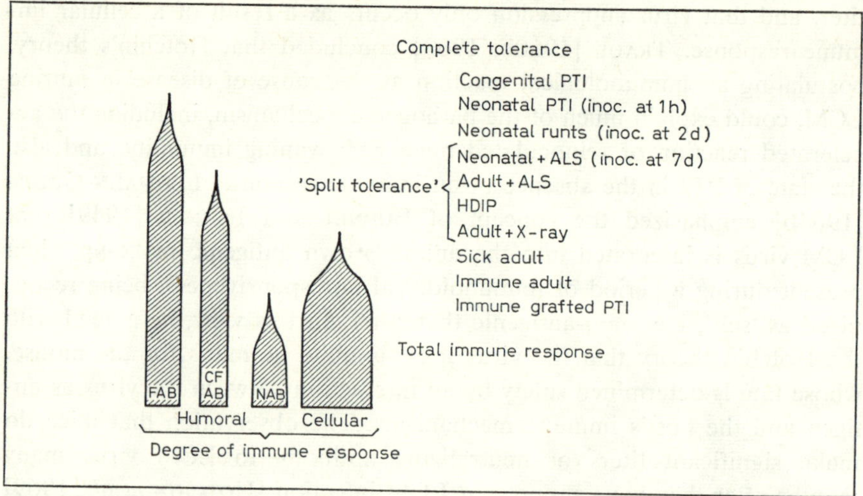

Fig. 19. Diagram of the possible 'spectral range' of immunological tolerance to LCM virus-induced antigens, and the types of antibody associated with the different levels of tolerance. The height of the columns for the different antibody types corresponds approximately with the levels of tolerance shown.

1963], X-ray protected mice [ROWE, 1956] and acutely sick animals (fig. 19). On this scale the hyperimmune lymph node graft recipients of VOLKERT [1963] with high neutralizing antibody would represent an extension of the spectrum beyond the range normally found. The suggestion of OLDSTONE and DIXON [1969], that LCM virus (or any other virus) cannot under any conditions induce immunological tolerance, becomes untenable in the face of all the evidence to the contrary. It is also noteworthy that the LCM model provided the primary example [BURNET and FENNER, 1949] which initiated the Burnet-Medawar tolerance concept.

It has become increasingly evident that the LCM cellular immune response is directed against a virus-induced new or transformed antigen in the infected cell surface (fig. 20), as originally proposed [HOTCHIN *et al.*, 1958] for influenza virus. This concept has been reviewed by ISACSON [1967], who postulated a mechanism whereby myxoviruses may induce autoimmunity, which is very similar to that outlined [HOTCHIN, 1962a] for LCM virus. A considerable weight of evidence now supports the concept that LCM virus induces the formation of a specific new antigen at the surface of the infected cell. Electron microscopy of LCM-infected

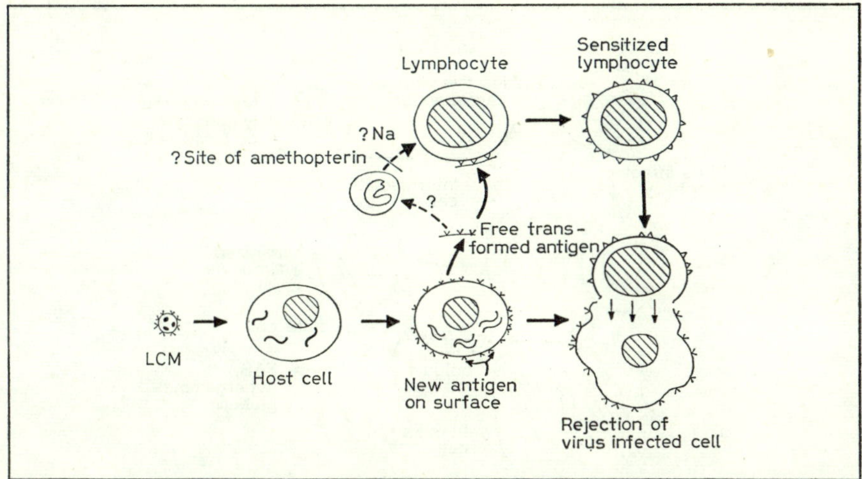

Fig. 20. Diagram of LCM virus infection showing the interaction between virus-induced tissue surface antigen and specifically sensitized lymphocytes.

cells [DALTON *et al.*, 1968] showed that virus particles are formed at the cell surface by budding, and ABELSON *et al.* [1969] used enzyme-labeled antibody to demonstrate surface LCM antigen. FAB staining of living LCM-infected cells shows[20] the presence of an LCM-induced antigen over most of the cell surface. The *in vitro* experiments on the immunologically specific cytotoxic reaction between LCM-infected cells and LCM-immune splenocytes first shown by BENSON [1962b] and confirmed by LUNDSTEDT [1969] and OLDSTONE *et al.* [1969] provided additional support for the homograft rejection of acute LCM. Further work is needed to determine whether the surface antigen is a single or a more complex entity, corresponding with soluble antigens or neutralizable antigen of the virion capsid, or both. It seems likely that the antigen involved both in virus neutralization and lymphocyte sensitization may be the A_1 fragment described by BARLOW and MUSTICO [1965]. Similarly, the precise nature of the antigenic stimulus for the cellular immune response is not known nor is it known whether this is a direct response or is mediated by another cell type via an intermediate messenger. It seems highly probable that the cellular response is mediated by an antigen which is different from soluble (CF) antigen, and that the response to the latter, by CF and 'internal staining' FAB, represents a cleaning up process for viral antigenic compo-

[20] J. HOTCHIN and L. BENSON, unpublished results.

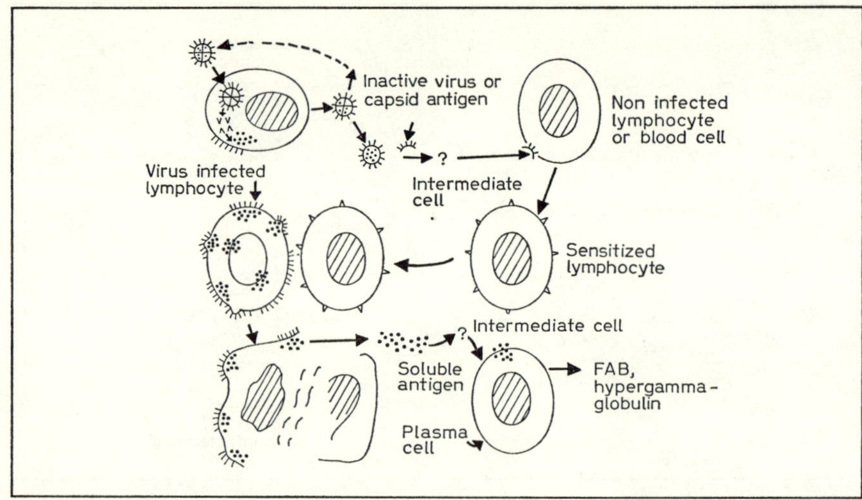

Fig. 21. Sequential events of persistent virus infection leading to cellular immune paralysis (high dose immune paralysis or split tolerance) and FAB production, sometimes with hypergammaglobulinemia.

nents liberated from infected cells lysed by the cellular immune response (fig. 21).

The results obtained by HANAOKA *et al.* [1969] on the destructive effect of LCM on lymphocytes normally responsible for the cellular immune response (see section on 'Lymphoreticular lesions') at first appeared to provide a new explanation for the HDIP effect, and probably for tolerance induction in the newborn. If the lymphoreticular lesions are due to a CPE of the virus, then it follows that LCM itself has an immune suppressive action, catalyzing its own tolerance. On this hypothesis, all lymphoreticular cells infected by LCM would be destroyed, and only those exposed to antigen (but not live virus) would become sensitized and capable of responding with cellular immunity or humoral antibody. This explanation seems adequate for acute disease but not for the PTI state, in which the majority of the lymphoreticular cells would have to be destroyed shortly after birth in order to enable the infection to persist. Such a state would virtually obliterate the normal immune capacity of the animal, a situation which is known not to occur, since in spite of temporary impairment, humoral immune capacity recovers after LCM infection [MIMS and WAINWRIGHT, 1968], and non-LCM cellular immunity is not severely affected in LCM tolerant mice[21]. Therefore, a simple lytic effect of LCM virus upon TDL appears untenable. A partial lysis is more possible, comparable to the partial CPE caused by LCM *in vitro* [BENSON, 1961] and this possibility cannot be ruled out. Surviving cells would be either persistently infected or sensitized, and both types would be immune to lysis, and would correspond at the cellular level with PTI or actively immune animals respectively.

Another explanation for the lymphoreticular destruction is that it is not a virus cytotoxic effect but represents the first result of cellular immune tissue rejection to occur in the infected animal. This explanation presumes that cellular immune response can begin as early as 2 days after infection, and that the first TDL which develop a mature LCM sensitization act upon their virus-infected neighbors before migrating elsewhere. This explanation seems eminently possible. Spleen and lymph nodes [VOLKERT and LARSEN, 1964] appear to be the only organs freed of detectable virus by transplantation of immune lymph nodes to PTI mice, notwithstanding the fact that the spleen and lymph nodes belong to the class of organs which in untreated tolerant mice have the highest virus titers. These titers are much higher than those found in lungs or liver, which are often not fully cleared by the transplantation. It seems likely that the edematous FP reaction of mice 7 days after FP inoculation may be due mainly to an obliterative immune response in the local lymph node. If both are caused by cellular immunity, this would explain the observation that the FP response is abolished by amethopterin [SIKORA and HOTCHIN, 1962] and by whole-body, but not local X-irradiation [BENSON, 1962a]. Both explanations require that persistently LCM-infected TDL are impotent to respond to LCM-induced antigen. The mechanism of this inhibition is unknown, but is intuitively feasible as an example of negative feedback, induced by the enormous concentration of antigen in the persistently infected cells. If the lymphocyte sensitization involves nucleic acid synthesis, this may be the site of action of amethopterin and other nucleic acid blocking agents, which prevent the cellular immune response and induce partial tolerance to LCM (fig. 20). Apparently LCM virus has greater specific depressive effect upon those immune cells responsible for the cellular immune response than those responsible for humoral antibody. This effect may be related to the impairment of immune response caused by leukemogenic viruses

---

[21] S. SUZUKI and J. HOTCHIN, unpublished results.

[CEGLOWSKI and FRIEDMAN, 1967; CHAN *et al.*, 1968], although the latter appear to effect humoral more than cellular immunity. It seems possible that leukemogenesis itself may be related to this phenomenon, whereby viruses with this property may possess ability partly to 'lysogenize' the cellular immune system, at the same time stimulating it to a fruitless hypertrophy. If the antigenic stimulus for humoral antibody production stems from 'soluble' intracellular antigen, as opposed to fixed cell surface antigen, then liberation of soluble antigen by lysis of infected cells must occur before humoral antibody can be produced. It follows that in the absence of such lysis, e. g. in congenital PTI mice, no humoral antibody stimulation would arise and none of the soluble antigen would be accessible to the host immune system. The converse situation, in which a partial cellular immune response causes significant lysis of infected cells, would induce a powerful soluble antigenic stimulus and prolonged high levels of humoral antibody, even though the cellular response was insufficient to suppress the infection. A diagram of this mechanism in shown in figure 22. The hypothesis proposes that the ratio between the proportion L_p of TDL which becomes persistently virus infected and the proportion L_s of TDL which becomes sensitized for vi-

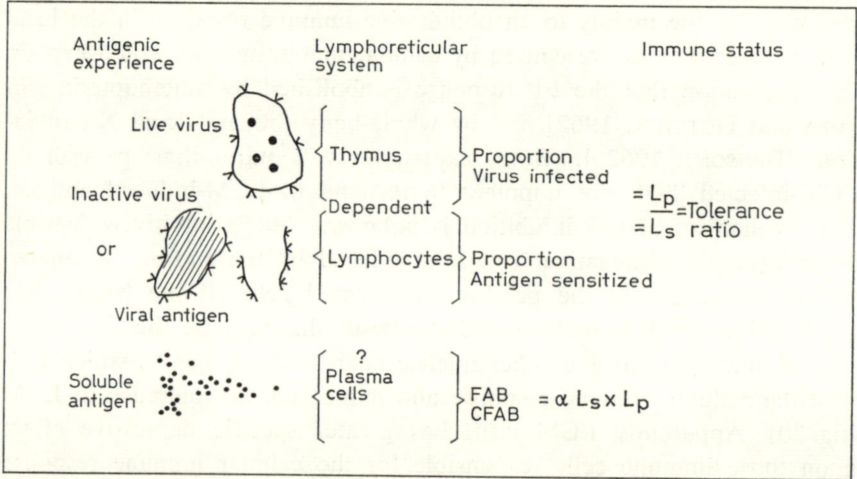

Fig. 22. Diagram of the hypothetical process determining the persistence-suppression choice of the lymphoreticular system. L_p = proportion of thymus dependent lymphocytes (TDL) persistently virus infected. L_s = proportion of TDL sensitized to viral antigen and available for virus suppression.

rus suppression by initial exposure to nonreplicative viral antigen will determine the immune status. This is referred to as the tolerance ratio, which can range from infinity in congenital PTI mice, to zero in virus-free, immune animals. It follows that the humoral antibody response which depends upon antigen liberated from infected cells by the sensitized TDL will be proportional to the product of L_p and L_s. This presupposes that L_p is proportional to the number of infected cells in the other tissues of the animal. The hypothesis conforms with the observed facts of tolerant and actively immune animals, and with the high levels of humoral antibody and antigen/antibody complexes found in states of partial or split tolerance. Presumably certain ranges of magnitude of L_p and L_s (and therefore of concentration of circulating antibody) will be most conducive to the production of antigen/antibody complexes, and, if these are the prime cause of glomerular damage, these magnitudes will also govern the incidence of glomerulonephritis. This concept would also explain LARSEN's [1969a] observation that CF antibody titer can be 100-fold higher in adoptively immunized mice than in freshly vaccinated or hyperimmunized mice; the value of $L_p \times L_s$ would be expected to rise to very high levels in adoptively immunized mice since L_p would start at maximal levels approximating the total number of cells in the animals, and L_s would progressively increase owing to multiplication of the grafted lymphocytes.

Production of LCM antibody in the acute disease has been found [BENSON and HOTCHIN, 1969] to be even more rapid after large virus doses leading to HDIP, than after lethal or small immunizing doses. This correlates with the impression that the main lesion induced by the virus and cellular immune response releases an extremely strong stimulus of liberated soluble antigen. The detailed immunofluorescent study by BROWN [1968] of the development of antigen in the lymphoreticular system suggested to him that the very rapid antigenic saturation of that system could be the cause of immunological suppression. There is some evidence that the humoral response produces mainly IgM[22] [POLLARD *et al.*, 1968a], but LARSEN [1969a] found the CF antibody in vaccinated and adoptively immunized mice to be IgG. The more extensive viremia found with viscerotropic LCM virus may explain the greater survival associated with this strain [HOTCHIN and BENSON, 1963] if, as would seem likely, high doses of viscerotropic virus cause a greater proportion of in-

[22] J. HOTCHIN, unpublished results.

fected lymphocytes in the thymus-dependent areas. These observations also suggest that the hypergammaglobulinemia of Aleutian mink disease may originate via a similar mechanism involving a relatively impotent cellular immune system and the production of extremely strong stimuli for humoral antibody formation. Since the humoral antibody-forming cells retain their ability to make antibody in spite of severe infection, it is likely that the specific cellular immune tolerance is caused by the development of virus-induced antigen on the surface of these cells. Presumably this would prevent or counteract their ability to become 'sensitized' to this antigen at the same location.

In summary, there appear to be three main categories of response to LCM virus [HOTCHIN, 1969]. These are as follows:

1. Normal acute response. Infection of the adult animal with a small inoculum dose is followed by complete suppression of virus in a short time (fig. 23). Some animals die during this suppression process. Fluorescent antibody studies [BENSON and HOTCHIN, 1969] showed that this situation is associated with a very rapid production of high serum titers of a specific antibody, detectable only by the reversed indirect FAB test. So-

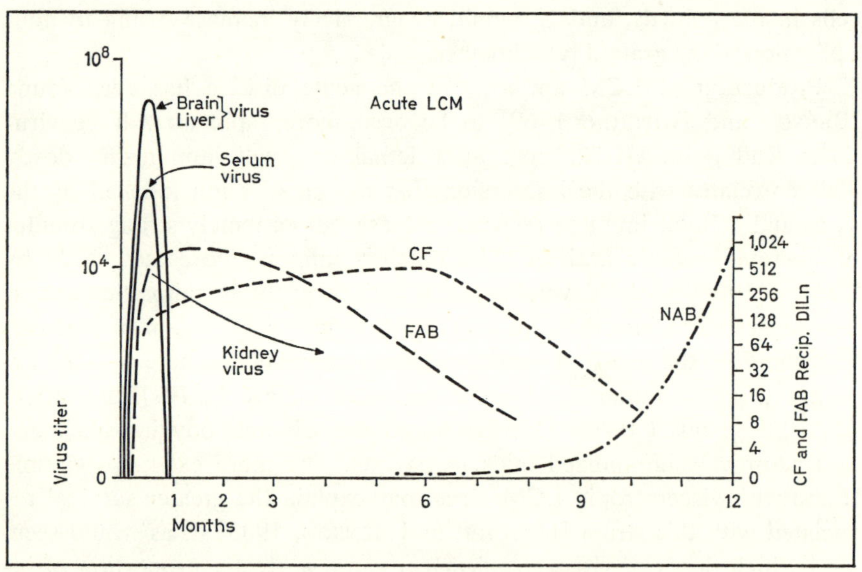

Fig. 23. Diagram of main virus and antibody levels after infection of the adult mouse with a small virus dose. NAB = neutralizing antibody.

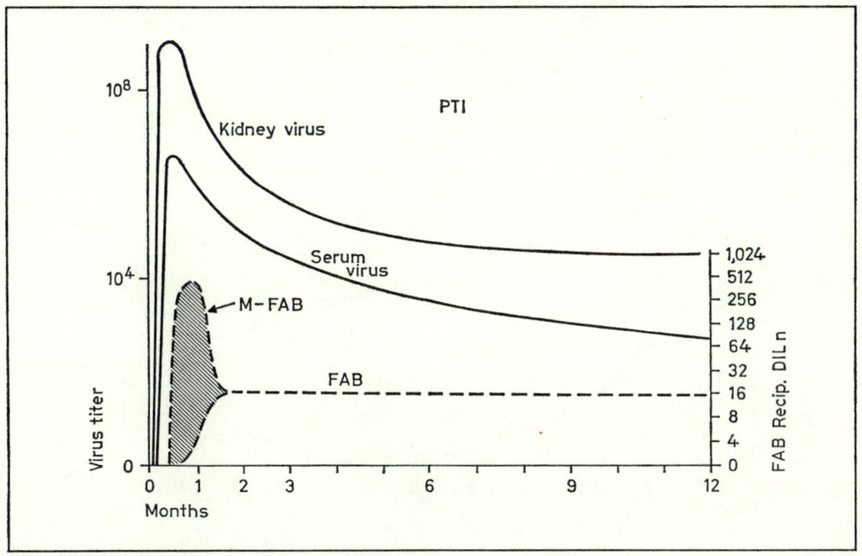

Fig. 24. Diagram of main virus and antibody levels in LCM-PTI mice. M-FAB = 'fluorescent antibody' of maternal origin.

mewhat later the CF antibody tests become positive and many months later significant titers of LCM neutralizing antibody appear.

2. Persistent tolerant infection (PTI). This condition results from the neonatal (or congenital) infection of mice with LCM virus (fig. 24). It is characterized by rapidly rising titers of virus throughout the animal in the few days immediately following infection. These titers maintain very high levels throughout the lifespan of the animal, which can reach 18 months or rarely 2 years. During this period, chronic glomerulonephritis develops and clinical signs of late disease begin at 7–10 months of age in most mouse strains. Study of the FAB levels in PTI mice [BENSON and HOTCHIN, 1969] revealed titers of 1/8 to 1/16 up to 12 months after neonatal infection. In the early weeks after infection, maternal antibody transferred via milk reached a titer of 1/64 in the PTI infants, but substitutions of mothers every 6 days with fresh uninfected ones prevented the appearance of FAB prior to weaning. The early titers of FAB in neonatal PTI mice are therefore of maternal origin (M-FAB).

3. Partial or split tolerance. The HDIP state following administration of large doses of viscerotropic LCM virus to the adult mouse by IC or IV inoculation results in a prolonged persistent infection in the presence

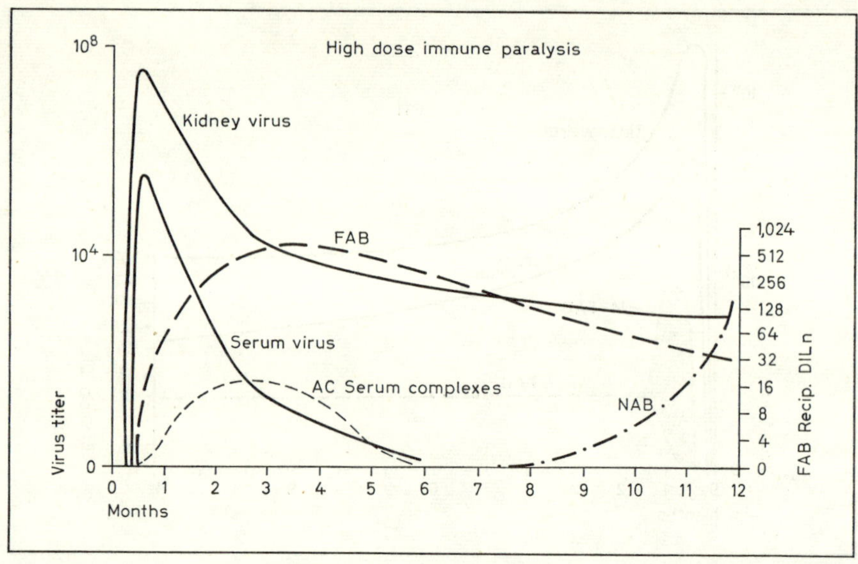

Fig. 25. Diagram of main virus and antibody levels in the high dose immune paralysis state (HDIP) following administration of large doses of viscerotropic LCM virus to the adult mouse via IC inoculation. AC = anticomplementary. NAB = neutralizing antibody.

of humoral, non-neutralizing CF and FAB (fig. 25). This condition imitates a state of immunological tolerance except that serum and organ virus titers gradually fall over a period of 3–10 months, at which time serum titers reach 0 and organ titers remain significantly high, especially in the kidney. The relationship between the persistent high kidney titers and the development of glomerulonephritis and LCM viruria [TRAUB, 1936c; UTZ, 1964] is not clear. The HDIP state is similar to the partial or temporary tolerance following adult LCM infection combined with immunosuppressive agents. In HDIP mice, FAB appears a few days after inoculation and is co-existent in the serum with high virus titers for many months. At the same time the CF antibody level rises and AC complexes are present in the serum. Kidney function is impaired throughout this period and glomerulonephritis may occur. In this condition LCM-induced paralysis or 'impotence' of the cellular immune system is fairly severe, since suppression of serum virus takes several months. This is presumably due to the high proportion of TDL which have become persistently infected, while plasma and reticulum cells appear to have largely escaped. Possibly the latter cells are more likely to receive an immunizing stimulus of soluble virus antigen prior to meeting virus than are lymphocytes (if the latter are sensitive only to viral envelope antigen), since the amount of soluble antigen liberated must be much greater than the amount of non-infectious viral envelope released. The HDIP state represents a halfway stage between the above two states of normal suppressive immunity or neonatal persistent tolerance. In the HDIP state, the cellular immune mechanisms which normally cause elimination of the virus-infected tissue operate in 'slow motion' and appear to be almost completely abolished. This cellular immune impotence to eradicate the virus is LCM-specific, since HDIP mice have unimpaired ability to reject homologous skin homografts[23], and the ability of the LCM-tolerant animal to suppress infection with influenza virus, SLE [HAAS, 1954] and EEE [TRAUB, 1960b] is unimpaired and neutralizing antibody is ultimately formed.

The two parameters, virus titer and FAB titer, can classify the three categories of LCM infection [HOTCHIN, 1969] (table VI). In the neonatal PTI state cellular immunity is absent, virus titer is high and FAB levels are very low; in the HDIP state cellular immune response is very slight, so virus titer is high but declines to zero in a period of months; FAB levels remain high. In the suppressive immunity after acute adult infection both cellular immune activity and FAB are high and virus has been eliminated.

The three categories of LCM infection which are outlined above are linked together by the variable rate at which the host reacts immunologically to the virus. This time variable is perhaps the most important single factor in explaining the different responses exhibited in the pathoge-

Table VI. Virus and FAB levels in the three major categories of LCM infection

Infection category	High virus titer	FAB
PTI	+	Low
HDIP	+[1]	High
Suppressed infection	–	High

[1] Falls to zero in 6–12 months.

[23] J. HOTCHIN and S. SUZUKI, unpublished results.

nesis of LCM. In this light, the PTI state can usefully be considered as a very protracted incubation period for the HDIP state, which in turn appears to be similar to a long drawn-out version of the acute infection, culminating in virus suppression. The different categories could theoretically be defined solely in terms of the rate of decline in virus titer. In this respect the PTI state would take many times the normal life span of the host before virus suppression was complete.

This model appears to be applicable to other persistent virus infections and will be referred to in the remaining sections of this monograph. It is hoped that it may serve as a working hypothesis in the study of the slow virus diseases and that variations of the model may explain a significant portion of the pathogenesis of this fascinating group.

Tacaribe-Machupo Group and Lassa Viruses

Tacaribe [Downs *et al.*, 1963], Machupo [Johnson *et al.*, 1965b; Webb *et al.*, 1967] and Junin virus [Parodi *et al.*, 1966] share a common CF antigen [Mackenzie *et al.*, 1965; Bruno-Lobo *et al.*, 1968] and appear to constitute important examples of tolerance-inducing persistent viruses. These viruses, which are responsible for Bolivian and Argentinian hemorrhagic fever in man [Johnson *et al.*, 1965a], can be isolated from lymph nodes for at least 48 days after inoculation of experimental guinea pigs, and it appears that this is the primary site of multiplication [Boxaca, 1961; Coto *et al.*, 1967; Bruno-Lobo *et al.*, 1968]. It seems clear that this group of ether-sensitive RNA viruses [Justines and Johnson, 1969] falls into the persistent class and that the mechanism may, like LCM, involve specific viral effects on the lymphoid cells normally responsible for suppression of virus infections. Machupo virus has been isolated from the blood and organs of apparently normal wild rodents [Johnson *et al.*, 1966], and Schmuñis *et al.* [1967] and Weissenbacher *et al.* [1969] were able to induce immunological tolerance to Junin virus by thymectomy of newborn mice. This virus induces fatal disease in the newborn mouse, but adult animals are able to suppress the agent without disease [Schmuñis *et al.*, 1967]. Tolerance is more complete in wild rodents, particularly *Calomys callosus* [Johnson *et al.*, 1965b; Justines and Johnson, 1969], and Kuns [1965] believes that human infection with Machupo virus is not arthropod-borne but follows contact with rodent excreta as in the case of human LCM. Experimental neonatal infection of *Calomys* by JUSTINES and JOHNSON [1969] has induced PTI lasting at least one year with an absence of neutralizing antibodies. Inoculation at 10 weeks of age caused similar PTI but some animals develop neutralizing antibodies and diminished virus titers.

It is clear that a very close parallel exists between LCM and the Junin-Machupo group of viruses. At the present time it seems likely that the pathogenic mechanism is identical, with variations in immunological responsiveness and virulence. Recent work on the morphology of Machupo and Tacaribe viruses by MURPHY *et al.* [1969] shows that they have the same morphology as LCM virus [DALTON *et al.*, 1968]. The authors have proposed that these viruses should form a single taxonomic group, with LCM as the type virus. Lassa virus, isolated by FRAME *et al.* [1970] and LEIFER *et al.* [1970] appears to belong to the same class [BUCKLEY and CASALS, 1970] and this virus shows some CF and FAB cross-reactivity with LCM (CASALS, personal communication) and possibly slight cross-reactivity with some members of the Tacaribe group.

Miscellaneous Persistent Viruses

African Swine Fever

African swine fever (ASF) virus is capable of causing a highly contagious fatal illness in domestic swine, but can also cause a carrier state with persistent infection both in the rare domestic animals that survive the acute disease [COWAN, 1961] and in wild wart hogs [DETRAY *et al.*, 1961]. The disease has been reviewed by DETRAY [1963] and SCOTT [1965a, b]. Acute ASF is characterized by fever, cyanosis of the skin and pronounced hemorrhages of the internal organs, particularly in lymph nodes, kidneys, and gastrointestinal mucosa. In the acute disease very high blood titers have been reported [MENDES and DASKALOS, 1955; VELHO, 1957]. BREESE and DE BOER [1966] have shown the virus to be a hexagonal particle of 175–215 nm diameter with a dense nucleoid 72–89 nm in diameter. It is extremely stable, and blood was reputed to be still infectious after 18 months at room temperature and after 6 years at 4° to 5° C, although it is inactivated at 60° C for 19 min [MONTGOMERY, 1921; DEKOCK *et al.*, 1940]. Infectious deoxyribonucleic acid (DNA) has been reported to be extractable from ASF virus [ADLDINGER *et al.*, 1966]; other analytical tests confirmed that only DNA could be detected in this virus [MOULTON and COGGINS, 1968a]. ASF causes hemadsorption followed by CPE in tissue cultures of pig cells [MALMQUIST and HAY, 1960]. Attachment of the red cells [BREESE and HESS, 1966] was of the cytohemadsorption type [HOTCHIN *et al.*, 1958].

Infection of the fetus of pigs carrying ASF can apparently occur and appears to be the cause of a congenital trembling disease associated with cerebellar hypoplasia and spinal hypomyelinogenesis in the newborn animals [HARDING *et al.*, 1966]. The primary histological lesions of ASF are in lymphoid tissues and the walls of arterioles and capillaries [MAURER *et al.*, 1958]. Severe necrosis of lymphoid cells, particularly mature lymphocytes, occurs and is apparently due to a direct effect of the virus. Simultaneously vascular damage leads to increased permeability of the capillaries with consequent edema, hemorrhage, occlusion, infarction and necrosis. A pronounced leukopenia follows [DeTray and Scott, 1957]. Plowright *et al.* [1968] found the greatest concentration of virus in recently infected pigs to be in the lymph nodes, especially those of the cephalic region, and in the spleen where titers commonly reached 10^8 to 10^9 HAD_{50}/g and exceeded the titers of the blood. Fluorescent antibody studies by Heuschele *et al.* [1966] showed that granular or globular deposits of antigen appeared in the cytoplasm of porcine kidney cells 10 h after inoculation *in vitro* and similar fluorescence was obtained with impression smears of organs after fatal infection with ASF virus. Both destructive and chronic hyperplastic lesions of the lymphoid system were described by Moulton and Coggins [1968b] in acute and chronically infected pigs with ASF; macrophages and reticular cells were primarily involved in the acute disease and lymphocytes were often the last cells to become involved. Colgrove *et al.* [1969] concluded that the virus replicated primarily in reticuloendothelial tissue. Heuschele [1967] found that the virus was first detected at one day postinoculation in the lymphoid tissues, including leukocytes circulating in the blood. De-Tray [1963] has pointed out that chronic cases frequently occur in pigs that have survived the acute disease with the carrier state remaining for a year or more. Such animals developed soft edematous swellings over the leg joints and under the mandible and became severely emaciated although joints appeared normal at necropsy. There was often a chronic pericarditis accompanied by consolidation and other changes of the lungs. During this period viremia has been reported; blood from apparently healthy wild hogs has also been reported to contain the virus [Steyn, 1932]. Neutralizing antibodies have not been demonstrated using a variety of different animals [De Boer, 1967a, b; De Boer *et al.*, 1969], although CF antibody is readily formed [Cowan, 1963] and a diagnostic precipitin test has been described [Coggins and Heuschele, 1966].

This virus disease appears to share several features of the LCM pathogenic mechanism outlined earlier. The absence of neutralizing antibody, persistent viremia and destructive effects on the lymphoid system suggest that specific paralysis of cellular immunity is related to persistence of the virus. The effects upon the fetus are reminiscent of rubella. De Boer [1967b] found that failure of swine to develop neutralizing antibody followed challenge with ASF virus and suggested that this indicates possible development of tolerance in these animals. In regard to the question of immunological tolerance of these animals, Coggins (personal communication) has pointed out that abundant precipitin and CF antibody, but little or no neutralizing or hemadsorption-inhibiting antibody, is produced even though the animal can be shown to be immune to a homologous challenge of virulent virus. STONE *et al.* [1968] followed antibody production in pigs after inoculation with ASF virus and found CF and precipitating antibody by 14 days postinoculation. At first mainly 19S antibody was produced but 7S was dominant by 35 days. Only pigs with both CF and precipitating antibody appeared to be immune to subsequent virus challenge. Challenge survivors showed no increase in antibody nor reversion to the 19S type. DETRAY [1957] showed that persistence of ASF virus occurred for as long as 456 days after inoculation of pigs, and both virus and circulating antibody could coexist. Resistance often appeared to depend on absence of antibody, and the presence of a persisting infection. Immunity to ASF is generally of low degree and can often be overcome by challenge with virulent ASF virus. A wide range of response to attenuated ASF virus is seen in pigs. The same material may immunize some animals, kill some, produce a state of chronic infection in others or fail to stimulate any apparent immunity at all. Killed vaccine provides very little protection [DE-TRAY, 1957, 1963; STONE and HESS, 1967]. DE BOER (1967b) and DE BOER *et al.* [1969] in an exhaustive study of antibody production, postulated a parallel situation between LCM and ASF and searched for neutralizing antibodies in the kidneys of ASF-reinfected sheep without success. In spite of the lack of neutralizing antibody production, affected animals produced high titers of CF and precipitating antibodies. MALMQUIST [1963] found that hemadsorption-inhibiting and precipitating antibodies coexisted with virus in the blood of swine which had survived ASF infection. Neutralizing antibody could not be found. This author also suggested that the situation was very similar to the tolerant immunity found in LCM. It would appear that there is a close parallel between the LCM-HDIP state and ASF, and that the antibodies produced in ASF reflect the response to the soluble antigens and not to mature virus particles.

Aleutian Mink Disease

Introduction

HARTSOUGH and GORHAM [1956] first described Aleutian disease of mink, which has recently been reviewed by GORDON *et al.* [1967], EK-

LUND *et al.* [1968] and GORHAM *et al.* (in press). KARSTAD and PRIDHAM [1962] suggested the name 'viral plasmacytosis'. Aleutian mink disease (AMD) is an important persistent virus infection [TRAUTWEIN and HELMBOLDT, 1962] which causes a particularly interesting series of slow clinical manifestations. It is a very widespread [RUSSELL *et al.*, 1963] and insidious disease occurring in mink, particularly those with the Aleutian (aa) gene, in all mink-raising areas of North America and Scandinavia. It appears as complete or partial sterility in affected animals, with slowly progressive anorexia, weight loss and fever. Renal involvement causes increased thirst. In addition, there is enlargement of lymph nodes and spleen, anemia and Bence-Jones proteinuria [OBEL, 1959] and bleeding from the gastrointestinal tract and mouth, with associated anemia, leukopenia and thrombocytopenia [THOMPSON and ALIFERIS, 1964; PHILLIPS and HENSON, 1966]. Death occurs after a few days to several months. PADGETT *et al.* [1967b] concluded that the incubation period was 5 to 6 months.

After inoculation into ferrets [KENYON *et al.*, 1966b], persistence of the virus of Aleutian disease was accompanied by viruria [KENYON *et al.*, 1963a] and lasted for at least 136 days. However, in hamsters similar inoculations only caused infection for 21 days. Neither species showed any illness, although some ferrets reacted with severe periportal lymphocytic infiltrations. A survey of ferrets from different mink ranches showed that similar lymphocytic infiltrates only occurred in ranches with the AMD-infected mink. KENYON *et al.* [1967] have described hypergammaglobulinemia in ferrets with lymphoproliferative lesions, which appeared to be identical to Aleutian disease. A similar disease of ferrets, regarded as lymphatic leukemia with hypergammaglobulinemia and lymphoid and thymic hypertrophy, has been described by KENYON and WILLIAMS [1967]. There is slight evidence that the disease can occur in man [WILLIAMS *et al.*, 1965; CHAPMAN and JIMINEZ, 1963] though some of this has been questioned by LEADER [1964].

Transmission

AMD is transmissible from mink to mink with crude organ suspensions and cell-free filtrates of diseased tissue [HENSON *et al.*, 1962; TRAUTWEIN and HELMBOLDT, 1962; HENSON *et al.*, 1963a; KENYON *et al.*, 1968]. Vertical transmission of AMD occurs from dam to offspring in mink [HENSON *et al.*, 1963b; GORHAM *et al.*, 1965] and there is a remarkable genotype responsiveness; transplacental transmission has also been shown to occur [PADGETT *et al.*, 1967]. GORHAM *et al.* [1964] showed that the agent of AMD could be transferred through 12 serial passages and was present in mink in whole blood, serum, bone marrow, spleen, feces, urine and saliva, but not in colostral milk. The agent was infective when given by mouth in feces or spleen or as an aerosolized spleen suspension. It appeared to be a virus and passed through filters of 450 mm [KARSTAD and PRIDHAM, 1962], although BUKO and KENYON [1967] claimed that filtration showed AMD virus was no larger than an albumin molecule; BASRUR *et al.* [1963] obtained a size of 10–50 nm. The agent is moderately stable to heat [KARSTAD and PRIDHAM, 1962; BURGER *et al.*, 1965] and to chemical agents including low concentrations of formalin [HENSON *et al.*, 1962; BURGER *et al.*, 1965]. It is resistant to ether [EKLUND *et al.*, 1968] and is not inactivated by proteolytic enzymes, DNase or RNase. TSAI *et al.* [1969] reported aggregates of virus-like particles seen on electron microscopy of the tissues of AMD-infected mink. The particles had a diameter of about 25 nm and were in crystalline array. No proof was obtained that these were in fact the virus of AMD although no similar particles were seen in control tissues. BASRUR and KARSTAD [1966] concluded that DNA extracted from spleens of mink with AMD could transmit the disease, but only in the absence of DNase. However, the DNA preparation did not produce clear-cut infection in tissue culture. Cultures of mink testis or kidney cells show specific morphological changes when inoculated with AMD [BASRUR *et al.*, 1963].

Pathological Changes

The pathological changes of AMD comprise a varied set of abnormalities which make the disease an attractive research model for a wide variety of human counterparts. In the mink, AMD is characterized by generalized lymphocytic and plasma cell proliferation with hypergammaglobulinemia, glomerulonephritis and necrotizing arteritis [HELMBOLDT and JUNGHERR, 1958; TRAUTWEIN, 1964; KARSTAD, 1965; GORDON *et al.*, 1967; EKLUND *et al.*, 1968; SAISON and KARSTAD, 1968]. Kidney changes are marked [THOMPSON and ALIFERIS, 1964; KARSTAD, 1965; HENSON *et al.*, 1966, 1967a, 1969; KINDIG *et al.*, 1967] and resemble those found in mice with persistent LCM virus infection [HOTCHIN and COLLINS, 1964; KARSTAD, 1967], NZB mice [HENSON *et al.*, 1968] and human systemic lupus erythematosus. The glomerular lesions begin as thickening due to the accumulation of eosinophilic material in the mesangial area. On electron microscopy, electron-dense granular material is found in the subendothelium and mesangium [HENSON *et al.*, 1967a, 1968]. The changes suggested that the glomerular alterations were initiated by the deposition of macromolecular material followed by secondary cellular proliferation. These workers believed that the deposit might be antigen-antibody complexes. Similar conclusions were drawn by KENYON *et al.* [1968] who found an association between severely damaged kidneys and the presence of an increased level of alpha$_2$-globulin in the serum mainly due to 19S macroglobulin. However, PORTER and LARSEN [1967], who found infectious virus antibody complexes in AMD-infected mink sera, felt that the relationship between antigen-antibody complexes and glomerular lesions has not yet been determined. The kidneys had apparently been damaged by proteinacious deposits in the glomeruli which had the character of amyloid. Immunofluorescent staining of the AMD-affected mink kidney occurred when the tissue section was exposed to rabbit anti-mink gamma globulin fluorescent antiserum [WILLIAMS, 1965; WILLIAMS *et al.*, 1966; GORDON *et al.*, 1967; PORTER and LARSEN, 1967; HENSON *et al.*, 1969]. Similar results have been obtained with the arteritic lesions [PORTER *et al.*, 1965; GORDON *et al.*, 1967]. HENSON *et al.* [1967] concluded that the glomerular lesions could be due to deposits of antigen-antibody complexes, by a mechanism similar to that found in LCM glomerulonephritis. As with other persistent infections causing slow onset of disease, a strong genetic factor operates in AMD affecting susceptibility. Mink which were homozygous recessive for the Aleutian gene were found to be significantly more susceptible to the experimental disease [HENSON *et al.*, 1962; LUTZNER *et al.*, 1966]. Such animals had large cytoplasmic inclusions in their leukocytes; they were photophobic and highly susceptible to infection and early death. This genetic syndrome is similar [PADGETT *et al.*, 1967, 1968] to the Chediak-Higashi syndrome of man [HIGASHI, 1954; SARAIVA *et al.*, 1959; PAGE *et al.*, 1962; KRITZLER *et al.*, 1964; PHILLIPS *et al.*, 1967].

Immunology

Immunological changes, particularly hypergammaglobulinemia [GOR-

DON *et al.*, 1967] are a prominent feature of AMD and have been studied extensively. Sera from AMD-affected mink have increased total proteins and gamma globulin, but decreased albumin as determined by electrophoresis [HENSON *et al.*, 1961; KENYON *et al.*, 1966a]. Detailed analysis showed an increase in the 7S components of euglobulin [KENYON *et al.*, 1963b]. This component could not be distinguished from normal mink 7S immunoglobulin on the basis of charge density, sedimentation or carbohydrate content. The level of euglobulin was found to parallel the degree of plasma cell infiltration in the organs of the affected animal. PORTER *et al.* [1965] and also KENYON *et al.* [1963b] found the globulin to be predominantly gamma globulin with a sedimentation coefficient of 6.4S. It had a shorter half-life than the normal gamma globulin; 9–17S and 22–25S complexes were also found in the serum, and were similar to the immune complexes found in rheumatoid arthritis. No reduction could be found in serum complement in AMD, and the gamma globulin did not neutralize the virus [GORHAM *et al.*, 1963, 1964; LEADER *et al.*, 1965; PORTER *et al.*, 1965]. Virus-free euglobulins from mink with AMD caused [KENYON, 1965] increased pathogenicity of infective tissue homogenates as shown by more pronounced clinical signs and earlier mortality. PORTER *et al.* [1969b] has shown that extraordinarily high titers > 1:100,000 of FAB rapidly develop in affected mink, and virus titers are high during the first 8–18 days after inoculation. It appears that the gamopathy of AMD represents an exaggerated non-neutralizing antibody response to a soluble AMD antigen and that the disease is very similar to the LCM state of HDIP or split tolerance. Coombs tests were found by SAISON *et al.* [1966] to become positive parallel to the development of plasmacytosis in experimentally infected mink, suggesting a possible autoimmune mechanism of pathogenesis. Antinuclear and LE cell tests were negative [PORTER *et al.*, 1965]. KENYON [1965, 1966] has found that AMD causes a diminished immunologic competency in infected mink. The maximum depression of antibody response (to *Brucella abortus*) occurred at the stage of rapid plasma cell infiltration. After approximately 6 months, response to the antigen had returned to almost normal. This immunosuppressive ability of AMD correlated with similar findings LCM virus infection of mice [MIMS and WAINWRIGHT, 1968] and may be related to the the ability of these viruses to persist KARSTAD *et al.* [1963] found formalin-inactivated ADM virus to be of no value as a vaccine for mink; this again parallels the LCM model.

Pathogenic Mechanism

An understanding of the pathogenic mechanism of AMD is clearly of considerable importance, since the disease is related to many poorly understood pathological processes found in man. Theoretical concepts of the pathogenesis of Aleutian disease have been discussed by LEADER *et al.* [1965]. KARSTAD and PRIDHAM [1962] considered that hypersensitivity of the host to products of Aleutian disease virus might be the responsible mechanism for the disease process. A parallel rate of development between histological lesions and hypergammaglobulinemia in mink with Aleutian disease was observed by HENSON *et al.* [1966], but evidence of a causal relationship is lacking. McKAY *et al.* [1967] have suggested that some of the lesions are due to intravascular coagulation with considerable removal of platelets from the circulation. PORTER and LARSEN [1967] and EKLUND *et al.* [1968] showed that mink affected with Aleutian disease have viremia which persists until death. The virus in the serum exists as a complex with immunoglobulin in which *in vivo* infectivity is still present. Removal of immunoglobulin G from infectious serum of affected mink markedly reduced the virus titer. In some species of mink viremia occurred 2 weeks after inoculation [EKLUND *et al.*, 1968] but in other breeds the response was erratic; some mink that remained healthy harbored virus in their mesenteric nodes for many months. The authors regarded the disease as a striking example of a pathologic process caused by a genetic defect in the host's defensive mechanism against viral infection. Possible pathogenic mechanisms of Aleutian disease were reviewed by KARSTAD [1967], who regarded it as a virus-induced autoimmune disease. KINDIG *et al.* [1967] felt that the similarities between morphologic lesions of Aleutian disease in the kidney and human lupus nephritis suggest a common pathogenic mechanism for the two entities, but PORTER *et al.* [1965] did not accept Aleutian disease as having an autoimmune mechanism. At the present time there appears to be good reason to believe that the main pathogenic lesion of AMD lies in the tolerance-inducing capacity of the virus for the immune system of the host coupled with (or causing) a distorted compensatory immunological response to viral products, which itself may cause much of the disease. The distortion could well be a relative paralysis of cellular immunity coupled with a hypertrophied humoralresponse which is impotent to eradicate the virus infection.

Creutzfeldt-Jakob Disease

An inoculation of a chimpanzee with human brain from a patient having Creutzfeldt-Jakob disease with severe status spongiosus was made by GIBBS *et al.* [1968]. This was followed after 13 months by the appearance of a subacute, progressive, noninflammatory, degenerative brain disease which was very similar to the human disease and showed similar neuropathological findings. The same fatal neurological syndrome was also reproduced in five more chimpanzees after incubation periods of 12 to 14 months [GIBBS and GAJDUSEK, 1969]. Each inoculum came from a different patient with Creutzfeldt-Jakob disease. Chimpanzee-to-chimpanzee transmission was successful, without reduction in the incubation period. Several other animal species, including spider monkeys, failed to succumb to disease up to 1 year following inoculation with the same material. Creutzfeldt-Jakob disease must therefore be caused by a transmissible agent which persists at least well enough in the brain of an appropriate case to succeed in transmission to a suitable host on the first attempt.

Chronic Polymyositis

Aggregates of myxovirus-like filaments were found by CHOU [1967] in muscle tissue biopsied from a patient with chronic polymyositis. The author concluded that the results provided presumptive evidence that a chronic persistent viral infection may be involved in the pathogenesis of chronic polymyositis in man.

Cytomegalovirus

Human cytomegalovirus (CMV) is a heat labile [KRUGMAN and GOODHEART, 1964] DNA virus which causes a CPE in tissue culture [MCALLISTER *et al.*, 1967]. Cytomegaloviruses have been reviewed by SMITH [1959] and more recently by HANSHAW [1968] in this series of monographs. The various diseases in man caused by CMV have been summarized [DREESMAN and BENYESH-MELNICK, 1967; STERN, 1968]. This virus group will be briefly considered from the point of view of its ability to induce persistence. The virus is extremely widespread in humans (as in animals) as revealed by sero-epidemiological study [JACK and MCAULIFFE, 1968]. It is capable of causing a fatal generalized infection [WYATT *et al.*, 1950; BIRDSONG *et al.*, 1956], mainly in the fetus or infantile period, in which the presence of characteristic inclusion-bearing cells is pathognomonic. The virus behaves as a necrotizing agent, causing gross damage in many different organs. In some cases [NAEYE, 1967] the congenitally-infected infant is small owing to a subnormal number of cells in many organs. Intrauterine CMV infection is a significant cause of fetal death and abnormality including mental retardation [WRIGHT, 1966; ANON., 1968]. There is evidence that the agent may be associated with indirect inguinal hernia [LANG, 1966].

Congenital human CMV infection may last as long as 54 months, accompanied by neutralizing antibody [WELLER and HANSHAW, 1962; MEDEARIS, 1964c]. There appears to be no detectable amount of interferon produced by congenital CMV infections, although the infants have normal interferon production due to a second virus [GLASGOW *et al.*, 1967]. Tissue cultures infected with CMV appear to become infected from cell to cell, with the virus not necessarily entering the fluid phase of the culture, and therefore not being susceptible to neutralizing antibody. This property may contribute to persistence or latency of the agent if a similar situation exists *in vivo*. Acute CMV infection of the adult is sometimes accompanied by a syndrome resembling infectious mononucleosis, where the serological changes are identical but there is no glandular enlargement [KLEMOLA *et al.*, 1967]. The immune response in the adult normally eliminates the agent; but, if the immune response is absent or suppressed [RIFKIND, 1965], generalized infection may occur. In these circumstances TEN BENSEL and ST. GEME [1968] concluded that infection is from an extraneous source rather than activation of latent virus in the salivary glands. An antibody response to the virus readily occurs in the adult [JACK and MCAULIFFE, 1968; HANSHAW *et al.*, 1968] and after congenital infection steadily increasing levels of gamma M globulin can be found [MCCRACKEN and SHINEFIELD, 1965; ALFORD *et al.*, 1967], but there is also evidence that the virus may impair capacity of the host for immunological response to it. Murine CMV was found to exert a suppressive effect on several components of the primary immune response during acute sublethal infection of 4-week-old mice [OSBORN *et al.*, 1968]. This is of interest in terms of the possibility that this lesion of the lymphoid system is like comparable events in LCM pathogenesis which may be closely related to the ability of a virus to induce persistent infection. CMV has been isolated from lymph node, blood [STULBERG *et al.*, 1966] or peripheral leukocytes [HARNDEN *et al.*, 1967; FOSTER and

JACK, 1968; JACK *et al.,* 1968; LANG and NOREN, 1968] in a wide variety of different human diseases. In congenital human CMV infection persistent viruria occurs [ROWE *et al.,* 1958; BENYESH-MELNICK *et al.,* 1964; STERN and TUCKER, 1965; FELDMAN, 1968], and LANG and NOREN [1968] reported the presence of CMV in the blood for as long as 5 months and in urine for over $1^{1}/_{2}$ years [DIOSI *et al.,* 1966]. Virus could only be recovered in blood specimens containing intact leukocytes and occurred in spite of the presence of circulating antibody. It seems clear that in the case of CMV, persistence is mainly dependent on intracellular virus. TEN BENSEL and ST. GEME [1968] failed to find CMV in the salivary glands in 100 normal subjects. They concluded that the susceptible host acquires the virus exogenously rather than from persistence in the salivary glands. Excretion of virus from the mouth and in urine occurred even when antibody had been present for a long time. Virus recovery was not related to the titer of serum CF antibody. ROWE *et al.* [1958] felt that the presence of the virus in urine suggested that the virus may propagate in the kidney during subclinical infection. This conclusion is supported by the high incidence of virus inclusions in the kidneys at autopsy when not present in other organs except the salivary glands [SEIFERT and OEHME, 1957]. Different human strains of CMV occur, but have overlapping CF antigens [DREESMAN and BENYESH-MELNICK, 1967]. Both early and late separable cytopathic effects occur in different phases of CMV multiplication [MCALLISTER *et al.,* 1967]. The possible relationship of these observations to cases exhibiting persistent virus is not yet clear.

In animals CMV infection appears to be almost always of a persistent or latent type [SMITH, 1959; DIOSI *et al.,* 1967], sometimes detectable by renal inclusions [MARKHAM, 1938] or by virus isolation in the absence of inclusions [KUTTNER, 1934]. Congenital infection with mouse CMV could not be produced by MEDEARIS [1964b], who concluded that if infection of the embryo did occur, it resulted in death; embryos born alive from persistently infected mothers were concluded to have escaped infection. Persistent infection could be initiated by MEDEARIS [1964a] following SC or IP inoculation of young adult mice. Infections lasted for more than 6 months and virus was readily recovered from the eye, throat swabs and urine, but not from feces. Neutralizing and CF antibodies were demonstrated in the sera of animals during this time. The CF exceeded neutralizing antibody in titer and persisted for a longer period. A positive correlation existed between the CF antibody titer, virus titer in the salivary gland and the inoculum dose. Congenital infection was not found in the offspring of animals which became pregnant during persistent infection. When methotrexate was administered in chronic infections, no change resulted, but if this was given before and during acute infection, it increased the extent of virus multiplication. A similar increase in severity of CMV infection after methotrexate treatment was observed by SMITH and VELIOS [1950]. The animal findings parallel the occurrence of generalized CMV disease in man when the cellular immunity is impaired; however, it appears that CMV is at the low end of the scale of viruses able to persist through induction of a specific immunological incompetence, and that an equally important factor is its ability to remain in a mature infections form inside cells, including leukocytes.

Equine Infectious Anemia

Introduction

The virus of equine infectious anemia (EIA), or swamp fever, can persist in the blood of an infected horse over a period of at least 18 years [ANON., 1914; FORTNER, 1944; STEIN *et al.*, 1955]. Virus is present at a high concentration in the blood during the febrile stage and can be recovered in decreasing amount after this time. The bone marrow, spleen, liver and lymph nodes of the abdominal cavity contain high concentrations of virus [ISHII, 1963]. The picture presented by this disease is suggestive of a pathogenic process closely related to the LCM model and other persistent virus infections, and it has been regarded by SQUIRE *et al.* [1969] as an immunoproliferative disease. However, although discovered by Lignéc as long ago as 1843 [ISHII, 1963], practical difficulty in using horses as experimental animals and lack of susceptibility of other species [MIURA *et al.*, 1947; PLACIDI and VERGE, 1953; MÖHLMANN, 1956] have so far prevented definitive experiments on the disease process and virology. EIA has been quite extensively reviewed in terms of virology by ISHII [1963], FRIEDMANN [1964] and briefly by TODD [1966] and HYSLOP [1966]. Clinical and control aspects have also been reviewed [DITCHFIELD, 1967; DITCHFIELD *et al.*, 1967; ISHITANI, 1966; NUSBAUM, 1967]. The disease has been widely reported in many parts of the world. In some regions it has been enzootic and tends to cause mild disease; in others it appears suddenly and tends to cause a severe epizootic infection with a high proportion of fatalities [Isнii, 1963]. The infection decreases in severity and sometimes becomes inapparent as the disease becomes more chronic. The natural infection appears to be restricted to animals of the genus *Equus*, and has been readily transmitted from horse to horse by inoculation of serum. It has been claimed that the virus can be grown in the mouse, where it causes fatal paralysis and can be re-transmitted to the horse using 10 % mouse brain [Yaoi *et al.*, 1958; 1959a, b]. Arakawa *et al.* [1952, 1953] have also claimed isolation of a mouse strain, but the evidence for this is slender and the isolation could not be repeated by others [Fortner and Ulbrich, 1952; Dreguss and Lombard, 1954; Yaoi *et al.*, 1959c]. Claims have also been made of transmission to rabbits [Yaoi *et al.*, 1960], sheep [Miura *et al.*, 1955; Möhlmann, 1956; Maramorosh, 1962], pigs [Soituz *et al.*, 1953; Stein and Songer, 1956] and possibly humans [Lührs, 1920; Peters, 1954a, b]. Similar unconfirmed reports of tissue culture growth of the virus have been made, both with [Watanabe, 1960; Kobayashi, 1961a, b, c, 1962; Saurino *et al.*, 1966] and without [Eli-Zein *et al.*, 1968] CPE. Precise data on EIA virus is lacking. There are reports of its filtration through Elford collodian membranes with pore diameters of 100 nm [Balozet, 1939], and several workers have reported particles in electron micrographs of tissue preparations from infected horses. However, by modern standards these appear to be without value. Möhlmann and Gralheer [1954] reported the size of the virus to be 60 to 95 nm by ultracentrifugation. It is reputed to remain viable for one year at –20 to –40° C and to be inactivated by 1 h at 60° C or when mixed with 2 % phenol [Isнii, 1963].

Persistence of Virus

Subcutaneous injection of EIA in the horse causes acute illness after an incubation period of 10 to 21 days [Isнii, 1963]. Thereafter, some animals undergo subclinical disease and become virus carriers. Others have acute disease with fatality as high as 80 %, with frequent remission and persistent infection in the survivors. Acute disease occurs as a sudden rise of temperature to 41–42° C with continual or remittent fever following. After the disappearance of fever, most animals enter a state of collapse which is frequently fatal. Intense anemia, jaundice and hemorrhage accompany the collapse. Septicemic complications may occur.

During chronic infection recurrent fever is the rule, occurring at 3 to 6 month intervals, with debility and anemia. Many surviving cases enter a final stage where there is persistence of the virus in animals which appear quite normal. The main histopathological changes occur in the reticuloendothelial system and walls of blood vessels [ISHII, 1963]. In the acute forms, there is hemorrhage and hyperemia of the splenic pulp with a pronounced histiocytic cellular reaction. The kidney often shows deposits in the glomeruli with lymphoid proliferation around the arterioles. In the more chronic forms, there is lymphoid proliferation; the albumin ratio changes with an over-all increase in gamma globulin. Virus has been demonstrated in the urine [ISHII, 1963], milk [LÜHRS, 1919; ISHII *et al.*, 1940; STEIN *et al.*, 1944], nasal discharge [SCOTT, 1924; BELLER and SCHWARZMAIER, 1940], tears, saliva and semen [ISHII, 1938; STEIN and MOTT, 1942] of infected horses during the febrile stage. Transmission of EIA in the natural state is believed to be due to passive transfer by bite of bloodsucking insects [ANON., 1914], and placental transfer of the virus with congenital infection of foals from infected mares has been reported [SATO, 1928; ISHII *et al.*, 1940; STEIN and MOTT, 1946].

Immunology

Although the serum of infected horses [DREGUSS, 1949] has been reputed to cause agglutination of chicken red cells, there was no parallel between the amount of virus present and hemagglutinating activity. Demonstration of neutralizing antibodies to EIA is of dubious definition [YAOI *et al.*, 1959b; ISHII, 1963]; STEIN and GATES [1950] reported some suggestive data without clear-cut results. ISHII [1963] concluded that the production of antibodies is less efficient with EIA virus than with other viruses in that none of the investigations proved the actual presence of neutralizing or CF antibodies although serum of affected animals can have AC activity. Various studies on the production of a vaccine have been made, none of which produced positive results [MARTIN, 1939; STEIN and OSTEEN, 1941; BANKIER, 1945; DREGUSS and LOMBARD, 1954; TABUCHI *et al.*, 1955]. CF antibody titer as a diagnostic method in EIA infection in horses was reevaluated by HENSON *et al.* [1967b] using an equine leukocyte tissue culture antigen [KONO and KOBAYASHI, 1966] which gave positive results in the early phase of the acute disease. These workers found an increase in gamma globulin in most infected horses and KOBAYASHI *et al.* [1969] found CF antibodies took 15–25 days to appear, while neutralizing antibody took 135 days. BOULANGER *et al.* [1969] found only a temporary nonspecific CF antibody response which they ascribed to the formation of autoantibody. A precipitin-based diagnostic test has been described [MOORE *et al.*, 1966] using serum from rabbits immunized with red cells from infected horses.

Pathogenic Mechanism

The older explanations of EIA pathogenesis included theories that the disease was essentially: (1) a disturbance of bone marrow with compensatory changes in the spleen [SEYDERHELM, 1914; ZIEGLER, 1924, 1925; SCHERMER, 1926]; (2) a virus infection which stimulated the mesenchymal system with changes of the reticuloendothelial system [DOBBERSTEIN, 1934]; and (3) an allergic phenomenon with perivascular cell infiltration of liver, spleen, lymph nodes, glomerulonephritis, increase in plasma cells, and an increase in circulating gamma globulin. The known facts of this disease appear to be compatible with current concepts of persistent virus infection with a severe disturbance of the immunological responses. There is clear evidence of persistent viremia, increased gamma globulin, circulating antigen-antibody complexes and glomerulonephritis, all reminiscent of the pathogenesis of Aleutian mink disease. Most of the histopathology of EIA appears to be explainable on the basis of a cellular immune response. At the present time it seems likely that the disease process will prove to be due to a protracted virus-induced disturbance of the mechanisms normally responsible for virus suppression, and that essentially the same concept proposed for LCM pathogenesis will explain the disturbances arising in EIA. However, the finding by SAURINO *et al.* [1966] of a protein peak in the serum of carrier animals raises the possibility that this is a virus-induced antigen, and that these animals are in a state of antigen excess more comparable to the PTI than to the HDIP state.

Kyasanur Forest Disease

PRICE [1966] has reported the initiation of persistent infection in mice inoculated with Kyasanur Forest disease virus. Although most inoculated animals died, approximately 2 % developed paralysis and survived up to 246 days. The mice remained abnormally small and ruffled, and most of them were found to carry persistent virus at titers of 10^2 or greater in their liver and brain. Although some of the animals with persistent infection showed neutralizing antibody, the majority showed no evidence of immunological response to the agent as judged by absence of CF, hemagglutination-inhibiting or neutralizing antibody. No virus, however, was found in the blood.

Lactic Dehydrogenase Elevating Virus

Lactic dehydrogenase elevating virus (LDV) qualifies very easily as an agent causing a persistent infection. Prolonged and very high titers occur in the blood and organs after inoculation of newborn or adult mice [RILEY, 1963a]. The behavior of this agent in mice has recently been reviewed by RILEY [1968] with particular reference to its interrelationship with neoplastic growths. The reader is referred to this review for the major features of the behavior and properties of the agent. Only those observations pertinent to the mechanisms of persistent virus infection will be considered here. Filtration indicates a size of 35 to 40 nm for the virus, but some experiments indicate the presence of a smaller infectious particle [RILEY, 1963b; ROWSON et al., 1963]. The virus was found to band sharply at a density equivalent to 1.168 g/ml [RILEY, 1968]. Ether treatment is reported [NOTKINS, 1964] to liberate an infectious RNA. Electron microscopy [DE-THÉ and NOTKINS, 1965] has shown the particle to be eliptical or oblong (36–42×45–75 nm) containing a nucleoid 26–29 nm in diameter. It infects only the mouse, and a high percentage of wild mice are carriers. The virus is commonly spread by biting and, since males are more aggressive than females, a higher incidence of infection is seen in males (100 % as opposed to 3 %). Cannibalism can result in infection, and the virus may also be spread by infected mothers to their offspring by suckling or by transplacental infection [NOTKINS, 1965]. The virus occurs in two different forms [ADAMS and BOWMAN, 1964], separable by centrifugation or chromatography. Both the small (S) and large (L) particles obtained from plasma of mice infected with LDV showed parallel inactivation with UV or ether treatment [CRISPENS, 1965c]. The virus induces increased enzyme formation and permanent benign impairment of the host mechanism for enzyme clearance from plasma [MAHY *et al.*, 1965, 1967; RILEY *et al.*, 1965] particularly affecting the lactic dehydrogenase (LDH) system [NOTKINS and SCHEELE, 1964]. There is an increased enzyme flux into the plasma of both cancer-free and tumorous hosts, but no obvious lesions or CPE in cell cultures have been observed [ANDERSON *et al.*, 1966; DUBUY and JOHNSON, 1968] although *in vitro* growth of the virus is possible [YAFFE, 1962; PLAGEMANN and SWIM, 1963a, b, 1966; RILEY, 1963b; EVANS and SALAMAN, 1965; ANDERSON *et al.*, 1966].

LDV appears to only replicate in macrophages or macrophage-like cells of spleen, liver, peritoneal cavity and lymph nodes [EVANS and SALAMAN, 1965]. Maximal growth occurs in liver and spleen [DUBUY and JOHNSON, 1966] and peak fluorescence of cells stained for LDV antigen is at 24 h post-infection. PLAGEMANN and SWIM [1966] found no CPE or increase in LDH of tissue cultures of mouse liver or other organs but FRANTSI and GREGORY [1969] found that an increase of LDH began in mouse liver cell cultures 4 h after infection with LDV. This was sometimes accompanied by CPE. The authors postulated that, if liver cells were destroyed by LDV *in vivo*, they could provide an influx of dehydrogenases; and, to the extent to which the liver might be involved in the removal of plasma enzymes, the clearance of these could simultaneously be impaired. Any virus causing similar damage to these cells would also release dehydrogenases. They point out that some LDH elevation has been noted following infection of mouse embryonic liver cell cultures with the Friend leukemia virus, in the absence of detectable CPE [FRANTSI, 1968]. Although LDV causes enhanced tumor growth when inoculated with a transmissible tumor [RILEY *et al.*, 1961], it appears to be capable of inducing partial protection for the host against some spontaneous tumors [RILEY, 1966]. When inoculated into young adult C_3H females, LDV protected them against Bittner virus and mammary adenocarcinoma [RILEY *et al.*, 1966]. LDV is claimed [RILEY, 1963c] to give some protection against X-ray induced anemias. In the serum, titers of 10^{10} or more per ml are readily reached 24 h after inoculation of adults [NOTKINS and SHOCHAT, 1963] and at this time LDV appears in urine, feces and saliva [NOTKINS and SCHEELE, 1963]; the plasma LDH enzyme titer was found by NOTKINS and SHOCHAT [1963] to be slower to rise, reaching a plateau at 72 h. Virus titers of around 10^5 or 10^6 were shown by ROWSON *et al.* [1966] and NOTKINS *et al.* [1966a] to persist in the host plasma for the lifetime of the infected animal in spite of circulating antibodies. These antibodies were active against LDV produced during the early stages of the disease but did not neutralize the later persisting virus which in other respects appeared to possess similar biological and infectious properties. NOTKINS *et al.* [1966b, 1968] have suggested that this 'sensitized virus' consists of infectious virus-antibody complexes since it is insensitive to the immune mouse serum but is neutralized by goat antimouse serum. PORTER *et al.* [1969a] have shown that non-neutralizing antibody with rapidly rising titers detectable only by the FAB technic was produced in LDV-infected mice 6 days after infection. This situation is remarkably similar to that in acute LCM infection of adult mice. After neonatal thymectomy, mice were shown by CRISPENS [1966] to fail to produce serum LDV antibodies to the normal extent and LDV titers were higher [CRISPENS and REY, 1967]. CRISPENS [1964b] has postulated two types of particle – one $MgCl_2$ resistant and antigenic and the other $MgCl_2$ sensitive and non-antigenic – to explain the persistent viremia and the permanent elevation of various plasma enzymes.

There is a marked synergism between *E. coccoides* and LDV [RILEY *et al.*, 1964], causing a substantial increase in the plasma LDH level, spleen enlargement and host anemia during dual infection [RILEY, 1964]. LDV was shown by MERGENHAGEN *et al.* [1967] and NOTKINS *et al.* [1966c] to have a tolerance suppressive action when given with an antigen (unaggregated human γ-globulin) which would have been tolerogenic when given alone. In this respect, LDV resembled bacterial endotoxin. In contrast to this, HOWARD *et al.* [1969] have shown that LDV infection temporarily decreases the cellular immune response to other antigens. An interesting relationship was found between interferon production and LDV serum titers by EVANS and RILEY [1968] who showed interferon production to be active during the highest phases of virus production but to drop to zero during the plateau of persistent viremia, from approximately 72 h after inoculation onwards. Subsequently, interferon production does not parallel virus growth [BARON *et al.*, 1964]. This virus appears to have significant similarities to LCM and pneumonia virus of mice [CRISPENS, 1965b], particularly in terms of: (1) Its capacity to induce persistence similar to the LCM-HDIP state; (2) the leukopenia following infection and growth in lymph nodes [DUBUY and JOHNSON, 1966]; (3) the ability of both LCM and LDV [NOTKINS and SCHEELE, 1963; GEORGII *et al.*, 1964; CRISPENS, 1964c, 1965a, 1967] to infect the embryo *in utero* and (4) the enhancing effect shown by *E. coccoides* on both agents.

Measles-Subacute Sclerosing Panencephalitis (SSPE)

Virus particles have been found [BOUTEILLE *et al.*, 1965; PERIER and VANDERHAEGHEN, 1966; TELLEZ-NAGEL and HARTER, 1966a; HERNDORN and RUBENSTEIN, 1968] within brain lesions of human cases of subacute sclerosing panencephalitis (SSPE), suggesting that this disease may be of viral origin, and that long-term persistence of the virus with ultimately slow onset of disease may occur [TELLEZ-NAGEL and HARTER, 1966b]. Attempts by ADELS *et al.* [1968] to transmit the disease to primates and to isolate a measles-related agent were unsuccessful, as were attempts [TELLEZ-NAGEL and HARTER, 1966a; HARTER and TELLEZ-NAGEL, 1968] to isolate an SSPE agent in cell culture. However, measles virus was successfully isolated from brain biopsy from cases of SSPE by CHEN *et al.* [1969] and by HORTA-BARBOSA *et al.* [1969], indicating the possibility that this condition is due to infection of the brain with measles. Serological evidence of measles virus as the causal agent has also been obtained [BERMAN *et al.*, 1968; CONNOLLY, 1968; GRIFFITH and KATZ, 1968; LENNETTE *et al.*, 1968; SEVER and ZEMAN, 1968; JABBOUR *et al.*, 1969]. However, in view of the difficulty with which measles may be isolated from the diseased tissue at the present time, it is not clear whether this condition qualifies as a persistent infection. It would appear that the infection is the result of a long-term latency or low level persistence of the virus, which either becomes activated to cause a slow progressively destructive lesion, or follows an exceedingly slow replicative pattern. SAUNDERS *et al.* [1969] found a striking increase in the transformation response of lymphocytes from an SSPE patient when they were exposed to measles antigen. Both the patient and a matched control had had measles, and both sets of lymphocytes reacted equally to phytohemagglutinin. The authors suggested that the destructive effect of SSPE is mediated by lymphocytes. It is possible that the progress of the lesions in the brain depends upon direct cell to cell transmission which could be expected to be both very slow and impervious to the presence of neutralizing antibody.

Rabies

Rabies appears to qualify as a persistent virus infection since long-term infection without symptoms can occur; the virus has been isolated from the brain of rats, rabbits and guinea pigs and rarely from the saliva of animals, including dogs and bats, for many months after infection [BELL, 1966; VEERARGHAVEN *et al.*, 1967; KAPLAN, 1969]. Infected insectivorous bats have been shown to excrete rabies virus in their saliva for as long as 16 months without showing clinical signs. Observable disease seems to be the usual outcome of infection in these animals [TIERKEL, 1959]; however, investigations into the pathogenesis of this virus disease have concentrated on its neurological manifestations at the expense of the systemic infection, partly due to the prevalence of the use of the IC inoculation route. *In vitro* studies by FERNANDES *et al.* [1964] showed that tissue cultures persistently infected [FERNANDES *et al.*, 1963] with rabies virus were lysed by antirabies virus serum in the presence of complement. Fluorescent antibody study showed that in the absence of complement only the surface of infected cells was stained [WIKTOR *et al.*, 1968]. The possibility that rabies falls into the LCM pathogenic mechanism class has important bearings on the practical aspects of vaccination. It seems to be a generalization that killed vaccines are virtually ineffective in the persistent virus group, and this attribute holds for rabies [HUMMELER and KOPROWSKI, 1969]. Although rabies induces much soluble CF antigen in infected tissue, the LCM-tolerance analogy suggests that this will not stimulate immunity, which would depend on a cellular response.

Rat and H Viruses

The picodnaviruses [MAYOR and MELNICK, 1966] (also called parvoviruses) including rat virus (RV), hamster osteolytic (H) virus, and AAV (adeno-associated virus) have been recently reviewed by TOOLAN [1968]. They are small heat- and ether-resistant DNA viruses about 20 nm in size with a 32-capsomere morphology. They hemagglutinate and have pathogenicity for newborn hamsters. Some of these agents induce temporary or more rarely, longterm persistence in some of their hosts. While RV causes a definite CPE [KILHAM and OLIVER, 1959], the related feline panleukopenia virus (FPV) only causes a slight, tansient CPE [JOHNSON, 1965]. In newborn hamsters dying of the infection with H [TOOLAN, 1960] or RV [KILHAM, 1961] agents, virus has been recovered from almost all tissues with highest titers usually in the kidneys and blood; virus was also present in the urine. The animals have been noted to have unusually small spleens. PORTELLA [1963] has observed that H-1 or H-3 virus can be isolated from blood clots of hamsters 31 days after infection but not at 38 days. FERM and KILHAM [1964, 1965b] suggested the possibility that the virus persists in the skull bones of neonatally infected hamsters and thereby causes the 'mongoloid' deformity which ensues. TOOLAN [1968] noticed that occasionally after neonatal inoculation of hamsters virus could be recovered from well-washed livers of old 'mongoloid' animals in spite of antibody titers in their sera as high as 1:20,000. However, it would appear that such levels of virus approximate a state of latency rather than persistent infection. In the adult hamster neutralizing antibody and suppression of the infection appears to follow the normal path of most acute virus infections [TOOLAN, 1965].

KILHAM and OLIVER reported the isolation of RV in 1959. These agents persist in and can readily be isolated from both animal and human sources [DALLDORF, 1961; TOOLAN, 1960; TOOLAN et al., 1960; KILHAM and MOLONEY, 1964; TOOLAN, 1964; MARGOLIS and KILHAM, 1968b]. They are very common in laboratory and wild rats [KILHAM, 1966] and have been quite extensively studied by KILHAM and other workers [ULE, 1952; BERNHARD et al., 1963; DALTON et al., 1963; BREESE et al., 1964; KARASAKI, 1966; KILHAM, 1966]. The rat viruses cause a broad spectrum of disease [KILHAM, 1966], including reproductive failure [MARGOLIS and KILHAM, 1965; MARGOLIS et al., 1967], teratogenic effect [FERM and KILHAM, 1965a], skeletal defects [FERM and KILHAM, 1965b] and a mongoloid type of deformity with associated dental deformities, cerebellar hypoplasia [KILHAM and MARGOLIS, 1964] and hepatitis [KILHAM and MARGOLIS, 1966b; RUFFOLO et al., 1966; MARGOLIS et al., 1968]. They are capable of causing death or dwarfism after IC inoculation of newborn mice [MATSUO and SPENCER, 1969]. KILHAM and MARGOLIS [1964] found that cerebellar hypoplasia and ataxia occur in hamsters 12 days after neonatal IC injection of RV and that death occurs some 3 to 4 weeks later. It can cause congenital infection and disease in rats [KILHAM and MARGOLIS, 1966b], and behavioral changes were found by LANDAUER et al. [1967] to be associated with neonatal RV infection of hamsters. KILHAM and MARGOLIS [1966a] showed that the group included a viral agent responsible for ataxia of cats [MARGOLIS and KILHAM, 1968]. Filtrates from the cerebellar tissue of 5 out of 18 ataxic kittens ranging in age from 5 weeks to 2 months have yielded an infectious agent which can cause the disease in kittens or ferrets. This agent has been called feline ataxia virus (FAV), and neutralizing antibodies develop against it in the ataxic animals. Although FAV has the same general physical and chemical properties as RV and H viruses, it is immunologically distinct from them. Collaborative studies [JOHNSON *et al.*, 1967] showed that spontaneous feline ataxia is due to the same virus as that which causes feline panleukopenia. KILHAM *et al.* [1967] reported that cerebellar hypoplasia was caused by persistent infection resulting from congenital infection of cats and ferrets with FPV. Maternal antibody to this virus is normally transmitted to kittens if the mother is immune to the virus [O'REILLY *et al.*, 1969]. Although this virus is in the same group as RV, it shows different immunological specifity. These viruses have selective affinity for mitotic cells and also cause nuclear inclusions [MARGOLIS and KILHAM, 1965]. The lesion in the cerebellum of the neonatal hamster induced by RV has been described [MARGOLIS and KILHAM, 1965, 1968] and the same lesion has been shown to be caused by a minute virus of mice which has properties similar to RV [CRAWFORD, 1966; MARGOLIS and KILHAM, 1968b]. RV also causes destruction of the cerebellar external layer after inoculation in neonatal kittens [KILHAM and MARGOLIS, 1966a]. However, neither normal nor spontaneously ataxic cats demonstrated hemagglutination-inhibition antibodies against RV. It is noteworthy that feline ataxia has hitherto been suspected to have a genetic basis. KILHAM *et al.* [1967] investigated congenital infection of rats and ferrets by FPV and showed that animals infected *in utero* can carry active virus for months after birth in various organs, especially the kidneys. These authors drew a parallel between congenital FPV infection of cats and rubella infection of man, but noted that neither rats nor cats develop immune tolerance as a result of congenital infection with this virus group. The fact that panleukopenia virus attacks white cells so vigorously suggests that it may achieve its partial persistence in the newborn by virtue of this destructive ability.

Reovirus

The reoviruses have some ability to induce in mice a persistent infection which is relatively short lived. This group has been reviewed briefly by STANLEY [1961a, 1964] and comprehensively by ROSEN [1968]. The name reovirus was given to an agent originally called ECHO Type 10 by SABIN [1959] who coined the term reovirus from the abbreviation of 'respiratory enteric orphan virus'. This virus was found to be larger than other enteroviruses and to have a different CPE [MALHERBE and HAR-

WIN, 1957; SHAVER *et al.*, 1958]. It was isolated by STANLEY *et al.* [1953] and STANLEY [1961b] from an aboriginal child and originally called hepatoencephalomyelitis virus. It was also isolated from human feces in Holland [TONGEREN, 1957] and from mice [STANLEY, 1961a]. SV 12 and SV 59 proved to be the same as reovirus types 1 and 2. STREISSLE and MARAMOROSCH [1963] have demonstrated a cross-reaction between reovirus and wound-tumor virus of plants. Reoviruses have a prolonged growth cycle in cell cultures and are not immediately cytocidal [HASHIMI *et al.*, 1966]. They appear to multiply in association with the mitotic apparatus of the affected cell [RHIM *et al.*, 1962; SPENDLOVE *et al.*, 1963; LERNER, 1964]. The ability of reovirus type 3 to induce persistent latent infection in human embryonic cells has been described [BELL and ROSS, 1966]. There was CPE only when the cells ceased to divide because of overcrowding.

Inoculation of reovirus into infant mice less than 5 days of age results in a runting syndrome [STANLEY and LEAK, 1963] showing retardation of growth, oily hair, diarrhea, alopecia, jaundice, an ataxic mincing gait and hunched posture. The condition resembles the runting syndrome following inoculation of immunologically competent lymphoid cells. Mice with reovirus runting syndrome showed focal necrotic, coagulative liver lesions; the thymus appeared normal [WALTERS *et al.*, 1963]. Reovirus types 1 and 2 infections in neonatal mice have caused some cases of chronic disease [WALTERS *et al.*, 1965]. However, infectious virus was not demonstrated in any tissue after the 42nd day. The viremia following SC inoculation of reovirus type 1 in newborn Swiss mice was studied by JENSON *et al.* [1966]. Virus appeared 4 days postinoculation and was found mainly in the buffy coat. Circulating leukocytes contained immunofluorescent antigen infrequently, but more often were found to contain membrane-bound structures inside vacuoles. KUNDIN *et al.* [1966] inoculated reovirus type 1 SC into suckling mice and found that a nonfatal pantropic infection ensued. Infectious virus was recovered from most of the tissues tested from 1 h to at least 20 days later. High titers were found in lymph nodes. The peak of infection occurred between day 6 and day 9 as judged by FAB staining. Virus could be isolated from an X-irradiated mouse 44 days after reovirus 1 inoculation. HASSAN and COCHRAN [1966] found that inoculation of pregnant mice with reovirus type 1 caused a high incidence of fetal resorption, death and malformation. WALTERS *et al.* [1965] were able to recover reovirus types 1 and 2 from the brains of adult mice 42 and 35 days, respectively, after infection. Hemagglutination-inhibiting antibody was formed. Reovirus type 2 could be isolated from the eyes of neonatally inoculated mice 2 weeks after infection at a time when blood showed no virus [KO-FENDER *et al.*, 1967]. More virus was found in the kidney than in the eye initially, but after 20 days virus was still present in the eye but not in the kidney. After 30 days, all tests were negative. HASHIMI *et al.* [1966] studied congenital infections with reovirus in mice born of mothers which had received reovirus type 2 IP at various times during the pregnancy. The authors concluded that some of the offspring had developed immunological tolerance to the virus with persistent infection, although ROSEN [1968] had pointed out that it was not shown that these antibody-free mice had ever been infected. However, the authors demonstrated viremia at 24 to 42 days after *in utero* infection in 4 of 16 mice which appeared healthy but were presumed to have been congenitally infected. Although HASHIMI *et al.* [1966] felt that reovirus type 2 may have initiated a similar state of tolerant infection to that described by HOTCHIN [1962a] for LCM virus, if this were so, the level of tolerance to reovirus was much less complete and its duration much shorter than that induced by LCM virus.

Type 3 reovirus was found by STANLEY *et al.* [1964] in the brain of suckling mice as long as 70 days after infection. STANLEY [1967] and JOSKE *et al.* [1967] considered that this reovirus can cause what appeared to be a chronic virus-free immunological disease following acute neonatal infection in mice. In the acute phase, virus multiplied in many parts of the animal and caused characteristic lesions, particularly in liver, central nervous system, heart, pancreas, salivary gland, lung, spleen and skeletal muscle. However, reovirus type 3 could not be found in the animals during this chronic phase and immunological tolerance did not apparently occur. A possible association of Burkitt's African lymphoma and reovirus type 3 has been suspected [ANON., 1966; STANLEY, 1966], since the virus has been isolated from a relatively large number of lymphoma biopsy specimens [BELL *et al.*, 1966]. It may be transmitted by mosquitoes from a vertebrate reservoir to man and is capable of inducing murine lymphomas [JOSKE *et al.*, 1966; KEAST and STANLEY, 1966; PAPADIMITRIOU, 1966; STANLEY and PAPADIMITRIOU, 1966; STANLEY *et al.*, 1966; KEAST et al., 1968] which have many similarities to Burkitt's lymphoma. STANLEY [1967] has suggested that the epidemiology of reovirus type 3 can fit the pattern of Burkitt's lymphoma as it occurs in Africa, New Guinea and possibly elsewhere. However, LEVY *et al.* [1968]

were unable to find a functional interaction between reovirus type 3 and EB virus, which is also associated with Burkitt's lymphoma. These authors concluded that its presence in these lymphomas may denote only an incidental passenger status. Complement-fixation tests by STANLEY and KEAST [1967] showed that reovirus-induced mouse lymphoma 2731/L shares an antigen with a cultured line of Burkitt's lymphoma and reovirus 3. The authors considered this to be further evidence supporting the reovirus 3 etiology of Burkitt's lymphoma and the murine lymphoma 2731/L [STANLEY and KEAST, 1967]. However, reovirus could not be isolated from this lymphoma. It seems clear that persistence is not a prerequisite of lymphoma induction by reovirus and that any persistence of virus caused by this group is relatively infrequent and short lived.

Rubella

Introduction

Congenital rubella infection in man appears to be a partial example of PTI in which the degree of tolerance induced by the virus upon the host is relatively low, resulting in only temporary persistence of the virus after birth of the fetus. In this respect, a parallel is probably more exact between congenital rubella in man and the LCM-HDIP state in the adult mouse. However, although noncytopathic in tissue and organ culture [BEST *et al.*, 1968], the rubella virus is capable of causing severe damage to the human fetus and is responsible for a wide variety of crippling birth defects. This ether-sensitive RNA virus replicates primarily in the cytoplasm [BROWN *et al.*, 1965] and is usually detected by its capacity to interfere with challenge virus. Diagnostic methods for confirmation of rubella and other infections of the newborn have been summarized by ALFORD *et al.* [1967], and congenital rubella has been extensively reviewed in recent years, e. g., by SCHIFF and SEVER [1966], MCCARTHY and TAYLOR-ROBINSON [1967], INGALLS *et al.* [1967], DUDGEON [1967b], ELIZAN *et al.* [1969] and RAWLS [1968].

Congenital Rubella

The scope and variety of congenital abnormalities caused by rubella virus is considerably wider than was at first thought [KORONES *et al.*,

1965; LAMBERT *et al.*, 1965; STRAUSS and BERNSTEIN, 1968]. It has become clear that rubella infection in the first trimester of pregnancy can pass from the mother to the fetus, causing an infection which is not necessarily fatal to the fetus. However, the infant may be born with a persistent infection lasting for months or even a few years [MENSER *et al.*, 1967b]. Typically, infants with congenital rubella present a syndrome consisting of growth retardation, generalized purpura (with thrombocytopenia), hepatosplenomegaly, encephalomyelitis and characteristic lesions of the long bones on X-ray. In addition to congenital heart and eye defects [RUDOLPH *et al.*, 1965], congenital deafness [KARMODY, 1968] and severe neurological disturbance [DESMOND *et al.*, 1967], including mental deficiency and schizophrenia, have been reported [MENSER *et al.*, 1967a]. Virus can be isolated in a high proportion of patients from throat swabs, rectal swabs, cerebrospinal fluid, liver biopsy, urine [MONIF and SEVER, 1966] and the lens of the eye (removed at operation for cataract) [RUDOLPH *et al.*, 1965; COTLIER *et al.*, 1966; HAMBIDGE *et al.*, 1966; REID *et al.*, 1966; MURPHY *et al.*, 1967]. Some infants excrete the virus in urine for many months after birth and contact infection is not uncommon [HAMBIDGE *et al.*, 1966]. Similar persistence of the virus has been reported in ferrets [RORKE *et al.*, 1968], rats [BOHIGIAN *et al.*, 1968] and monkeys [PARKMAN *et al.*, 1965]. The general development of the rubella syndrome has been summarized by WELLER *et al.* [1965], who stressed the close similarity with the comparable situation in congenital cytomegalovirus infection where the period of hepatosplenomegaly extends to approximately 18 months and the ensuing residual damage is confined to the nervous system. The pathological changes found in congenital rubella have been summarized by DUDGEON [1967a] as shown in table VII.

The mechanism of the teratogenic [ELIZAN *et al.*, 1969] and the degenerative effects of rubella virus is not understood, but WAY [1967] believes that studies of the cardiovascular defects indicate the basic lesion is damage to the endothelium. RAWLS [1968] has pointed out that rubella virus infection during the first few weeks of intrauterine life does not apparently produce immunological tolerance, since serological studies of children with rubella demonstrated rubella antibody long after the loss of maternal antibody [PLOTKIN *et al.*, 1963; ALFORD *et al.*, 1964; DUDGEON *et al.*, 1964; WELLER *et al.*, 1964]. Many infants have been shown to produce high levels of IgM which may persist for many months [SOOTHILL *et al.*, 1966; HANCOCK *et al.*, 1968] while the production of

Table VII. The pathological changes found in congenital rubella[1]

Changes due to retardation or inhibition of cell growth	Changes due to cell necrosis
Intrauterine growth retardation	Focal and diffuse necrotizing myocarditis
Small size of thymus, adrenals, brain, eye, lens, lack of development of primary lens fibers	Hemorrhages and inflammation in stria vascularis; focal meningo-encephalitis; necrosis of paraventricular white matter; dystrophic calcification
Malformations of heart, organ of Corti and lens	Thickened alveolar septa; necrotizing bronchiolitis; splenic fibrosis

[1] DUDGEON [1967a].

IgG may be normal or suppressed. Some cases of hypogammaglob-ulinemia have resulted [SOOTHILL *et al.*, 1966; PLOTKIN *et al.*, 1966]. The globulins are readily detectable [BAUBLIS and BROWN, 1968] by the indirect FAB method of BROWN *et al.* [1964], and VESIKARI and VAHERI [1968] have shown that the IgM antibody possessed hemagglutina-tion-inhibiting activity. DENT *et al.* [1968] concluded that the persistence of rubella virus is an immunological paradox, in which the presence of circulating 19S rubella-virus-neutralizing antibody shows that an immune response has been provoked by the virus. This in turn indicates that tolerance in the usual sense of the word is not present, but nevertheless a defect in cellular immune function appears to be a cause of the underlying failure of the tissues of some infants to terminate virus excretion. However, JACK and GRUTZNER [1969] have shown that the viremia is due to leukocyte-associated virus which is apparently rendered detectable when the neutralizing antibody is removed. Rubella has been reported by MENSER *et al.* [1967c] to cause not only con-genital kidney defects but also apparently a slowly resolving nephritis. It is not clear whether this was antibody mediated or a primary effect of the virus upon the kidney. It therefore seems extremely likely that some degree of split tolerance to this virus occurs, probably similar to the HDIP state with LCM virus infection of adults. Studies on the function-al role of the different types of rubella antibody are needed, since it appears likely that this virus differs from some of the other persistent vi-ruses by being so constructed that antibody against its soluble antigenic component has neutralizing activity. Immunoglobulin levels remain high [KENRICK *et al.*, 1968] in adults who have recovered from congenital rubella. Most of the rubella research has utilized human infections but a start has been made on experimental congenital infections in rabbits. LONDON *et al.* [1969] reported that after inoculation of rabbit fetuses early in gestation, high levels of hemagglutinating antibody develop in the doe. Only low titers occurred in the newborn offspring, and these titers dropped to zero by 35 days. Increased stillbirths and underweight infants occurred but no malformations were found.

Effects of Rubella Virus on Lymphocytes

OLSON *et al.* [1967] and WHITE *et al.* [1968] showed that lymphocytes from infants with congenital rubella failed to undergo blastogenesis when stimulated by phytohemagglutinin. This finding fits the concept that the virus causes a lesion of lymphocytes in which they are prevented from developing their normal maturative response when stimulated by foreign antigen. However, it is necessary to postulate that an immunologically specific lesion is caused by the virus in order to explain the persisting infection since there appears to be no evidence of a concomitant persistence of other pathogens due to the lymphoid lesion, and affected infants possess a functional delayed hypersensitivity reaction [OLSON *et al.*, 1967]. The decreased phytohemagglutinin response occurs mainly in the first few months of life; as the infant improves, the responsiveness of the lymphocytes returns to normal. A similar effect can be obtained *in vitro* [MONTGOMERY *et al.*, 1967]. DENT *et al.* [1968] concluded that the specific rubella lesion of lymphocytes is caused by an inability of these cells to undergo the metabolic changes requisite to their recruitment for immunological functions. This lesion could explain the lack of ability of such cells to suppress a rubella virus infection competently by means of the homograft response. SINGER *et al.* [1969] found that 8 of 11 infants with congenital rubella below two years of age had precocious lymphoid maturation, correlating with elevated serum IgM. SIMONS and FITZGERALD [1968] found that lymphocytes from congenital rubella babies could be stimulated by phytohemagglutinin but that the response was inhibited by prior exposure of the lymphocytes to rubella virus. An impairment of lymphocyte function is evident even after virus could no longer be recovered from patients [WHITE *et al.*, 1968] and is also caused by rubella infection of normal human leukocytes *in vitro* [OLSON *et al.*, 1968]. Such cells showed decreased synthesis of normal nucleic acids and structural proteins, and the virus infection abrogated the enhanced DNA synthesis induced by pokeweed and specific antigen stimulation. The effect was only caused by live rubella virus and not by ultraviolet irradiated virus. The authors noted that similar inhibitory effects were caused on normal lymphocytes by other RNA viruses including mumps and poliovirus. This finding appears to weaken somewhat the explanation of persistent infection in terms of the PHA-inhibiting effect of virus, and suggests that the key inhibitory event enabling viral persistence to occur must involve a high degree of specificity for the virus concerned. Rubella virus was isolated [SIMONS and JACK, 1968] from lymphocytes taken from venous blood of three babies with congenital rubella at 24, 51 and 196 days after birth.

Persistence of Virus and Pathogenesis

It is well established that rubella virus can induce a persistent infection of the fetus [SELZER, 1963; KAY *et al.*, 1964; ALFORD, 1965; HORSTMANN *et al.*, 1965; PHILLIPS *et al.*, 1965; COOPER and KRUGMAN, 1966] which is maintained for a considerable time in spite of the presence of antibody to the virus [ALFORD, 1965; BELLANTI *et al.*, 1965; PHILLIPS *et al.*, 1966; SOOTHILL *et al.*, 1966]. As many as 47 % of therapeutic abortions of clinically diagnosed rubella in the first trimester of pregnancy contained the virus [ALFORD *et al.*, 1964] and the number was even higher during a rubella epidemic year. The development of clinical disease and virus persistence appear to be more closely associated with high levels of virus growth than with infection very early during gestation. Studies of the duration of virus persistence as determined by virus excretion showed that after the first few months of life virus was usually recovered only from cerebrospinal fluid or throat swabs [PHILLIPS *et al.*, 1965]. The proportion of infants excreting virus apparently falls from about 60 % to about 7 % during the first year after birth [LINDQUIST *et al.*, 1965; COOPER and KRUGMAN, 1967], although RAWLS [1968] found a slower decay with 5 % excreting virus at 18 months; one infant was positive at 30 months. The situation is similar to congenital persistent LCM infection in mice except that the time period is very much foreshortened in rubella. Interferon production in congenital rubella could not be detected, although congenitally infected infants were able to respond to live measles virus vaccination with interferon production. The virus was sensitive to human interferon in acutely infected tissue culture cells but not in chronically infected cells [DESMYTER *et al.*, 1967]. Congenital rubella infants often are found to have low birth weights and fail to gain weight or thrive after birth. A significant correlation between virus excretion and failure to thrive has been reported [RAWLS *et al.*, 1967]. This situation parallels the runting found in neonatal LCM and reovirus infections. NAEYE and BLANC [1965] showed that the organs of infants with congenital rubella contained a smaller number of cells than normal, although cells present were normal in morphology and size. BOUÉ and BOUÉ [1969] have suggested that the retardation of growth *in vivo* may be due to cell death from the large number of chromosome breaks which they have shown to occur *in vitro* in human cell cultures persistently infected with rubella virus. Immunofluorescence studies of tissue sections of infants with congenital rubella [WOODS *et al.*, 1966] have shown very few cells containing rubella antigen. Positive cells which did occur were found to be scattered in small foci suggesting that a clone of infected cells had arisen from a single infected parent cell. The cells containing rubella antigen were morphologically normal when stained with hematoxylin and eosin. Assay of the number of infectious centers in a suspension of fetal cells from human *in utero* infected embryos [RAWLS *et al.*, 1968] revealed that only 0.1 % of the fetal cells contained infectious virus and that the noninfected cells were fully susceptible to rubella virus. Chronically infected cells from tissues of infants with congenital rubella were studied by RAWLS and MELNICK [1966] and found to have a reduced growth rate and a shortened life span. The carrier cultures could not be cured by rubella antibodies. These workers related their findings to the *in vivo* state of persistently rubella-infected cells and postulated that the same mechanism might explain the viral persistence in congenital rubella. The authors compared the situation with congenital LCM infection of mice where all the cells contain viral antigen or are resistant to superinfection by the virus. It was felt that the lower incidence of infected cells in rubella might be due to the later onset of infection in the case of rubella than to transovarial infection which is believed to occur with LCM virus. It also seems likely that rubella has less ability than LCM to induce a cellular immune paralysis. RAWLS [1968] has pointed out that destruction of thymus cells would not seem to provide an adequate explanation for viral persistence, and there appears to be no evidence of destruction of thymus cells by rubella virus [TONDURY and SMITH, 1966; SINGER *et al.*, 1967]. It may be relevant that rubella in the adult frequently causes palpable enlargement of peripheral lymph nodes, suggesting a more severe effect on these organs than many other acute virus infections of man.

Serum Hepatitis

It is well established that human serum hepatitis (SH) virus can persist in the blood of healthy carriers for periods of several years. The history of this important disease has been well summarized by ZUCKERMAN [1969]. However, satisfactory isolation and identification of a causative agent for this condition has yet to be accomplished; the subject has been recently reviewed by HERSEY and SHAW [1968]. DEINHARDT *et al.* [1967] have apparently been able to transmit the agent to marmoset monkeys, although there is evidence [MELNICK and PARKS, 1968] that a marmoset virus may be responsible for these results. Transmission of human hepatitis via blood or other tissues from apparently healthy carriers of the virus is well known and has been reviewed by ALLEN and SAYMAN [1962]. The disease bears some resemblance to infectious equine anemia, and chronic human cases are suspected [GALLAGHER and GOULSTON, 1962]. There is some evidence that giant cell hepatitis may result in the newborn from transmission of serum or infectious hepatitis (IH) from mother to infant [ALTERMAN, 1963]. STOLLER and COLLMANN [1965] have implicated human maternal hepatitis as a cause of early intrauterine damage to the ovum resulting in congenital Down's syndrome in the newborn infant. Detailed investigation of the relationship between human hepatitis and persistent virus infection awaits the development of adequate virus detection and assay procedures.

Recent work on the Australia antigen (first found in the blood of an Australian aborigine) by BLUMBERG [1964, 1966]; BLUMBERG *et al.* [1965, 1967a, b, 1968]; SUTNICK *et al.* [1968] and LEVENE and BLUMBERG [1969] appears to be opening a new field of hepatitis research since there is increasing evidence [BAYER *et al.*, 1968; PRINCE, 1968a] that the antigen is associated with the virus or may be a part of it [PRINCE, 1968b; MILLMAN *et al.*, 1969]. Using the immunological technic developed by PRINCE [1968a], ZUCKERMAN and TAYLOR [1969] reported evidence that the virus can cause persistent infection in man for nearly 20 years. PRINCE [1968a] found the antigen to be present in SH but not in IH and this was confirmed by GILES *et al.* [1969]. GOCKE and KAVEY [1969] have also described an acute phase hepatitis antigen. The relationship between Australia antigen, SH and the acute hepatitis antigen appears to be very close but has yet to be precisely worked out. BLUMBERG *et al.* [1966] have estimated that tens of millions of humans carry persistent SH infection, though in the United States Australia antigen is found in only 1 in 1,000 normal people. It has an incidence as high as 6 or 7 % in Asia and Oceania, where it apparently persists for at least 8 years without causing disease. The antigen has been found in primates including chimpanzees, African green monkeys and squirrel monkeys, but not in some 30 other species tested including *Macaca mulatta*. The antigen was found by BAYER *et al.* [1968] to be about 20 nm in diameter with knob-like subunits on the surface; this coincides with the size estimated for SH virus [McCOL-LUM, 1952]. The test for its presence can be used as a screening method for SH carriers [BLUMBERG *et al.*, 1969]. Several workers [BLUMBERG and RIDDELL, 1963; BLUMBERG and MELARTIN, 1966; CHAUVEAU *et al.*, 1962] have raised the question of a possible hereditary immunological defect in certain classes of individuals with persistent SH infection, including those with mongolism and lepromatous leprosy. BLUMBERG *et al.* [1968] have drawn attention to the fact that patients with lepromatous leprosy have generalized impairment of delayed tissue hypersensitivity; this would render them less able to eradicate any virus infection by a tissue-rejection mechanism. It will be most interesting to see whether such a defect turns out to be truly hereditary or whether the effect is specifically induced by a virus acquired by prenatal or early neonatal infection. However, the results of BLUMBERG *et al.* [1968] indicate that the Australia antigen is not the cause of Down's disease (in which it is readily found) but results from infection of these patients as a consequence of institutionalization, and that these patients have a true hereditary immunological defect rendering them more susceptible to SH infection. The agent was also found in a high proportion of leukemia, including patients who had not received transfusions or radiation therapy. It remains to be seen whether the hepatitis virus is responsible for both hepatitis and some forms of leukemia.

Suckling Mouse Cataract Agent

The suckling mouse cataract (SMC) agent was isolated by CLARK [1964] in mice, from ticks removed from a dead rabbit. This agent is a possible candidate for consideration as a persistent virus, since it remains in adult mouse brain for as long as 827 days after inoculation [CLARK and KARZON, 1968a]. The virus also induces cataracts in rats [CLARK, 1969]. After inoculation of the newborn mouse, virus was consistently isolated from brain, liver, spleen and eye up to 5 weeks, with titers peaking at approximately 37 days [CLARK, 1964]. Apparently the virus is somewhat persistent in the newborn, but not truly persistent in the adult, and may occupy a place comparable to rubella virus, which also shares with SMC virus the ability to cause cataracts [OLMSTED *et al.*, 1966]. SMC grows on the chorioallantoic membrane of fertile chicken eggs, is ether-sensitive and is of intermediate size [CLARK, 1964]. CLARK and KARZON [1968a] showed that peak titers were reached in suckling mice in all tissues 7 to 15 days after infection with SMC agent. However, virus titers slowly decreased thereafter, disappearing from liver, spleen and eye tissues by 60 days but persisting indefinitely (up to 827 days) in the brain. Neutralizing antibody could not be detected in infected or hyperimmunized mice. In most of the eye tissues, virus titers correlated with the degree of inflammation [CLARK and KARZON, 1969], but in the lens the disease process continued even after the virus titer had declined. Virus was not found in viscera or blood stream [CLARK, 1967; CLARK and KARZON, 1968a]. In spite of this, the offspring of these congenitally persistently infected mice were found by CLARK and KARZON [1968b] to be protected against neonatal challenge with virus by a mechanism which was believed by the authors to be due to transfer of maternal antibody. The protective agent was transferred via the milk [CLARK and KARZON, 1968c]. This generation of protected mice which had resisted challenge with SMC virus failed to transmit protection to their offspring [CLARK and KARZON, 1968b].

The Visna, Maedi Group

Visna and maedi, two slow virus diseases of sheep, were both cited by SIGURDSSON [1954] as prime examples in his original description of slow virus disease. They are concluded to be due to different pathogenic responses to the same agent and will be considered together. In visna the effects are neurological, while in maedi the lung is the target organ. Visna is usually insidious in onset, with an abnormality of gait presenting as the first sign [THORMAR and PÁLSSON, 1967]. This progresses to paraplegia, particularly of the hind legs, culminating in total hindquarter paralysis and sometimes in paralysis of all limbs of the affected sheep. Animals retain full consciousness, occasionally developing blindness, and can live for a considerable time if cared for. There are few other signs of disease, and the temperature is normal or very slightly increased. The duration between first signs and complete paralysis varies from several months to several years. Remissions are rare and the disease is invariably fatal [SIGURDSSON *et al.*, 1957; SIGURDSSON and PÁLSSON, 1958].

Maedi [SIGURDSSON *et al.*, 1952; SIGURDSSON, 1954a] is also insidious in its onset, loss of condition usually being the first sign. The sheep become dyspneic after any exertion and the condition progresses to death in 3 to 8 months. Remissions or recoveries do not appear to occur. Maedi virus can also cause the neurological lesions found in visna [GUDNADÓTTIR and PÁLSSON, 1967]; the two diseases have been reviewed by THORMAR [1966b] and by GUDNADÓTTIR *et al.* [1968].

Properties of Visna Virus

Visna was initially found to be a transmissible disease [SIGURDSSON *et al.*, 1953, 1957; SIGURDSSON and PÁLSSON, 1958] with an incubation period of 1–2 years. It can be induced by intrapulmonary inoculation as well as by the IC route [GUDNADÓTTIR and PÁLSSON, 1965]. The chemical and physical properties of visna and maedi viruses were found by THORMAR [1960, 1965a, b] to be almost identical. Both were sensitive to ether, chloroform, metaperiodate and trypsin, with similar rates of inactivation by 0.04 % formaldehyde, UV light, heat (57° C for 28 min) and pH. However, at pH 4.2 maedi virus was inactivated 3 times more rapidly than visna virus. Propagation and CPE of both viruses was inhibited by 5-bromodeoxyuridine. Neither virus showed hemagglutination nor hemadsorption. Electron microscopy showed them to be spherical particles averaging 85 nm in diameter and having a dense core; they seemed to be formed by budding of the external cell membranes [THORMAR 1961, 1967]. Negative staining showed a myxovirus-like structure [THORMAR and CRUICKSHANK, 1965]. Fluorescent antibody technics showed that viral antigen was produced in the cytoplasm and later became concentrated at the cell surface [THORMAR, 1969]. Both are RNA viruses as judged by acridine orange staining [THORMAR, 1966c]; antimetabolite experiments indicate a DNA-dependent RNA virus [THORMAR,

1965c]. In this respect the virus is similar to Rous sarcoma virus [TE-MIN, 1963, 1964; BADER, 1964, 1965]. Both visna and maedi are relatively resistant to UV radiation [THORMAR, 1965a], being 10 times more resistant than Newcastle disease virus, herpes and polioviruses. This again is similar to Rous sarcoma virus [RUBIN and TEMIN, 1959]. THORMAR and PÁLSSON [1967] suggested that visna virus may be related to the avian leukosis viruses. However, cross-neutralization tests do not show any relationship [THORMAR, 1966a]. Visna virus was found by THORMAR and PETERSEN [1964] to be relatively sensitive to photodynamic inactivation, and was comparable in this respect to vaccinia virus. It can be cultivated *in vitro* in sheep [SIGURDSSON *et al.*, 1960; THORMAR, 1963b; HARTER *et al.*, 1967], human [THORMAR and SIGURDARDÓTTIR, 1962], porcine and bovine tissue cultures [HARTER *et al.*, 1968], usually causing complete cell destruction [THORMAR, 1966a] but sometimes only destroying a proportion of cells [SIGURDSSON *et al.*, 1960]. A plaque assay is available [HARTER and CHOPPIN, 1967a]. Specific immunofluorescence showed the viral antigen to appear in the perinuclear area of infected cells [HARTER *et al.*, 1967] with the formation of polykaryocytes; these may be formed even with cells in which visna virus does not replicate [HARTER and CHOPPIN, 1967b]. Similar transmission [SIGURDSSON *et al.*, 1953] and tissue culture growth [SIGURDARDÓTTIR and THORMAR, 1964] have been reported for maedi virus. The detailed behavior of visna and maedi in tissue culture has been reviewed by THORMAR [1966a]. Although causing a slow disease, the virus has a latent period of only 22–30 h *in vitro* with large inocula, though with smaller ones CPE may take 14 to 20 days. Virus particles are formed by budding and have never been observed inside cells [THORMAR and CRUICKSHANK, 1965]. After 35 tissue culture passages, visna virus did not seem to gain access into the CNS of any sheep inoculated intrapulmonarily with the virus [THORMAR and PÁLSSON, 1967], although neutralizing antibodies appeared 3 to 12 months after inoculation and virus could also be isolated from the sheep.

Immune Response

Neutralizing antibody for visna virus can be detected by tissue culture assay [THORMAR, 1963a] and occurs in high titer (up to 1/2048) in visna-infected sheep at the same time that virus can be recovered from the blood, where it is apparently attached to leukocytes [GUDNADÓTTIR and Pálsson, 1966]. In maedi, a prolonged leukocytosis precedes the onset of disease [Sigurdsson *et al.*, 1953]. Antibody is detectable 2 to 3 months after experimental infection and remains at high levels for several years [Gudnadóttir, 1965, 1966; Gudnadóttir and Pálsson, 1965, 1966, 1967; Gudnadóttir and Kristinsdóttir, 1967]; neutralizing antibody is also found in sheep flocks naturally affected with maedi [Sigurdardóttir and Thormar, 1964; Gudnadóttir, 1965, 1966; Thormar *et al.*, 1966; Gudnadóttir *et al.*, 1968]. Comparative cross neutralization tests between visna and maedi showed partial cross-reaction between the two with considerable quantitative variation from one strain to another [Thormar and Helgadóttir, 1965]. A rise in titer of CF antibody occurs during the first few weeks after experimental infection with visna and maedi viruses, but neutralizing antibody could not be found for 2 months after inoculation [Gudnadóttir and Kristinsdóttir, 1967]. In some cases of maedi, no neutralizing antibody could be found. This aspect of maedi appears to bear some resemblance to the HDIP state in LCM infection of mice.

Pathogenesis

The pathological lesions of visna [Sigurdsson and Pálsson, 1958; Sigurdsson *et al.*, 1962] have received more study than those of maedi [Thormar and Pálsson, 1967], due to their apparent significance for the pathogenesis of the human demyelinating diseases. The lesions are in the brain and spinal cord and in most cases are detectable only by microscopic examination. There is infiltration and proliferation of reticuloendothelial cells with perivascular infiltration of lymphocytes predominating. Widespread demyelination occurs around the ventricles as well as in the white fibers of the spinal cord [Sigurdsson *et al.*, 1957; Sigurdsson and Pálsson, 1958; Pette *et al.*, 1961; Sigurdsson *et al.*, 1962]. In maedi, pathological changes are confined to the thoracic cavity; the weight of lungs and tracheobronchial lymph nodes increases up to four times the normal value and the lungs are uniformly thickened. The changes are due to extreme proliferation of mesenchymal cells with thickening of the alveolar septa. Ultimately, the lungs lose their characteristic histological structure and consist mainly of mesenchymal tissues with the air spaces reduced to small openings in the otherwise solid tissue [Sigurdsson *et al.*, 1952; Sigurdsson, 1954a]. During the very long preclinical period of visna, the only indication of infection is a marked cerebrospinal pleocytosis [THORMAR and PÁLSSON, 1967] which appears one to two months after inoculation, and persists during the preclinical and clinical phases of the disease in both natural and experimental visna. Some animals develop progressive paralysis [SIGURDSSON *et al.*, 1957] 1 to 2 years after inoculation; others recover without showing any signs of disease. The recovery is more common in those animals showing mild pleocytosis. GUDNADÓTTIR and PÁLSSON [1966] followed the development of disease in sheep inoculated IC with tissue culture-grown visna virus. In spite of a strong antibody response, virus was grown repeatedly from blood and CSF, but not from feces. Occasionally it was found in saliva or nasal secretion. Some sheep showed viremia between 2 months and 4 years after infection. Virus was present in most of the organs tested, including choroid plexus, spleen, mediastinal lymph node, lung, salivary gland, and rarely kidney. Blood virus appeared to be bound to the leukocytes. Lesions indistinguishable from both visna and maedi were found in 7 of 12 sheep, all of which developed neutralizing antibodies. Most of the tissues of visna-infected sheep were apparently healthy. In a series of experiments by SIGURDSSON *et al.* [1962] clinical disease and antibody titer were followed in visna-inoculated sheep for 6 years. In several animals the onset of clinical disease coincided with the appearance of neutralizing antibody. GUDNADÓTTIR and PÁLSSON [1966] believed that the neurological lesion may involve a demyelinating process, which is caused by an antigen-antibody reaction on the surface of infected glial cells, with the neutralizing antibody present in the CSF causing the destructive process. HARTER and CHOPPIN [1967b] also have suggested that the mechanism of demyelination in visna may be due to a change in the cell membrane produced by the virus parallel to its ability to induce giant cell formation. They suggest that it may be significant that viruses which are associated with 'postinfection' encephalomyelitis in man, such as measles, mumps, varicella, smallpox and vaccinia, possess a common feature in the form of a lipid-containing envelope which is probably derived, at least in part, from the cell membrane.

Viruses Similar to Maedi or Visna

In 1957 SIGURDSSON [1958] described experimental transmission of infectious adenomatosis of sheep (Jaagsiekte) which, like other slow viruses, appeared to have been imported into Iceland by sheep brought from Germany in 1933 [DUNGAL *et al.*, 1938; SIGURDSSON, 1954a]. In this disease anatomical lesions are found in the lungs only, and consist of widespread epithelial proliferations which increase the weight of the lungs two- or three-fold. Cross-neutralization tests with sera from maedi-affected sheep were all negative [THORMAR, 1966a] but sera from Montana, Scottish and Bulgarian sheep affected with chronic progressive pneumonia [SIGURDSSON *et al.*, 1952; MARSH, 1958] neutralized maedi to a low titer and visna to a high titer [THORMAR, 1966a]. Sera from Dutch sheep affected with Zwoegerziekte [KOENS, 1943; BOS, 1951; RESSANG *et al.*, 1968] also neutralized maedi virus, some of them to a titer as high as 1/360. From these results it appears that maedi and visna viruses are similar to those causing progressive pneumonia of sheep and Zwoegerziekte while infectious adenomatosis of sheep is due to a separate entity. Occasionally Zwoegerziekte has been reported to cause CNS lesions similar to those of scrapie [RESSANG *et al.*, 1966]. The sheep diseases, La bouhite (France) [LUCAM, 1942] and Graft-Reinet (South Africa) [KOCK, 1929] are apparently also in the same class as maedi. KENNEDY *et al.* [1968] have pointed out that the Montana chronic pulmonary disease was transmitted in 1936 by CREECH and GOCHENOUR [1936] by inoculating sheep with a suspension of lung and mediastinal lymph nodes from infected Montana sheep. Successful transmission was also made by DURAN-REYNALS *et al.* [1958]. KENNEDY *et al.* [1968] described isolation of a virus having properties comparable to maedi, in tissue culture from Montana sheep affected with natural or experimental progressive pneumonia. They conclude that this virus is closely related to maedi. DE BOER (personal communication, 1968) noted that the indirect FAB technic showed antibodies in the maedi-like diseases at a much earlier phase than other technics, occurring about one month post-infection.

The Spongiform Encephalopathies

This group includes the agents of scrapie, encephalopathy of mink, rida and kuru. They appear to be closely related but their precise nature and interrelation is at present unclear.

Scrapie

Introduction and History

The clinical aspects of scrapie have been admirably described by
ZLOTNIK and STAMP [1961] and the disease has been the subject of several reviews [PLUMMER, 1946; PALMER, 1957, 1959b; STAMP, 1958,
1962, 1967; EKLUND *et al.*, 1963; HOURRIGAN, 1966; McDANIEL and
MOREHOUSE, 1966], none of which have been exhaustive. Since this
agent provides what is perhaps the most perfect example of persistent
infection, it is considered here in some detail. It should be emphasized
that as a virus scrapie is most exceptional and its precise nature, manner
of replication and pathogenic processes are almost completely unknown.
These facts, coupled with its apparent ability to replicate without containing nucleic acid, qualify the scrapie agent to be regarded at the present time as one of the most fascinating enigmas of microbiology.

Since the early part of the present century scrapie has possessed a remarkable capacity to induce controversy [McGOWAN, 1918], particularly concerning whether the disease is due to an infectious agent or not.
Contradictory and violently held views have been repeatedly expressed
from that time on. The earliest definite record of the occurrence of scrapie in sheep in England was in 1732, and by 1755 the disease had apparently become very prevalent [McGOWAN, 1918; STAMP, 1958]. Scrapie has been transmitted via pedigree sheep [STAMP, 1958] to various
parts of the world where it did not previously exist, including places as
remote as the Indo-Tibetan border in the Himalayan mountains [ZLOTNIK
and KATIYAR, 1961]. The disease has been known by at least 34 different names in different nationalities [PALMER, 1959b]. Some of the British terms are of interest since they include such expressive names as
Euky Pine, Goggles, Rickets, Trotters, Scratchie, Rubbers, Shaking,
Shrew Croft, Cuddie Trot and the Rubs, mainly derived from rubbing
and scratching which are salient clinical features of the disease [STAMP,
1967]. It is interesting to note that one name for scrapie was La tremblante [PLUMMER, 1946] which is very similar in meaning to the closely
related human disease called kuru, which means shivering in the local
Fore language.

As early as 1869 DAMMANN attempted without success to transmit
scrapie by inoculation. Similar failures were experienced by McFADYEAN
[1918a] and BERTRAND *et al.* [1937]. Many widely differing views have

been held on the origin of scrapie; McFADYEAN [1918a] believed that the disease was due to the multiplication of 'some parasite in the sheep's body' and in 1919 BIGOTEAU suggested that scrapie was due to infection with *Corynebacterium ovis*. This conclusion was based on post-mortem lesions and could not be proved experimentally. McGOWAN [1914] believed that sarcosporidia was a cause of scrapie. This theory was attacked in 1926 by several workers, including McFADYEAN [1918a, b]. STOCKMAN [1926] suggested that scrapie was not hereditary but rather a congenital infection. However, he was unable to prove this. In France in 1928, VERDIER, quoted by BERTRAND *et al.* [1937], thought that 'La tremblante' was due to a virus but that special soil was necessary to create 'hereditary' conditions needed for the virus to become infective. Ten years later came the brillant but unnoticed investigations of CUILLÉ and CHELLE [1936, 1938a, b, c, 1939a, b], who were able to transmit the disease and establish its infectious nature. These findings were confirmed by GREIG [1940a, b]. The first reported cases of scrapie in the United States occurred in 1947 [THORP *et al.*, 1952]. Since then scrapie has spread to many parts of the country. It was introduced into New Zealand in 1952 [BRASH, 1952].

Research on scrapie was greatly handicapped by the need to use sheep as the sole experimental animal. A major advance occurred when scrapie was transmitted to mice by CHANDLER [1963c]; this vastly increased the volume and accuracy of experimental work with this agent.

The Nature of Scrapie Virus

Filterability

The scrapie virus was found by WILSON *et al.* [1950] to pass a 410 nm gradacol membrane. EKLUND *et al.* [1963] found the size to be of the order of 50 nm by filtration studies, while HAIG and CLARKE [1965] reported a particle size of less than 40 nm. GIBBS and GAJDUSEK [1966] demonstrated filtration through 43 nm APD but not through 27 nm APD and suggested a particle size of 17–27 nm. A report was made by PATTISON and SANSOM [1964] that scrapie virus was dialyzable through visking cellophane tubing, with an average pore diameter of 2.4 nm. A portion of the activity was repeatedly found by goat inoculation tests on the outside of the membrane after some days of continuous dialysis. However, the conclusion that scrapie virus is dialyzable is very much weakened by several features of the experimental technic as admitted by the authors, e. g., that the radioactive-iodinated protein test of the dialysis membrane indicated a 2% leakage and 25% of the sacs were defective. In early experiments using sheep, titrations of the material were rarely if ever made, and concentration of the agent was estimated solely by the length of the incubation period. The experiments clearly suffered from the limitations imposed by the use of very small numbers of experimental animals and the lack of quantitative methods. Electrodialysis [PATTISON and JONES, 1967a] produced conflicting results with some evidence that scrapie virus had migrated through visking tubing with average pore diameter of 0.4 nm. In contrast, exhaustive simple dialysis and continuous counter-current dialysis of tissue suspension from scrapie cases by MOULD and DAWSON [1968] using mouse brain virus and mouse titration showed that no transmission of virus across the dialysis membrane had occurred; both visking tubing and collodion shells were used. MACKAY [1968] pointed out that when the technic of dialysis was modified, it reduced the chances of contamination. It is evident that when careful, quantitative methods are used scrapie virus does not pass through a dialysis membrane.

Stability to Physical and Chemical Agents

a) Heat

Early studies of the nature of scrapie virus indicated that it remained viable in the desiccated state at 0 to 4° C for at least 2 years. MACKAY *et al.* [1960] found that scrapie tissue which had been boiled for 30 min could still infect sheep by SC inoculation, but all activity was destroyed by autoclaving. Titrations were not performed. Using Seitz filtered material, EKLUND *et al.* [1963] found that the agent did not withstand a temperature of 99.5° C but did withstand 80° C for 30 min. The observation that scrapie virus was resistant to boiling was confirmed by GIBBS *et al.* [1966] and also by WILSON [1954] and HARTLEY [1967]. Heat inactivation was also studied by HUNTER and MILLSON [1964a], who used mouse titrations to show that progressive inactivation occurred above 75° C for 1 h, although some infectivity still remained after heating at 100° C for 1 h; the critical temperature for rapid heat inactivation appeared to be 87.5° C. ZLOTNIK and RENNIE [1967] reported that boiling scrapie virus caused both a loss in titer and also modified the behavior of the virus on subsequent mouse passage.

b) Formalin

Scrapie virus has remarkable stability to formalin. Initially it was found to retain activity in 35 % formalin for many months [GORDON, 1946; GREIG, 1950; STAMP *et al.*, 1959]. PATTISON [1965b] tested pieces of brain tissue, which had been in formalin of various strengths ranging from 0.25 to 20 % over a period of 18 to 28 months, by inoculation into goats or mice. None of the treatments entirely removed the scrapie activity, although there was some evidence, based on the length of the incubation period of the disease, that increasing time of exposure and strength of formalin caused progressive loss. The agent withstood 20 % formalin for 18 h and 12 % for 28 months.

c) Lipid Solvents

DARCEL *et al.* [1963] found that scrapie virus survived extraction for 18 h with diethyl ether, or Soxhlet extraction for 24 h with 95 % ethanol containing 2.0% of 4M HCl. The mouse strain was found by HUNTER and MILLSON [1964b] to be inactivated by acetone and ether. Its sensitivity to lipid solvents was confirmed by EKLUND *et al.* [1963] and MOULD *et al.* [1965a]. Ultrasonic treatment had a similar inactivating effect to that of ether [MACKENZIE *et al.*, 1968a].

d) Ionizing and UV Radiation

An experiment of crucial importance was carried out by ALPER *et al.* [1966], who investigated the radiation sensitivity of the scrapie agent in the dry state. Significant inactivation by ionizing radiation was only obtained by extremely high doses. The Do value proved to be 4.3 Mrads, which indicated a molecular weight of 15×10^4 and a target size of about 7 nm. Equivalent values for other comparable agents are shown in table VIII from ALPER *et al.* [1966]. In similar experiments utilizing ultraviolet light at 2,537 Å there was no significant loss in activity of the scrapie agent up to doses of 2.4×10^4 erg/mm², a level more than 10 times that which reduced bacteriophage T3 to 1 % of its previous activity. The presence or absence of oxygen during UV radiation was found [ALPER and HAIG, 1968] to have less effect on scrapie virus than other viruses tested in the dry state. The authors concluded that if the radiation target were a nucleic acid, its molecular weight was unlikely to be greater than about 2×10^5, which would be equivalent to approximately 800 bases; this is equivalent to an implausibly small piece of nucleic acid coded information. Further experiments on the effect of UV light on scrapie by

Table VIII. Comparative estimates of the target size of scrapie virus and other agents, derived from their radiation sensitivity[1]

Material	Do megarads	Ref.	Target size (LEA, 1946) molec. wt. $\times 10^{-4}$	Independent estimate molec. wt. $\times 10^{-4}$	Ref.
Ribonuclease	22	1	3	1.27	6
Lysozyme	33	2	1.8	1.7	6
Trypsin	25	2	2.5	2.38	6
Deoxyribonuclease	{ 17	2	3.9		
	7.8	3	8	6.3	6
Scrapie virus	4.3		15		
Marker, transforming principle	{ 1.6		45		
	2.7	4	29		
Bacteriophage R17 (RNA phage)	0.78	5	92	100	7
Bacteriophage ΦX 174 (free DNA irradiated)	0.34	5	220	170	8
Bacteriophage T3	0.08		*diameter* 28 nm	*diameter* head 47 nm DNA 34 nm	9

[1] From ALPER *et al.* [1966].

References

1. HUNT, TILL and WILLIAMS [1962].
2. BRUSTAD [1961].
3. OKADA and FLETCHER [1960].
4. TANOOKA and HUTCHINSON [1965].
5. GINOZA [1963].
6. DIXON and WEBB [1964].
7. ZINDER [1965].
8. SINSHEIMER [1959].
9. ADAMS [1959].

ALPER *et al.* [1967] and HAIG *et al.* [1969] strengthened their previous conclusion that scrapie virus is most unlikely to depend upon a nucleic acid moiety for its replicative ability (fig. 26). These data did not give conclusive evidence on whether or not the agent might be associated with a protein. After irradiation, scrapie virus was assayed by 10-fold serial dilutions, each of which was inoculated IC into 7 or 8 mice. The authors believed that if free exposed nucleic acid were at risk within the organism it was most unlikely that the doses they used would have failed to affect the agent. Other systems which were included in the tests are

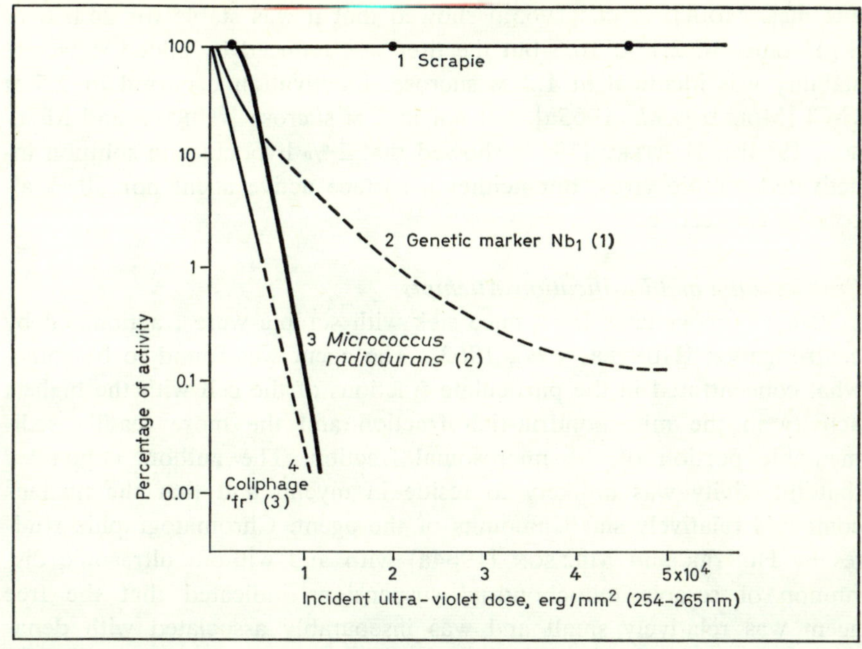

Fig. 26. Effects of ultra-violet light in the range 254–265 nm on some test systems. (1) Scrapie virus (●). (2) Effect of extracellular irradiation of transforming DNA, *H. influenzae,* on genetic marker for resistence to novobiocin, after repair by recipient cell. The dashed line is an extrapolation of data according to the exponential dose law (1). (3). Survival curve, *M. radiodurans,* which has effective intracellular repair mechanisms (2). (4) Inactivation of single-stranded RNA coliphage 'fr'. The dashed line is an extrapolation of Winkler's data (3) according to the exponential dose law. (1) PATRICK and RUPERT [1967]; (2) SETLOW and DUGGAN [1964]; (3) WINKLER [1964]. Reproduced from ALPER *et al.,* 1967, by permission of the editor and authors.

known to be highly resistant to UV light and to have very efficient intracellular repair mechanisms, but these still showed considerable inactivation when exposed to the high doses which did not affect scrapie. At the present time, the available evidence indicates that scrapie is caused by a replicating virus in which the nucleic acid is present in very small amount or in a highly stabilized state.

e) Chemical Agents and pH

The scrapie virus was reported by HAIG and CLARKE [1965] to be resistant to a wide range of pH levels and to be unaffected by proteolytic enzymes. MOULD *et al.* [1965a] showed that it was stable for 24 h over a pH range of 2.1 to 10.5 but the titer was reduced by added salts. pH stability was identical in 1.2 M sucrose. Inactivation occurred in 2.5 M CsCl [MOULD *et al.*, 1965a], but not in 2 M sucrose [HUNTER and MILLSON, 1964b]. HARTLEY [1967] showed that 2 % hypochlorite solution inactivated scrapie virus, but neither a surface active agent nor 50 % alcohol was effective.

Fractionation and Purification Attempts

Brain homogenates from mice sick with scrapie were fractionated by centrifugation [HUNTER *et al.*, 1963]. The agent was found to be somewhat concentrated in the particulate fractions of the cell with the highest activity in the mitochondria-rich fraction and the more readily sedimentable portion of the microsomal fraction. The authors concluded that infectivity was unlikely to reside in myelin and that the nucleus contained relatively small amounts of the agent. Chromatographic studies by HUNTER and MILLSON [1964a] with and without ultrasonic disruption of scrapie mitochondrial suspensions indicated that the free agent was relatively small and was inseparably associated with denatured proteinaceous material. Differential centrifugation and sucrose density gradients were used [HUNTER *et al.*, 1964] to fractionate homogenates of scrapie-infected mouse brain tissue. Most of the infectivity was associated with heavy particulate fractions containing mitochondria and possibly lysosomes. However, only the 'top layer' of soluble material gave significantly different results from the other layers, all of which had very similar titers. MOULD *et al.* [1965b] concluded that no particular cellular fraction of the brain appears to be involved in the replication of the virus, which was associated with tissue debris in all density gradient fractions. Only slight success was obtained in purification attempts using calcium phosphate columns [MOULD *et al.*, 1964] or fluorocarbon, detergent and salt solutions [HUNTER, 1965; HUNTER and MILLSON, 1967]. Treatment with fluorocarbon increased the sensitivity to papain [HUNTER *et al.*, 1967b] and scrapie was destroyed at room temperature by 6 M urea, 50% phenol, 6 M LiCl and 0.01 M periodate at pH 4 [HUNTER *et al.*, 1967b] but not by DNase or RNase [HUNTER and MILLSON, 1967]. Slight loss of titer was caused by 0.5 % Beta propiolactone [GIBBONS and HUNTER, 1967a]. PATTISON and JONES [1967a] applied the technics used to purify the encephalitogenic factor (EF) of allergic encephalomyelitis to scrapie-infected brain, but most of the scrapie activity was lost during the procedure and material discarded at every step showed high infectivity. The stability of scrapie virus to chemical and physical agents as summarized by GIBBONS and HUNTER [1967a] is shown in table IX.

Table IX. Stability of scrapie virus[1]

Treatment	Significant titer loss	Reference
Ionizing radiation	–	1
UV	–	1
100° C for 60 min	+	2, 3
80° C for 60 min	–	2, 3
Fluorocarbon at 4° C	–	4
80° C for 20 min after fluorocarbon	+	
Ether at room temperature	+	5, 6, 7
pH 2.5–10.5	–	6, 8, 9
Strong acid or alkali	+	6, 8, 9
Formalin 18%	–	10, 11
Beta-propionolactone 1%	–	9
0.01 M periodate at pH 4 and room temperature	+	
6–8 M urea	+	3
90% phenol	+	3
6 M salt solutions	+	4, 8
Detergents	–	2, 4
Proteolytic enzymes	–	4, 6
Proteolytic enzymes after fluorocarbon	+	4, 6
DNase, RNase, lipase, phospholipase *a* and *c*, neuraminidase, Beta-glucuronidase	–	4, 3

[1] Modified from GIBBONS and HUNTER [1967a].

References

1. ALPER *et al.* [1966, 1967].
2. HUNTER and MILLSON [1964a].
3. MOULD [referred to in GIBBONS and HUNTER, 1967a].
4. HUNTER and MILLSON [1967].
5. HUNTER and MILLSON [1964b].
6. HAIG and CLARKE [1965].
7. EKLUND *et al.* [1963].
8. MOULD *et al.* [1965a].
9. HAIG and CLARKE [referred to in GIBBONS and HUNTER, 1967a].
10. PATTISON [1965b].
11. GORDON [1946].

Electron Microscopy

Extensive electron microscopical examination of crude tissue homogenates, centrifuged deposits and chromatographic fractions for evidence of a scrapie virus have been consistently negative [MOULD *et al.*, 1965b].

Hypothesis on the Nature of the Scrapie Agent

Recent studies on the nature of the scrapie agent have mainly adhered to an orthodox virus concept as proposed by EKLUND *et al.* [1963]. Nevertheless its unusual chemical stability, radiation resistance and other properties have stimulated intense speculation that it may be a radically different entity from all familiar life forms. HUNTER and MILLSON [1964a] concluded that scrapie could be a small arbovirus with unusual surface properties. HUNTER [1965] suggested that the agent was in the 20 to 40 nm size range with a double-stranded nucleic acid component, probably DNA, and GIBBONS and HUNTER [1967a, b] also suggested that scrapie may result from an alteration in the basic three-dimensional configuration of a commonly occurring membrane structure. They pointed out that double-stranded nucleic acid molecules react very slowly with formaldehyde and that polyoma virus is relatively resistant to this chemical. In their view scrapie virus could have a formalin-resistant outer surface, similar to some protein and many carbohydrate molecules. HUNTER *et al.* [1967b] suggested that carbohydrate was probably a component of the scrapie structure. ADAMS and CASPARY [1967] proposed that scrapie consists of a small nucleic acid core enclosed in a mucopolysaccharide or even a polysaccharide coat which would stabilize the nucleic acid by covalent bonding with the sugar residues in the coat. A model of this type would be very stable and probably non-antigenic. ADAMS and CASPARY [1967] suggested that enough coded information could be carried by a small nucleic acid core for the small amount of protein which may be present in the coat structure. GAJDUSEK [1967b] concluded that scrapie may prove to be a small (6–7 nm) nucleic acid moiety enclosed by a stable protein capsid of small diameter (15–20 nm), and might also belong to the group of defective viruses. ALPERS *et al.* [1967] leaned towards a polysaccharide structure. PATTISON and JONES [1967a] concluded that the agent may be a small basic protein, possibly analogous to the encephalitogenic factor of experimental allergic encephalomyelitis. GRIFFITH [1967] concluded that mathematical models of protein replication are compatible with scrapie as a protein that replicates by inducing a gene which codes the normally re-pressed scrapie agent. BOSQUANET *et al.* [1956], PARRY [1957, 1960, 1962] and DRAPER and PARRY [1962] have taken refuge in semantic mysticism by doggedly maintaining that scrapie is caused by a 'genetical-ly determined provirus, which is artificially transmissible'. Their views appear to apply more appropriately to the transmission of susceptibility to scrapie, rather than its causal agent. In terms of the possibility that scrapie could be largely an oligosaccharide or glycoprotein, GIBBONS and HUNTER [1967a] point out that three carbohydrases have been reported to be present in scrapie brain, which lends support to the carbohydrate concept [MILLSON, 1965; FIELD, 1966; HUNTER *et al.*, 1967a; GIBBONS and HUNTER, 1967b]. Other highly speculative and untested concepts have been proposed such as those of ADAMS and FIELD [1968].

Review of the hypotheses on the molecular nature of scrapie virus forces the impression that most of the obvious speculative concepts have been invoked to fill the hiatus of precise knowledge. PATTISON [1967] has justifiably claimed that speculation on the nature of the scrapie agent has far outstripped precise experimental data. It must be remem-bered that, whatever the composition of scrapie should turn out to be, its genetic qualities must include both replicability and variation of host range and clinical disease type. For the present it seems reasonable to conclude that scrapie virus could still be a very small 'ordinary' virus possessing an unusually small, highly stabilized nucleic acid genome and a poorly antigenic capsid.

The Genetic Concept of Scrapie

In spite of the many observations showing that scrapie is a transmis-sible disease due to an infectious agent, the genetic view of its origin as stated by DRAPER as recently as 1963 has persisted with remarkable ob-stinacy. STAMP [1958] expressed the opinion that the genetic hypothesis of the origin of scrapie was based on the reports initiated by MCGOWAN [1918] and developed by BOSANQUET *et al.* [1956] that muscle damage constituted the primary lesion of scrapie, coupled to a loose analogy (cautiously evaluated by WALTON [1956]) with human muscular dystro-phy. PARRY [1960, 1962, 1966] has defended the genetic view and on epidemiological evidence states that scrapie is due to a single autoso-mal recessive gene; PARRY [1962] also states 'the genetic disease is arti-ficially infectious by inoculation'. These mutually contradictory concepts appear to arise from confusing the cause of the disease with the genetic control of host susceptibility to it. DICKINSON *et al.* [1966c, 1968a, b] have provided evidence for the genetic control of susceptibility of sheep and mice to scrapie.

Growth in Tissue Culture

Scrapie virus appears to be maintained and produced in an infective form for many months in tissue cultures from organs of scrapie-infected animals [GUSTAFSON and KANITZ, 1965a; BROTHERSTON *et al.*, 1966; STAMP, 1967], but culture of the agent in normal tissue *in vitro* has not yet been definitely established. Cell cultures of the thalamus and mid-brains of scrapie-infected sheep were found by GUSTAFSON and KANITZ [1965a] to retain their ability to induce scrapie in mice for 30 months. BROTHERSTON *et al.* [1965, 1966] failed to cultivate the virus in tissue culture, although it survived for 16 days in spleen cultures from infected mice, and for 48 days in cultures of normal mouse tissue inoculated with infected mouse brain. After $10^{1}/_{2}$ months, these cultures failed to produce scrapie in mice; no CPE was observed. HAIG and CLARKE [1965] reported doubtful survival of scrapie in mouse embryo cells after 5 to 7 passages and since then have reported more definite *in vitro* multiplication [CLARKE and HAIG, 1970]. In 1966 GORDON reviewed the progress in tissue culture of scrapie virus and found no definite reports of tissue culture passage of the agent. GUSTAFSON and KANITZ [1966] reported that after 34 subcultures lasting some 30 months, scrapie-affected sheep cells had a different appearance and characteristics than similar subcultures of normal sheep cells. Mice developed scrapie when inoculated with media from the scrapie culture harvested 3 and 5 weeks after initiation, and stored 9 months prior to use. Similar results were obtained with scrapie mouse brain cultures [GUSTAFSON and KANITZ, 1965b]. Explants obtained from scrapie mice were found by FIELD and WINDSOR [1965] and HAIG and PATTERSON [1967] to grow more rapidly than similar explants from normal mice.

The Transmission of Scrapie

Strain Differences

Different strains of scrapie cause characteristic clinical and pathological features in goats, mice [PATTISON and MILLSON, 1961a; ZLOTNIK and RENNIE, 1963] and sheep [PATTISON, 1966]. Major strains in goats are termed 'drowsy' and 'scratching' according to the clinical signs [PATTISON, 1966]. Strain differences involving the length of incubation period in mice have been described by DICKINSON and MEIKLE [1969] and DICKINSON and FRASER [1969b].

Transmission in Sheep

In 1938 CUILLÉ and CHELLE [1936, 1938a, b, c, 1939a, b] were the first workers to transmit scrapie by IC, intraocular, SC and intradermal inoculation of sheep with infected spinal cord. Though unable to infect rabbits, CUILLÉ and CHELLE [1939b] succeeded in reproducing the disease in goats as well as sheep. They showed by filtration through a Chamberland L-filter that the agent was a filterable virus with an incubation period of 5 months to several years. The incubation period was shorter after IC than after peripheral inoculation. This brilliant work was ignored for many years. The results of CUILLÉ and CHELLE were accidentally confirmed [GORDON *et al.*, 1940; GORDON, 1946, 1957; GREIG, 1950] as a result of an outbreak of scrapie following inoculation of sheep with a scrapie-contaminated 'louping-ill' vaccine. The transmissibility was not confirmed experimentally until 1950 by WILSON *et al.*, using inocula filtered through a 0.41 μ gradacol membrane, and in 1959 by STAMP *et al.*, who showed that the agent could be transmitted from brains, spleen, lymph gland or CSF of scrapie-infected sheep but not from their offspring. STAMP *et al.* [1959] found that the scrapie agent could be recovered from the brains of naturally-infected animals but not from offspring of such sheep nor from the brains of normal sheep. In their hands, scrapie was not transmitted by ingestion. PALMER [1959a] was unable to transmit the disease using semen from an affected ram. In 1961 CHANDLER [1961, 1963a] transmitted the disease to mice, thereby initiating quantitative research with scrapie virus.

As a result of field observations and experiments, GREIG [1940a] concluded that scrapie was transmitted by the environment of the pasture itself. STOCKMAN [1913] and McFADYEAN [1918a] presented circumstantial evidence that scrapie could spread among sheep at pasture without mating between infected and noninfected sheep. CHELLE [1942] found that scrapie was apparently transmitted to a goat which had been in contact with scrapie-infected sheep. SIGURDSSON [1954] noticed that rida appeared in a group of sheep placed on farms where it had previously existed but from which the original sheep had been cleared. In an experiment by PATTISON [1964] scrapie did not occur in any of 17 sheep held indoors for 55 months in direct physical contact with a succession of sheep and goats infected with experimental scrapie. Neither did the disease occur in 192 goats maintained in the scrapie environment for up to 60 months.

GORDON [1966b] reviewed the possibility that scrapie could be spread from affected to susceptible sheep and concluded that it could, but only in animals at pasture. Field observations are complicated by the fact that sheep, unlike other sensitive species, exhibit marked variation in susceptibility to scrapie [GORDON, 1966a]. BROTHERSTON *et al.* [1968] demonstrated the transmission of natural scrapie from sheep to goats but not to sheep, although sheep-to-sheep contact transmission occurred during a 5-year period with natural scrapie. The use of IC inoculation in the experimental disease may explain the failure to induce contact infection, since EKLUND and HADLOW [1963] and EKLUND *et al.* [1965, 1966, 1967] demonstrated less peripheral spread of virus after IC than after peripheral inoculation. FITZSIMMONS and PATTISON [1968] failed to transmit scrapie by nematode parasites from infected animals. DICKINSON *et al.* [1966b, e] gathered some evidence that scrapie may be transmitted maternally to the offspring in sheep but not in goats.

Host Range

In 1874 BÉNION reported the occurrence of scrapie in goats, and in 1939 CUILLÉ and CHELLE [1939b] demonstrated this by inoculation. The susceptibility of goats [PATTISON *et al.*, 1959; MACKAY and SMITH, 1961; PATTISON and MILLSON, 1960, 1961b, 1961c, 1962; PATTISON, 1965a; ZLOTNIK and RENNIE, 1965], hamsters [ZLOTNIK and RENNIE, 1965; ZLOTNIK, 1966b], rats [ZLOTNIK and RENNIE, 1965] and mice [CHANDLER, 1961, 1962, 1963b; ZLOTNIK and RENNIE, 1962, 1963; MORRIS and GAJDUSEK, 1963; GIBBS *et al.*, 1966; ZLOTNIK, 1966b], but not monkeys [DICK *et al.*, 1965] has more recently been amply confirmed. The first transmission to mice by CHANDLER [1961] was an extremely important advance for the experimental study of scrapie, with reduction of the incubation period to between 20 and 40 weeks [MORRIS and GAJDUSEK, 1963; DICKINSON and MACKAY, 1964]. Only the drowsy type of goat-passed scrapie (not the scratchy type) initially caused disease. Scrapie was readily transmitted from mouse to mouse by inoculation [CHANDLER, 1962]. Signs in mice were described by MORRIS and GAJDUSEK [1963]. They began with hyperexcitability, rapid jerky movements and increased speed in normal activities, particularly grooming. The animals tended to run, jump and execute circular movements changing irregularly from clockwise to counterclockwise direction. Vibration or touch stimulation resulted in excessive response in the affected mice. There was some indication of behavior similar to that of infected sheep, attributable to itching. Excoriation of the ears, lumbosacral regions and snout occurred, with frequent loss of hair, scabbing and ulceration. Hyperextension of the neck, waddling gait and tail stiffness were common, followed by emaciation and decreased hyperexcitability. Behavioral changes have been described [SAVAGE and FIELD, 1965], some occurring 10 weeks prior to obvious clinical signs [HEITZMAN and CORP, 1968]. Urinary and fecal incontinence and persistent priapism were often present. Histological examination revealed marked astrogliosis and moderately severe loss of neurones with some vacuolated neurones similar to the findings of scrapie in other animals.

Scrapie is not known to induce disease in primates [GAJDUSEK, 1967b] and high-titered mouse scrapie failed to cause disease in rhesus and cynomologus monkeys after an incubation period of 3 years.

Incubation Period

The incubation period of scrapie in sheep is reported by WILSON *et al.* [1950] as 4 to 36 months and also as 18 months to 5 years. Breeds of sheep vary widely in their susceptibility [EKLUND *et al.*, 1963]. Common breeds of dairy goats are more uniformly susceptible but the incubation period has been reported to be as long as 4 years and 11 months [PATTISON, 1965c]. In the mouse, this period shortens to about 7 to 12 months depending on virus and mouse strain. The incubation period in the mouse was found by DICKINSON and FRASER [1969a] to be inversely related to the early growth rate of virus in the spleen. PATTISON and SMITH [1963] reported a significant shortening of the incubation period of scrapie in goats by pre-treatment with goat brain. They believed that in some way this had sensitized the goat to scrapie.

Inoculation Routes

While most animal inoculation of scrapie virus has been made via the IC route, both oral and contact transmission in goats, mice and sheep have been described [GREIG, 1940a; PATTISON and MILLSON, 1961b; ZLOTNIK and RENNIE, 1963; DICKINSON *et al.*, 1964, 1966d; HUNTER, 1965; MORRIS *et al.*, 1965]. Unfiltered milk, saliva, urine or feces from infected animals did not cause the disease [PATTISON and MILLSON, 1961b].

Accidental Transmission of Scrapie

Scrapie infection has occurred in supposedly normal, uninoculated or normal-tissue inoculated animals sufficiently frequently [CHELLE, 1942;

PATTISON and MILLSON, 1960, 1961c; MACKAY and SMITH, 1961; DARCEL et al., 1963; PATTISON, 1965a; PATTISON and JONES, 1968] to stimulate several workers to investigate the phenomenon. DICKINSON et al. [1966d] reported 2 cases of scrapie in mice which had not been inoculated but had apparently acquired scrapie by cannibalism of cage mates which had been inoculated with a mouse-adapted strain. PATTISON [1964] found that scrapie occurred in 15 of 49 mice held in direct physical contact with successive batches of scrapie-inoculated mice. He concluded that scrapie spread from mouse to mouse by ingestion of tissue fragments during periods of fighting between the animals. Similar contact transmission of scrapie was reported by DICKINSON et al. [1964] and ZLOTNIK [1968] who obtained scrapie infection of mice after injecting human biopsy material from a case of multiple sclerosis. However, the mice used were of the Moredun stock, developed in a scrapie laboratory, and the isolation was performed in a scrapie environment, lending some weight to the author's admission that multiple sclerosis isolation attempts should not be made in scrapie laboratories. Scrapie was shown by MORRIS et al. [1965] to be capable of natural transmission between control mice housed in different cages but in the same animal room as scrapie-infected animals. The disease occurred in only $3^1/_2$ % of control mice with incubation periods of 16 to 22 months after initial exposure. PATTISON and JONES [1968] and ZLOTNIK [1968] reported the occurrence of scrapie in mice inoculated with normal mouse brain, and a small proportion of cases in mice inoculated with normal tissue from sheep, goats or humans. Although the presence of a low grade infection in the Compton strain of mice could well explain the results obtained, the authors concluded that their work showed the presence of a scrapie agent in normal mice. In view of the known properties of scrapie, it seems likely that in a laboratory where scrapie work has been performed for many years, mouse colonies may well become infected with the virus, initially at a low level. MACKAY [1968] pointed out the case of recipients in which the injection of 'normal' material gave rise to scrapie. The incubation periods cited were shorter than those reported [PATTISON, 1964; PATTISON et al., 1964; DICKINSON et al., 1964; ZLOTNIK, 1968] for contact transmission between mice in the same cage and were also shorter than the period required for scrapie to spread between mice in separate cages in the same room [MORRIS et al., 1965]. This suggests that the affected 'normal' animals had already acquired scrapie virus prior to their injection, and had come from contaminated stock. It is clear that these results have important implications for experiments using mice to test for

scrapie-like agents in human or other tissue, such as those reported by
FIELD and RAINE [1966].

Titration

PATTISON and MILLSON [1961a] found an inverse relationship between
length of incubation period and titer of scrapie virus inocula. HUNTER and
MILLSON [1964b] found that titration results based on the length of the
incubation period after IC inoculation were comparable with results
based on serial dilution end points. Many workers used the incubation period method to avoid the need for large numbers of animals. However,
the significance of results based on this method is open to serious doubt
and certainly lacks the conviction of serial dilution end point titration. It
was pointed out by BUTLER and SMITH [1960] and MOULD and SMITH
[1962a, b] that early experiments were often marred by inadequate titration methods. DICKINSON and FRASER [1969] showed that the incubation
period of a given scrapie strain can be modified by physical treatment
such as heat. This clearly implies that the incubation period assay method
is unreliable, particularly for stability tests. In a study of the accuracy and
reproducibility of scrapie titrations in mice, MOULD *et al.* [1967a] concluded that with 10 mice/dilution, titers should differ by at least 0.8 log
10 units to be significant.

Pathology

The pathological histology of scrapie has been reviewed by ZLOTNIK
[1966a] and STAMP [1958] and has been extensively studied in sheep by
WIGHT [1960, 1961], ZLOTNIK [1958, 1962a] and others [BESNOIT and
MOREL, 1898; CASSIRER, 1898; BERTRAND *et al.*, 1937; BROWNLEE,
1940; HOLMAN and PATTISON, 1943] and in goats in a classical study by
HADLOW [1961] and also by ZLOTNIK [1961, 1962a, b]. The pathology of
scrapie-affected mice and rats has also been studied [ZLOTNIK and REN-
NIE, 1962; EKLUND *et al.*, 1967; PATTISON and JONES, 1967b; FRASER and
DICKINSON, 1968]. Up to 1956, scrapie was confused with what was regarded as a degeneration of skeletal muscle [ANONYMOUS, 1956]. The
crucial importance of the presence and number of vacuolated neurones,
first described by BESNOIT and MOREL [1898] was emphasized by
BROWNLEE [1940] and confirmed by HOLMAN and PATTISON [1943] and
later by ZLOTNIK [1957a, b, 1960] and ZLOTNIK and RENNIE [1957]. Sig-

nificant pathological findings are now regarded as being largely confined to the nervous system, which typically shows degeneration of nerve cells, prominent astrocytosis, and a spongy alteration of the neuroparenchyma [HADLOW, 1959a; EKLUND *et al.*, 1963]. MACKENZIE and WILSON [1966] examined the brains of control and scrapie mice and found significant accumulations of neutral fat in the gray matter. Electron microscopy of scrapie-infected rat brains by CHANDLER [1967a, b, 1968] showed an encephalopathy involving neurons, nerve fibers and astrocytes. The changes consisted of nonspecific degeneration that could be due to a variety of causes and resembled those reported by FIELD and RAINE [1964] and FIELD *et al.* [1967] in scrapie-affected animals. These workers described the apparent formation of dense bodies within degenerating mitochondria in the cytoplasm of sheep nerve cells affected with scrapie. Inside the dense bodies were seen filamentous structures showing a helical or stacked disc appearance, with a central rod-like core. The filaments were about 120 Å apart and the turns of the helix about 50 Å apart. Similar structures were seen in normal sheep neurone-dense bodies, but their frequency in scrapie was claimed to be much greater. Particles and rods were also seen by DAVID-FERREIRA *et al.* [1968] in electron micrographs of enlarged cell processes in scrapie-affected mouse cerebral cortex. However, the authors concluded that the particles did not represent the scrapie agent since similar particles were found in other diseases of animals and man. In the mouse, hypertrophy and proliferation of astrocytes is by far the most conspicuous microscopic change produced by the scrapie agent [EKLUND *et al.*, 1967]. The disease is characterized by the absence of both acute neuronal degeneration and inflammation, which usually typify acute virus diseases of the CNS. EKLUND *et al.* [1967] considered that the course of events in scrapie resembled that of a malignant neoplasm or chronic degenerative disease rather than an infectious process as customarily conceived. These authors pointed out that in scrapie high titers of virus are produced in the CNS without acute cellular destruction and that the long-continued presence of large amounts of virus in the CNS seems to be a prerequisite of clinical disease. They stressed that the cell types which support growth of scrapie in the CNS are unknown, but suggested that replication of virus in astrocytes may be the key feature, with resultant hypertrophy and proliferation of these cells and impairment of their function; this could lead to injury and death of nerve cells with which they are intimately associated metabolically.

A slow, progressive decrease in brain weight was noted by KIMBERLIN and MILLSON [1967] in scrapie-affected mice, which began 40 to 50 days after inoculation. Just before the first clinical signs of disease appeared, this process was greatly accelerated and was accompanied by a decrease in total body weight. There was no apparent change in cell numbers within the brain in spite of a 10 to 20 % decrease in physical size. The respiratory activity of brain homogenates from clinically-affected scrapie mice decreased in parallel with the reduced cell size but was not otherwise impaired. MOULD et al. [1967b] found good correlation between body weight of scrapie-affected animals and the degree of neuronal vacuolation and spongy degeneration. In affected brains, total dry matter, protein and sodium concentrations remained constant but there was a 5 % decrease in potassium concentration. A rise in acid proteinase activity appeared at the same time as minimal lesions, but reached a maximum before widespread lesions were present. FRASER and DICKINSON [1967] reported that lesions were the same in different mouse strains, but that spleen virus caused a different distribution of brain lesions from that of brain virus in mice. Efforts by MOULTON and PALMER [1959] to demonstrate the agent of scrapie in the brains of experimentally infected goats by the FAB method were unsuccessful.

Pathogenesis

Knowledge of the pathogenesis of scrapie in large animals is incomplete, but progress has recently occurred by using mice for scrapie virus titrations. PATTISON and MILLSON [1961a] showed that scrapie became widely distributed in the tissues of the goat prior to the onset of clinical illness and DICKINSON et al. [1966a] showed that peak titer occurred at 3.5 years of age in sheep. Scrapie virus has been isolated from sheep in the brain [WILSON et al., 1950], spleen and lymph nodes [STAMP et al., 1959]. In the goat it has been isolated from brain, pituitary gland, adrenal glands, spleen, pancreas, and liver [PATTISON and MILLSON, 1960]. Peak titers occurred in goat brain 17 weeks after inoculation. Neurohistological changes were noted at 25 weeks and clinical signs did not appear until about 34 weeks. Virus was irregularly present in cerebrospinal fluid, but was not detected in blood or urine [EKLUND et al., 1967]. FRASER [1969] has described the progressive development of nerve fiber degeneration in mice after scrapie inoculation and prior to the onset of clinical signs.

In the mouse, brain titers were found by HUNTER and MILLSON [1964b] to be higher than those of the spleen. This was confirmed by ZLOTNIK [1966b], who reported titers to be approximately 10^6 in the brain and 10^3 in gut or spleen homogenates. ZLOTNIK [in GARDINER and MARUCCI, 1969] is reported to have found maximum spleen titers by 3–4 weeks post-infection. The mechanism of localization of scrapie appeared to FIELD [1967] to be similar to that of poliomyelitis, since inoculation of mice in either the fore- or hindlimb caused the earliest reaction in the nervous system in the corresponding area of the same side of the spinal cord. EKLUND et al. [1963, 1967] provided an excellent quantitative study of the pathogenesis of scrapie virus in the mouse. These workers inoculated large numbers of mice SC with a 10^{-2} dilution of scrapie-infected mouse brain suspension containing $10^{5.7}$ mouse LD_{50} of the virus. Thereafter mice were sacrificed at intervals and titrations of their organs were made. The over-all results are shown in table X. It is noteworthy that the EKLUND study showed that scrapie multiplied extensively in the animal before invasion of the nervous system occurred. The earliest stage of invasion was in the spleen, where virus was detected one week after infection. This virus was concluded to be part of the initial inoculum, since 2 weeks later no virus was detected in any tissue. After 4 weeks virus reappeared in peripheral lymph nodes and spleen at a low titer which rapidly increased. Virus was detectable in the thymus 8 weeks after inoculation. At the same time, virus appeared in the submaxillary salivary gland and remained at high titer for 32 weeks and then began to decline. This decrease is important since it shows that some mechanism exists for diminution of virus titer in the infected host. The salivary gland growth of the virus may also provide a mechanism of contact infection via saliva. In the spinal cord virus appeared at low titer after 12 weeks and increased to a maximum, where it remained after 24 weeks. Virus appeared in the brain 12 weeks later than in the spinal cord. The authors concluded that virus replication in the CNS was slower than in lymphocytic tissue or submaxillary salivary gland. In other tissues, only intestine and bone marrow contained appreciable amounts of virus, and in kidney, liver and uterus virus titers were very low. No virus whatsoever was detectable in blood clot, serum or testes. Similar inability to detect scrapie in blood was reported by PATTISON et al. [1964], but GIBBS et al. [1965] found scrapie virus to be present in sheep serum; this was confirmed by GIBBONS and HUNTER [1967a] and by CLARKE and HAIG [1967] who found scrapie in the serum of mice and rats. RENWICK and

Table X. Temporal distribution of scrapie virus in Swiss mice inoculated subcutaneously with $10^{5.7}$ LD_{50} of virus[1]

Weeks after inoculation	1	4	8	12	16	20	24	28	29[2]	32	36	42
Percent of surviving mice sick with scrapie							6.8	26	40	60	63	25
Percent of total mice dead of scrapie								4.5	6.9	25	61	73
Tissues examined[3]												
Spleen	4.5[4]	3.5	5.6	5.6	6.2	6.2	5.5	5.5	5.7	5.6	5.2	5.5
Peripheral lymph nodes		3.4	5.6	4.7	4.7	5.2	4.5	4.8	5.4	5.5	5.6	4.6
Thymus			4.2	4.8	5.5	5.0	5.4	4.5	0.85[5]	5.2	5.6	4.5
Submaxillary salivary gland			5.8	5.5	6.5	5.2	6.2	6.0	6.4	5.6	3.4	2.5
Lung				3.5	3.4	3.2	3.2	2.4	2.5		2.2	3.8
Intestine				2.2	2.2	3.4	5.3	5.5	4.6	5.4	5.2	4.5
Spinal cord				1.4	5.6	4.5	6.6	6.5	7.4	7.4	6.7	6.6
Brain					4.4	3.2	5.7	6.3	6.7	6.5	7.2	7.4
Bone marrow (femur)							1.7	2.8	4.8	3.5	5.0	3.6
Uterus						+[6]			+		+	+
Liver	← Not examined →							+	+	+	+	+
Kidney	← Not examined →										+	+

[1] EKLUND *et al.* [1967].

[2] From the 29th week on, only sick mice were examined.

[3] Blood clot, serum, and testis were also examined but virus was never detected in them.

[4] Negative $\log_{10}$ of dilution of tissue suspension that contained 1 LD_{50}/0.03 ml when inoculated intracerebrally into mice. Blank spaces indicate virus was not detected in any dilution.

[5] Questionable whether thymus was removed.

[6] Virus was detected in 10^{-1} dilution only and not all mice were affected.

ZLOTNIK [1965] reported the isolation of scrapie in mice, from one apparently normal 18-week-old lamb born of a scrapie-affected mother. Although the mice used were of the Moredun strain, which were shown by FIELD [1966] to be possibly contaminated with scrapie, the fact that all 10 inoculated mice developed scrapie while 10 controls remained normal shows the isolation to be genuine. This provides evidence for the congenital transmission of scrapie virus from the mother.

Biochemistry of Scrapie-infected Tissue

Considerable effort has been expended on chemical investigations of scrapie-infected tissue. Although scrapie-induced changes have been reported, their significance remains unclear. Enzyme activity associated with scrapie infection of mouse brain was found by SLATER [1965b] to be unchanged with respect to succinic dehydrogenase, cytochrome oxidase and acid phosphatase, but MILLSON [1965] reported a 2–3-fold rise in the level of β-glucuronidase and deoxyribonuclease activity. The increased enzyme activities were detectable before the appearance of histologically identifiable lesions in the brains. No change in acid phosphatase could be found during the period of incubation of the disease, neither were there any detectable differences between normal and control mice in terms of β-glucuronidase levels in the spleen or liver. This was confirmed with implication of other lysosomal enzymes by HUNTER and MILLSON [1966]. CHANDLER and SMITH [1968] found the activity to be localized in small neuronal cells rich in dense bodies. This appeared to indicate that lysosomes were involved in the replicative mechanism of the scrapie agent. However, it was then found that many other lysosomal enzymes were not affected by scrapie infection. These included lipase, phospholipase a, arylsulphatase A and arylsulphatase B and also the cytoplasmic enzyme glucose-6-phosphate dehydrogenase. The authors concluded that enzymes responsible for the degradation of mucopolysaccharides were specifically activated in scrapie infection of mouse brain. Detailed histochemical study in the brains of scrapie-affected rats, sheep, and goats by MACKENZIE *et al.* [1968a] confirmed these biochemical investigations and showed that the abnormal enzyme activity was demonstrable at least as early as vacuolation and astrocytic reactions. HEITZMAN [1968] investigated the levels of uridine diphosphate glucose pyrophosphorylase and uridine diphosphate glucose-4'-epimerase, both of which increased significantly 18 weeks after scrapie infection. HEITZMAN suggested that the increase might result from the gross pathological changes in the brains. GAJDUSEK [1967b] has drawn attention to the possible relevance of the syndrome described by BIGNAMI and PALLADINI [1966] produced by the enzyme ouabain in rats. This condition arises as a result of an enzyme inhibition-induced pathology similar to the status spongiosus seen in human kuru, experimentally transmitted scrapie and naturally occurring mink encephalopathy. The normal effect of ouabain is to specifically inhibit the membrane ATPase system which controls brain cell membrane permeability to Na⁺ and K⁺ ions. GAJDUSEK postulated that a slow virus might progressively deplete the supply or interfere with the action of an enzyme and produce this type of pathological response.

Protein synthesis of brain tissue was reported by CASPARY and SEWELL [1968] to be increased by scrapie infection with the finding that uptake of labelled lysine into nuclear histones was greater in scrapie-affected animals but only after the onset of positive histology at 4 months. It was not determined whether this was a primary or secondary effect of the disease process. In contrast MILLSON and HUNTER [1968], using different methods, reported that protein synthesis was unaffected by scrapie infection. No differences in nitrogen metabolism due to scrapie could be detected by SLATER [1965a]. Water and sodium content were reported by FIELD et al. [1966] to be changed in mouse brain with advanced scrapie. Several of the studies on the pathogenic aspects of scrapie infection of the mouse have been performed during terminal stages of the disease and also in the absence of comparable data on other neurological virus diseases. The significance of such results is rendered somewhat obscure because of this. However MACKENZIE et al. [1968b] compared enzyme changes in mouse brains infected with scrapie or with other viral encephalitides including louping ill, yellow fever and herpes simplex. Similar qualitative changes were found, but the pattern of these varied with the different viruses and only scrapie caused alteration in β-glucuronidase and N-acetyl-β-D-glucosaminidase. Tissue sections of scrapie brain contained deposits of PAS positive material believed to contain glycolipids since it was only found in cryostat sections and disappeared from paraffin sections. Other chemical tests of scrapie-affected mice have failed to reveal significant change in esterified cholesterol in the CSF [MOULD and DAWSON, 1965] or in the general biochemistry of CSF, blood [MILLSON et al., 1960] or liver function [DARCEL et al., 1963]. No significant abnormalities were found by chromatographic analysis by KASTING and DARCEL [1963] of the brain or urine of scrapie-infected sheep. MOULD and SLATER [1966] have reviewed the biochemistry of scrapie tissue. KIMBERLIN and HUNTER [1965, 1967] studied the DNA metabolism of scrapie-affected mouse brain utilizing IC injections of thymidine and measuring its incorporation into DNA. They found that an enhanced synthesis of DNA was detectable in the later stages of development of scrapie in affected mice. The authors concluded that synthesis of DNA is not a primary feature of the reduplication of scrapie virus. No controls were used with other RNA or DNA viruses. KIMBERLIN [1968] found the RNA metabolism to be normal in mouse brain even in the late clinical stages of scrapie. Increased DNA synthesis in scrapie-infected brain was concluded by KIMBERLIN and ANGER [1968] to be due to increased activity in the nuclei of the sub-ependymal cells in the region of the lateral ventricle and glial cells. It appeared that both oligodendrocyte and astrocyte nuclei were carrying out DNA synthesis. WILCOX and NUSSBAUM [1968] found scrapie in mice caused a diminution of cells in metaphase in the spleen, compared with controls of the same age.

Some attempt has been made to implicate interferon in scrapie infection. In a study of experimental mixed infection with scrapie and Friend virus, CHANDLER [1965] found no significant interaction, although there were indications of a reduction in the extent of Friend virus tumor production in the scrapie-inoculated animals. GRESSER and PATTISON [1968] found that the administration of interferon to scrapie-infected mice had no effect upon the course of the disease.

Immunity

So far scrapie infection has defied analysis by immunological technics, since no antibody response to the agent has been detected [STAMP, 1967; GIBBS, 1967]. CHANDLER [1959] used 10 different serological procedures in an unsuccessful attempt to detect antibody in the sera of scrapie sheep and goats. GIBBS *et al.* [1965, 1966] failed to demonstrate antibody against the scrapie agent using neutralization, CF and direct and indirect FAB tests. Similar negative results have been obtained by other workers [GARDNER, 1965; CLARKE and HAIG, 1966; EKLUND *et al.*, 1967] using different sera from scrapie-affected animals hyperimmunized with the scrapie agent over a period as long as 5 months. However, it is necessary to bear in mind that the mechanism of genetic variation in susceptibility to scrapie is quite unknown, and at present an immune reaction in these animals has not been excluded. At present it would appear that the persistence of scrapie infection occurs less as a result of virus-induced tolerance than as the outcome of an infection with an agent which is non-antigenic. It is difficult to escape the impression that this unique occurrence is likely to be related to the other exceptional properties of the agent. GIBBS *et al.* [1966] attempted to determine whether scrapie could induce immunological tolerance, but no difference in incubation period nor disease was found when scrapie was injected shortly after birth or in adult animals. CLARKE [1968] has investigated the antibody response of mice to sheep red cells administered from 1 to 168 days after IP scrapie inoculation. The response was identical to that of control mice, indicating that scrapie had no detectable effect upon humoral antibody formation. Similar results were obtained by GARDINER and MARUCCI [1969] using sheep red cells, which induced the same immune response in scrapie-infected and normal mice; a diminution in immune response to bovine serum albumin was noted in both scrapie-infected mice and controls inoculated with normal mouse brain.

Rida

Rida appears to be a variant of scrapie, affecting Icelandic sheep. SIGURDSSON [1954b] described rida in one of his classical papers on slow virus disease. It caused a chronic encephalitis of sheep in which the main signs consisted of spastic movements, uncoordinated gait and tremors. In advanced stages the animals lost interest in food and water and progressed rapidly to emaciation and death. The incubation period appeared to be 8 to 18 months. Farmers believed the condition to be contagious. The limitation of the disease to northern Iceland, where it is enzootic in a few mountain valleys, bears a remarkable resemblance to the behavior of kuru in the Fore tribe of New Guinea. Anatomical lesions of rida in sheep were conspicuous in the hemispheres of the brain, particularly in the frontal lobes. Marked changes similar to those of scrapie were also found in the cerebellum, thalamus, mesencephalon, pons and medulla oblongata. Rida was transmitted artificially to healthy sheep by IC inoculation of extracts of diseased brains. The agent passed through a Berkefeld N2 bacterial filter and was concluded to be a filter-passing virus.

Encephalopathy of Mink

A disease of mink very similar to scrapie and believed to be due to a very similar virus strain [HADLOW and KARSTAD, 1968] has been named encephalopathy of mink by HARTSOUGH and BURGER [1965] and BURGER and HARTSOUGH [1966]. It has an incubation period of 7 months or more, and causes degenerative changes of the brain similar to those described in scrapie-infected sheep. Mink developed a typical disease syndrome after being injected by the intramuscular (IM) or alimentary route with brain suspensions from a natural case of mink encephalopathy [BURGER and HARTSOUGH, 1965]. After IM inoculation the incubation period was approximately 5 months, and after alimentary infection was 8 months. The agent in unfiltered brain suspension was resistant to boiling for 15 min, to 0.3 % formaldehyd for 12 h at 37° C and to diethyl ether. These properties resemble those of scrapie virus, and there was evidence that mink could transmit the disease by cannibalistic ingestion of flesh from diseased mink. Encephalopathy of mink has been transmitted by ZLOTNIK and BARLOW [1967] to the goat which developed a high-stepping gait, circling and apparent blindness. Its brain was found to have histological lesions similar to those found in scrapie.

Kuru

Kuru is a fascinating and important example of a persistent virus infection of man which is confined to one area of New Guinea. The disease has reached the attention of the rest of the world largely as a result of the work of GAJDUSEK and ZIGAS [1959], who showed it to be a slow disease of the nervous system largely confined to the cerebellum. In distribution, kuru is entirely confined to one small area in the Eastern Highlands of New Guinea, mainly in the Fore linguistic group, where it appears to have been present only for the past 60 years [GLASSE, 1962, 1963]. During this period its distribution has changed in a way which suggests that transmission is due to cannibalism which has been largely suppressed in recent years. Its confinement appears to show that the disease only occurs in the genetically susceptible population found in this area [BENNETT *et al.*, 1959; BENNETT, 1962a, b; GAJDUSEK, 1963; ALPERS, 1965; ALPERS and GAJDUSEK, 1965; MATHEWS, 1965]. The clinical signs are due to neuronal degeneration of the cerebellum and the pathology of kuru mainly consists of astrocytic proliferation and hypertrophy, and status spongiosus [FOWLER and ROBERTSON, 1959; GAJDUSEK and ZIGAS, 1959; KLATZO *et al.*, 1959; NEUMANN *et al.*, 1964; KAKULAS *et al.*, 1967]. Demyelination is a secondary phenomenon and signs of inflammation are absent. The disease appears to be a human counterpart of scrapie, and HADLOW's [1959b] original observation of this fact gave great stimulus to the investigation of the possible infectious nature of kuru. The name kuru derives from a local word meaning shivering; it is interesting that this name parallels the name rida, which means tremor [BECK and DANIEL, 1965], since rida is believed to be due to an Icelandic strain of scrapie. The similarity in the nomenclature represents one of the many strange features shared by these animal and human slow virus diseases. HADLOW [1959] compared kuru and scrapie and noted that the following characteristics are shared by them both: similar natural history and clinical manifestations, insidious onset, lack of febrile signs, relentless progression ending fatally within 3 to 6 months after onset, very rare remissions, ataxia, tremors, behavioral changes, and lack of significant abnormalities in the blood or CSF. Remarkably similar neuropathological changes include widespread neuronal degeneration, hyperchromia of the cell body, vacuolation of the cytoplasm, astrocytic gliosis and minimal degeneration of myelin. 'Soap-bubble' vacuoles in the cytoplasm, rarely seen in other conditions, are characteristic of both diseases. A remarkable breakthrough in the understanding of chronic human neurological disease occurred in 1966 when GAJDUSEK et al. [1966, 1967; GAJDUSEK, 1967a] demonstrated that kuru could be transmitted to chimpanzees by IC inoculation of brain from human patients. GAJDUSEK began the long-term study of kuru in 1962 and based it on the slow virus infection concept using scrapie as a model [GIBBS and GAJDUSEK, 1967]. The program has been described in detail [GAJDUSEK and GIBBS, 1964]. In chimpanzees the incubation period ranged from 18 to 30 months after IC inoculation with a single 0.2 ml dose of 10 %/o brain tissue suspension. Similar suspensions from 6 different kuru patients caused kuru in 7 of 8 animals [GAJDUSEK et al., 1966]. The chimpanzees suffered a progressive syndrome of fatal ataxia, incoordination, withdrawal and terminal inanition lasting from 3 to 9 months before the animals were killed in the late stages of the disease. The disease itself was essentially similar to kuru in man [KLATZO et al., 1959]; its neuropathology has been studied in detail by BECK et al. [1966]. The only difference was a significant increase in the extent and severity of status spongiosus, particularly in cerebral cortex. The disease could be transmitted serially to other chimpanzees [GAJDUSEK et al., 1967] with a reduction in the incubation period from about 24 months on first passage to about $11^1/_2$ months on second passage. This constituted the first successful example of the transmission of chronic human neurological disease to animals. Susceptibility was initially restricted to chimpanzees, although many other appropriate laboratory animals, including mice, were tested and found unresponsive. Kuru has been reported by FIELD

[1968] to be transmissible to mice, but, as in the case of a similar report that human multiple sclerosis was transmissible to mice [FIELD, 1966], these results could be due to contamination by scrapie virus of the mouse strain used.

Up to 1968, 7 cases of kuru had occurred in chimpanzees out of 8 inoculated with human kuru-infected brain, although at that time Koch's postulates had not all been fulfilled [GAJDUSEK, 1967b]. More recently kuru has been passed by GAJDUSEK *et al.* [1968] from the chimpanzees to two spider monkeys *(Ateles geoffreyi)* with the production of kuru after incubation periods of 23 and 26 months. It is unclear at the present time whether the spider monkey is fully susceptible to human kuru or whether partial adaptation to this species occurred by virtue of chimpanzee passage of the human agent. Although the spider monkey is a more convenient animal than the chimpanzee, at present this animal has the disadvantage of a longer incubation period.

In recent years there has been an impressive change in the distribution of kuru among the Fore with a significant fall in the incidence of the disease in children [GAJDUSEK and ALPERS, 1966]. The Fore are known to have been ardent cannibals and they commonly ate kuru victims, including their brains [GLASSE, 1963]. ALPERS [1968] pointed out that children may have become infected either from an *in utero* infection or by eating human flesh. He regarded it significant that women were the main eaters of dead relatives and originally the incidence of kuru was highest in women and children. HOTCHIN [1966] reviewed kuru as a persistent virus infection and suggested it might have arisen as a human pathogenic variant of scrapie imported into the country and possibly transmitted via the pigs which are housed with the female Fore.

As an explanation of how kuru arose in the Fore, GAJDUSEK [1967] has suggested that, rather than a particular genetic susceptibility building up in the kuru region, it is more satisfactory to envisage a widespread, latent virus with the sudden production of a neuropathogenic variant. In this hypothesis, cannibalism would explain the restriction of kuru to this particular ethnic group. MATHEWS *et al.* [1968] considered that kuru was spread in the Fore entirely by cannibalism with an ensuing incubation period of 4 to 20 years before disease occurred. They suggested that in the absence of cannibalism, kuru should disappear within the next few decades.

There is clearly a remarkable similarity between scrapie, encephalopathy of mink and kuru in man. The pathology of all these diseases is almost uniquely similar and the clinical disease is almost identical. The three diseases are very host-specific, with strong elements of genetically controlled susceptibility, and while the mode of transmission of scrapie in the natural state is entirely unknown, the transmission of encephalopathy of mink and kuru are both suspected to be associated with the cannibalistic habits of their hosts.

Multiple Sclerosis

Experimental work on inoculation of animals with human brain suspension from cases of multiple sclerosis (MS) have caused come workers to conclude that this condition may be related to scrapie in sheep in spite of the pathological differences between the two conditions. At present the significance of the observations is in doubt, since the scrapie agent is extremely stable and can readily contaminate an experiment performed in a laboratory where scrapie has been used. FIELD *et al.* [1962] and PÁLSSON *et al.* [1965] reported that Icelandic sheep inoculated IC with brain suspension from an acute human MS case developed a disease histologically indistinguishable from scrapie. FIELD [1966] has also tentatively reported the occurrence of scrapie in mice inoculated with biopsy material from a human case of multiple sclerosis. However, scrapie virus had been in use in the laboratory concerned and the mouse strain had originated from a scrapie center. No data were given to indicate that the mouse strain was scrapie-free. Scrapie is known to be transmitted among mice in separate cages [DICKINSON *et al.*, 1964, 1966d; PATTISON, 1964; MORRIS *et al.*, 1965; PATTISON and JONES, 1968; ZLOTNIK, 1968], and in Field's experiments the scrapie incubation period was shorter than normal, suggesting that infection had been prior to the time of inoculation. MACKAY [1968] has pointed out that this suggests that the mouse stock is contaminated with scrapie. Reports that scrapie has appeared in mice [RENWICK and ZLOTNIK, 1965; PATTISON and JONES, 1968], goats [PATTISON and MILLSON, 1960, 1961c; PATTISON, 1965a; PATTISON and JONES, 1968] or sheep [DARCEL *et al.*, 1963] after inoculation with supposedly normal tissue throw further doubt on human scrapie isolations (see section on scrapie accidental transmission). In a study by DICK *et al.* [1965], human MS material was inoculated into approximately 20 lambs or sheep. No evidence of any scrapie-like condition was found. The authors noted that in experiments performed by Field *et al.* [1962] and Pálsson *et al.* [1965] 4 out of 4 Icelandic sheep succumbed to a scrapie-like infection after inoculation with brain from the same patient, but Icelandic sheep inoculated with control human brain from a case of subacute encephalitis [Campbell *et al.*, 1963] showed an incidence of 3 out of 4 with a similar scrapie-like condition. Dick *et al.* [1965] suggested that the Icelandic sheep may have carried rida, and IC inoculation may activate this agent. Pálsson *et al.* [1965] performed a series of experiments in which brain material from SELL, a very acute case of MS, was inoculated in England and Iceland into a variety of breeds of scrapie-susceptible sheep with a total of 47 experimental animals and 40 controls. A scrapie-like illness occurred in 6 out of 14 Icelandic sheep after inoculation with the MS brain. Four Icelandic control sheep remained normal. A second passage from the sick sheep caused a scrapie-like disease in 5 of 5 inoculated sheep. These workers concluded that their experiments were significant, and indicated that human MS could infect sheep. However, the more recent data on accidental transmission of scrapie tends to undermine these conclusions. Furthermore it appears (Pálsson, personal communication) that the brain specimen causing the positive inoculations had been sent to Iceland via the scrapie research laboratoy at Moredun, where it had been transferred to a different container. It is clear that this would not prevent contamination with scrapie virus even if the specimen was preserved in formalin. Since there is evidence [Renwick and Zlotnik, 1965; Field, 1966] that the Moredun mice may be contaminated with scrapie, it is possible that similar contamination of the SELL specimen could explain the isolation results. Any laboratory which has worked extensively with scrapie prior to knowledge of its unique viral stability obviously runs a high risk of being extensively contaminated. Thormar and Von Magnus [1963a] attempted to isolate a possible visna-like virus from cases of MS by inoculating a total of 73 specimens of cerebrospinal fluid into tissue cultures derived from human embryonic brain tissue. No evidence of CPE was obtained in any of the cultures. The program was derived from observations made in the course of research on visna infection of sheep. Although human sera did cause some inactivation of visna virus [Thormar and Von Magnus, 1963b], it was found that there was no significant difference between the sera of normal persons and MS cases. It was concluded by the authors that a heat stable substance in human sera which was able to inactivate visna virus was most likely to be a non-specific inhibitor. Webb [1967] has discussed the possibility that MS is due to a virus similar to scrapie; he sees the neuronal degeneration as secondary to a neuronal abnormality induced by a tumor-like virus. Webb's concept seems to be similar to the hypothesis of virus transformation of nerve cells coupled with a cellular immune response against the new antigen outlined by HOTCHIN [1967]. A possibility that measles virus is involved in MS has been considered [ADAMS and IMAGAWA, 1962] and GUDNA-DÓTTIR *et al.* [1964] isolated a herpes-like virus from an MS case and found evidence of specific antibody in other MS patients. ROSS *et al.* [1965] also found increased antibody levels to varicella-zoster in MS patients. It is clear that the importance of MS warrants more carefully controlled work to determine whether a scrapie-like agent or other slow virus is responsible, but it is equally clear that the weight of evidence points to scrapie-contaminated test animals as the explanation for the positive scrapie virus isolation results to date.

A Comparison of the Properties of Persistent Viruses

An examination [HOTCHIN, 1970a] of the pathogenic behavior of many of the persistent and slow animal viruses provides rather convincing evidence that many, but not necessarily all of them, fit the general concept of pathogenesis outlined earlier for LCM virus. It may be that these constitute a heterogeneous, functionally similar group. The relevant data derived from a review of the literature are shown in table XI. The available information showed a high level of positive correlation between the properties of the different viruses listed. It seems likely that this correlation will increase for many of the agents, and no doubt the opposite will occur with others.

The ability to grow in lymphoid tissue may be a key property of persistent viruses causing the induction of some form of specific cellular and/ or humoral immunological incapacity. The induction of non-neutralizing antibody, of the type detected by immunofluorescence, is an important feature of chronic LCM infection of the adult mouse (HDIP); it also appears from the work of PORTER *et al.* [1969b] to be a paramount feature of Aleutian mink disease. The LCM-HDIP state may prove to be a model for many persistent viruses where there is a specific partial tolerance, or incapacity of the immune system.

The ability of neonatal thymectomy to predispose to tolerance rather than disease upon subsequent virus challenge appears to be a good test of the persistent property. However, only a few examples have been tested in this way. Temporary nonspecific virus-induced changes in the immune response have received insufficient attention to allow much generalization but this property appears to be closely related to antigenic enhancement and also to the effects of leukemia viruses. Although the absence of effective neutralizing antibody would appear to be a prerequisite for virus persistence, non-neutralizing FAB may be produced and reach abnormally high concentrations, sufficient to constitute a gamopathy. Perhaps any monoclonal gamopathy should be considered as a pos-

Table XIa. Properties of persistent viruses

Virus[1]	Congenital infection	Persistence	Growth in lymphoid tissue	Thymecto-my-induced tolerance	Nonspecific immuno-suppression	Poor NAB
LCM	+ (1, 2, 3)	+ (1, 4, 5, 6)	+ (7, 8, 9, 10, 11)	+ (12, 13, 14, 15)	+ (16)	+ (6, 17, 18, 19, 20, 21, 22)
LDV	+ (23, 24, 25)	+ (26)	+ (27, 28)	+ (29)	+ (30)	+ (26)
AMD	+ (31)	+ (32)	+ (33, 34)		+ (35, 36)	+ (37)
Vis		+ (38)	+ (38, 39, 40)			− (38, 41)
EIA	+ (42, 43)	+ (44)	+ (45)			+ (45, 46, 47, 48)
SH		+ (49, 50)				+ (51)
Rubella	+ (52)	± (53, 54, 55)				
SMCA		+ (56)	+ (56)			+ (56)
CMV	+ (57, 58)	± (59, 60)	+ (61)		+ (62)	
ASF	+ (63)	+ (64, 65)	+ (66, 67, 68, 69)			+ (70, 71, 72)
Reo	+ (73)	± (73, 74)	+ (75, 76)			
RV/FPV	+ (77, 78)	± (78)	+ (78, 79)			
Jun		+ (80, 81)	+ (82, 83)	+ (84, 85)		+ (81)
Scrapie	+ (86, 87)	+ (88, 89)	+ (90)		− (91)	+ (89, 92, 93)
Rabies		+ (94, 95, 96)				

[1] LCM = Lymphocytic choriomeningitis virus; LDV = Lactic dehydrogenase virus; AMD = Aleutian mink disease virus; Vis = Visna/Maedi viruses; EIA = Equine infectious anemia; SH = Serum hepatitis virus; SMCA = Suckling mouse cataract agent; CMV = Cytomegalovirus; ASF = African swine fever virus; RV = Rat virus; FPV = Feline panleucopenia virus; Jun = Junin/Machupo.

References

1. HOTCHIN [1962a].
2. TRAUB [1936c].
3. TRAUB [1960c].
4. HOTCHIN [1958].
5. TRAUB [1939].
6. WEIGAND and HOTCHIN [1961].
7. BROWN [1968].
8. DANĚS *et al.* [1963].
9. HANAOKA *et al.* [1969].
10. TRAUB [1960b].

Table XIa (continued)

11. WILSNACK and ROWE [1964].
12. EAST *et al.* [1964].
13. FÖLDES *et al.* [1964].
14. HOTCHIN and SIKORA [1964].
15. ROWE *et al.* [1963].
16. MIMS and WAINWRIGHT [1968].
17. HAAS [1954].
18. ROWE [1954].
19. SMADEL and WALL [1940].
20. TRAUB [1936b].
21. TRAUB [1960a].
22. VOLKERT *et al.* [1964].
23. CRISPENS [1964a].
24. GEORGII *et al.* [1964].
25. NOTKINS and SCHEELE [1963].
26. RILEY [1968a].
27. DU BUY and JOHNSON [1966].
28. EVANS and SALAMAN [1965].
29. CRISPENS and REY [1967].
30. HOWARD *et al.* [1969].
31. HENSON (Personal communication).
32. PORTER and LARSEN [1967].
33. GORHAM *et al.* [1964].
34. PORTER *et al.* [1969b].
35. KENYON [1965].
36. KENYON [1966].
37. GORHAM *et al.* [1963].
38. GUDNADÓTTIR and PÁLSSON [1966].
39. SIGURDSSON [1954a].
40. SIGURDSSON *et al.* [1952].
41. GUDNADÓTTIR and KRISTINSDÓTTIR [1967].
42. ISHII *et al.* [1940].
43. STEIN and MOTT [1946].
44. STEIN *et al.* [1955].
45. ISHII [1963].
46. KOBAYASHI *et al.* [1969].
47. MYERS *et al.* [1969].
48. STEIN and GATES [1950].
49. BLUMBERG *et al.* [1966].
50. ZUCKERMAN and TAYLOR [1969].
51. GILES *et al.* [1969].
52. RUDOLPH *et al.* [1965].
53. BLATTNER [1966].
54. HAMBIDGE *et al.* [1966].
55. PHILLIPS *et al.* [1965].
56. CLARK [1964].
57. NAEYE [1967].
58. WRIGHT [1966].
59. MEDEARIS [1964c].
60. WELLER and HANSHAW [1962].
61. STULBERG *et al.* [1966].
62. OSBORN *et al.* [1968].
63. HARDING *et al.* [1966].
64. STEYN [1932].
65. DETRAY *et al.* [1961].
66. DETRAY [1963].
67. HEUSCHELE [1967].
68. MAURER *et al.* [1958].
69. PLOWRIGHT *et al.* [1968].
70. DE BOER [1967a].
71. DE BOER [1967b].
72. MALMQUIST [1963].
73. HASHIMI *et al.* [1966].
74. WALTERS *et al.* [1965].
75. JENSON *et al.* [1966].
76. KUNDIN *et al.* [1966].
77. KILHAM and MARGOLIS [1966b].
78. KILHAM *et al.* [1967].
79. KILHAM [1966].
80. JOHNSON *et al.* [1965a].
81. JUSTINES and JOHNSON [1969].
82. BRUNO-LOBO *et al.* [1968].
83. COTO *et al.* [1967].
84. SCHMUNIS *et al.* [1967].
85. WEISSENBACHER *et al.* [1969].
86. DICKINSON *et al.* [1966a].
87. RENWICK and ZLOTNIK [1965].
88. EKLUND *et al.* [1967].
89. PALMER [1957].
90. STAMP *et al.* [1959].
91. CLARKE [1968].
92. CLARKE and HAIG [1966].
93. GIBBS *et al.* [1965].
94. BELL [1966].
95. HUMMELER and KOPROWSKI [1969].
96. KAPLAN [1969].

Table XIb. Properties of persistent viruses

Virus[1]	Circulating Ag/Ab	Glomerulo-nephritis	Gamopathy	CPE	Viruria	Ineffective killed vaccine
LCM	+ (97, 98)	+ (1, 11, 99, 100, 101, 102, 103)	+ (98, 102)	± (104, 105, 106)	+ (2, 107)	+ (108, 109, 110, 111, 112)
LDV				± (113, 114)		
AMD	+ (115, 116)	+ (117, 118, 119)	+ (120, 121)		+ (33, 122)	+ (123)
Vis	+ (38)			± (124)		
EIA	+ (45)	± (45)	+ (45, 125)			+ (126, 127, 128)
SH						
Rubella		+ (129)	+ (130, 131)	± (132)		
SMCA						
CMV			+ (133, 134)	+ (135)	+ (136, 137, 138, 139)	
ASF	+ (140, 141)					+ (142)
Reo				+ (143)		
RV/FPV				± (144)	+ (145)	
Jun					+ (81, 146)	
Scrapie						
Rabies				± (147, 148)		

[1] LCM = Lymphocytic choriomeningitis virus; LDV = Lactic dehydrogenase virus; AMD = Aleutian mink disease virus; Vis = Visna/Maedi viruses; EIA = Equine infectious anemia; SH = Serum hepatitis virus; SMCA = Suckling mouse cataract agent; CMV = Cytomegalovirus; ASF = African swine fever virus; RV = Rat virus; FPV = Feline panleucopenia virus; Jun = Junin/Machupo.

References

97. HIRSCH *et al.* [1968].
98. HOTCHIN (Unpublished observations).
99. HOTCHIN and COLLINS [1964].
100. OLDSTONE and DIXON [1969].
101. OLDSTONE and DIXON [1967].
102. POLLARD *et al.* [1968a].
103. POLLARD *et al.* [1968b].
104. BENSON [1959].
105. BENSON [1960a].
106. HOTCHIN and CINITS [1958].
107. UTZ [1964].

Table XIb (continued)

108. MILZER and LEVINSON [1949].	129. MENSER *et al.* [1967c].
109. MILZER and LEVINSON [1946].	130. HANCOCK *et al.* [1968].
110. STOCK and FRANCIS [1943].	131. SOOTHILL *et al.* [1966].
111. TRAUB [1937].	132. MAES *et al.* [1966].
112. TRAUB [1938].	133. ALFORD *et al.* [1967].
113. FRANTSI and GREGORY [1969].	134. McCRACKEN and SHINEFIELD [1965].
114. PLAGEMANN and SWIM [1966].	
115. KENYON *et al.* [1963b].	135. WELLER and ROWE [1964].
116. LEADER [1964].	136. BENYESH-MELNICK *et al.* [1964].
117. HENSON *et al.* [1969a].	137. FELDMAN [1968].
118. HENSON *et al.* [1967a].	138. ROWE *et al.* [1958].
119. KINDIG *et al.* [1967].	139. STERN and TUCKER [1965].
120. GORDON *et al.* [1967].	140. COLGROVE *et al.* [1969].
121. HENSON *et al.* [1963a].	141. DeTRAY [1957].
122. KENYON *et al.* [1963a].	142. STONE and HESS [1967].
123. KARSTAD *et al.* [1963].	143. BELL and ROSS [1966].
124. SIGURDSSON *et al.* [1960].	144. JOHNSON [1965].
125. HENSON *et al.* [1967b].	145. TOOLAN [1960].
126. BANKIER [1945].	146. JOHNSON *et al.* [1965b].
127. STEIN and OSTEEN [1941].	147. FERNANDES *et al.* [1963].
128. TABUCHI *et al.* [1955].	148. FERNANDES *et al.* [1964].

sible end result of a persistent virus-induced immunoproliferative lesion. Viruria and glomerulonephritis appear to be secondary effects of the persistent tolerant state. The evidence for ineffectiveness of killed vaccine as a general property of this group is not strong, but, if the conclusion is valid, it may be related to the key role of the cellular immune response in suppressing this type of infection. It is conceivable that the class of viruses which cause the induction of new surface antigens in infected cells are only suppressed by a cellular immune response. Standard vaccines may lack sufficient concentration of the relevant cell surface antigen.

Several of the viruses listed in table XI do not readily fit the LCM model. Visna differs from it in terms of the free virus which is only present in association with lymphocytes [GUDNADÓTTIR and PÁLSSON, 1966], and true persistence (defined as the ability to demonstrate significant titers of free virus in blood or organs over a period of months) appears to be relatively short-lived in most visna-affected sheep. Persistence is also short-lived in infection with rubella, suckling mouse cataract

Table XIc. Properties of persistent viruses

Virus[1]	High CFAB or FAB	Virus-induced surface antigen	Persistence *in vitro*	Similar to HDIP
LCM	+ (149)	+ (150, 151)	+ (106, 152, 153, 154)	+
LDV	+ (155)		+ (28, 114, 156, 157)	+
AMD	+ (34)			+
Vis	+ (41)	+ (158)	+ (124)	−
EIA				+
SH				+
Rubella			+ (159, 160)	±
SMCA				
CMV				±
ASF	+ (72)			+
Reo			+ (143)	
RV/FPV			± (144)	±
Jun		+ (161)	+ (161)	+
Scrapie				−
Rabies		+ (162)	+ (147, 148, 163, 164)	

[1] LCM = Lymphocytic choriomeningitis virus; LDV = Lactic dehydrogenase virus; AMD = Aleutian mink disease virus; Vis = Visna/Maedi viruses; EIA = Equine infectious anemia; SH = Serum hepatitis virus; SMCA = Suckling mouse cataract agent; CMV = Cytomegalovirus; ASF = African swine fever virus; RV = Rat virus; FPV = Feline panleucopenia virus; Jun = Junin/Machupo.

References

149. Benson and Hotchin [1969].
150. Abelson *et al.* [1969].
151. Hotchin and Benson (to be published).
152. Benson [1961].
153. Lehmann-Grube [1967].
154. Traub [1961a].
155. Porter *et al.* [1969a].
156. Anderson *et al.* [1966].
157. Plagemann and Swim [1963a].
158. Thormar and Cruickshank [1965].
159. Rawls *et al.* [1968].
160. Rawls and Melnick [1966].
161. Murphy *et al.* [1969].
162. Wiktor *et al.* [1968].
163. Love *et al.* [1964].
164. Wiktor *et al.* [1964].

agent, cytomegalovirus, or reovirus. Scrapie virus may well be in a special class but data are lacking on its exact nature. It is possible that generalized asymptomatic rabies infection of bats may fit the model, but definitive data are lacking.

The nature of the process whereby persistent infection of immune cells renders them tolerant or paralyzed remains conjectural. The idea that intracellular production of high concentrations of antigen could readily induce immunological paralysis is both plausible and simple, but the exact molecular events may be much more complex and have yet to be determined. Virus-induced shut down of both host and viral components may be involved, and the tolerogenic lesion may occur at a different locus or in different cells with different viruses or different strains of the same virus. The exact intracellular mechanism whereby induction of the specific viral immune response is prevented is a fascinating subject for future study. The lesion may be closely related to the cause of some types of leukemia, which may take the form of an 'impotent' cellular immune response. The possible alternative effects of serum hepatitis virus in causing hepatitis, an asymptomatic carrier state, or leukemia [BLUMBERG *et al.*, 1968] may be relevant in this respect. Infection with Aleutian mink disease virus has been observed by KENYON (personal communication) to be associated with leukemia instead of gamopathy in some cases.

Finally, the ability of persistent virus infections to cause disease by gradual damage to target organ cells must not be overlooked. This type of effect appears to be caused by scrapie and kuru, and may be involved in visna and other slow virus diseases. It appears that virus-induced cellular deterioration as well as virus-induced autoimmunity may be involved in the aging process of animals and man [HOTCHIN, 1970b]. As an incentive for slow virus research, the elimination of an ubiquitous human agent causing accelerated senility would surely be a powerful candidate. After all Noah lived for 950 years[24].

[24] Bible: Genesis 9:29.

References

ABELSON, H. T.; SMITH, G. H.; HOFFMAN, H. A., and ROWE, W. P.: Use of enzyme-labeled antibody for electron microscope localization of lymphocytic choriomeningitis virus antigens in infected cell cultures. J. nat. Cancer Inst. *42:* 497–515 (1969).

ACKERMANN, R.: Über die Züchtung des Virus der lymphocytären Choriomeningitis in Mäuseembryo-Zellkulturen. Arch. ges. Virusforsch. *10:* 183–194 (1960).

ACKERMANN, R.; SCHEID, W. und JOCHHEIM, K. A.: Der Einfluss der Lagerung auf die neutralisierenden Fähigkeiten von Seren gegenüber dem Virus der Lymphozytären Choriomeningitis. Zbl. Bakt. Parasitkde *185:* 343–354 (1962).

ADAIR, C. V.; GAULD, R. L., and SMADEL, J. E.: Aseptic meningitis, a disease of diverse etiology: Clinical and etiologic studies on 854 cases. Ann. intern. Med. *39:* 675–704 (1953).

ADAMS, M. H.: Bacteriophages, p. 40 (Interscience Publishers, Inc., New York 1959).

ADAMS, D. H. and BOWMAN, B. M.: Studies on the properties of factors elevating the activity of mouse-plasma lactate dehydrogenase. Biochem. J. *90:* 477–482 (1964).

ADAMS, D. H. and CASPARY, E. A.: Nature of the scrapie virus. Brit. med. J. *iii:* 173 (1967).

ADAMS, D. H. and FIELD, E. J.: The infective process in scrapie. Lancet *ii:* 714–716 (1968).

ADAMS, J. M. and IMAGAWA, D. T.: Measles antibodies in multiple sclerosis. Proc. Soc. exp. Biol., N. Y. *111:* 562–566 (1962).

ADELS, B. R.; GAJDUSEK, D. C.; GIBBS, C. J., jr.; ALBRECHT, P., and ROGERS, N. G.: Attempts to transmit subacute sclerosing panencephalitis and isolate a measles related agent, with a study of the immune response in patients and experimental animals. Neurology, Minneap. *18:* 30–51 (1968).

ADLDINGER, H. K.; STONE, S. S.; HESS, W. R., and BACHRACH, H. L.: Extraction of infectious deoxyribonucleic acid from African swine fever virus. Virology *30:* 750–752 (1966).

ALFORD, C. A., jr.: Studies on antibody in congenital rubella infections. I. Physicochemical and immunologic investigations of rubella neutralizing antibody. Amer. J. Dis. Child *110:* 455–463 (1965).

ALFORD, C. A., jr.; NEVA, F. A., and WELLER, T. H.: Virologic and serologic studies on human products of conception after maternal rubella. New Engl. J. Med. *271:* 1275–1281 (1964).

ALFORD, C. A.; SCHAEFER, J.; BLANKENSHIP, W. J.; STRAUMFJORD, J. V., and CASSADY,

G.: A correlative immunologic, microbiologic and clinical approach to the diagnosis of acute and chronic infections in newborn infants. New Engl. J. Med. *277:* 437–449 (1967).

ALICE, F. J. and McNUTT, S. H.: A study of lymphocytic choriomeningitis virus. Amer. J. vet. Res. *6:* 54–60 (1945).

ALLEN, J. G. and SAYMAN, W. A.: Serum hepatitis from transfusions of blood. Epidemiologic study. J. amer. med. Ass. *180:* 1079–1085 (1962).

ALPER, T. and HAIG, D. A.: Protection by anoxia of the scrapie agent and some DNA and RNA viruses irradiated as dry preparations. J. gen. Virol. *3:* 157–166 (1968).

ALPER, T.; HAIG, D. A., and CLARKE, M. C.: The exceptionally small size of the scrapie agent. Biochem. biophys. res. Comm. *22:* 278–284 (1966).

ALPER, T.; CRAMP, W. A.; HAIG, D. A., and CLARKE, M. C.: Does the agent of scrapie replicate without nucleic acid? Nature, Lond. *214:* 764–766 (1967).

ALPERS, M. P.: Epidemiological changes in kuru, 1957 to 1963. NINDB Monograph No. 2. Slow, latent and temperate virus infections, pp. 65–82 (US Dept. of Health, Education and Welfare, Washington, D. C. 1965).

ALPERS, M. P.: Kuru: Implications of its transmissibility for the interpretation of its changing epidemiologic pattern; in The central nervous system. International Academy of Pathology Monograph No. 9, pp. 234–251 (The Williams & Wilkins Co., Baltimore 1968).

ALPERS, M. and GAJDUSEK, D. C.: Changing patterns of kuru: Epidemiological changes in the period of increasing contact of the Fore people with Western civilization. Amer. J. trop. Med. Hyg. *14:* 852–879 (1965).

ALTERMAN, K.: Neonatal hepatitis and its relation to viral hepatitis of mother. Amer. J. Dis. Child *105:* 395–416 (1963).

American Ass. for Lab. Anim. Sci.: Laboratory infection bibliography, pp. 1–49 (1966).

ANDERSON, H. C.; RILEY, V.; FITZMAURICE, M. A.; LOVELESS, J. D.; WADE, P., and MOORE, A. E.: Quantitative study of the lactate dehydrogenase-elevating virus in mouse embryo cultures. J. nat. Cancer Inst. *36:* 89–95 (1966).

ANDREWS, C. H. and HORSTMANN, D. M.: The susceptibility of viruses to ethyl ether. J. gen. Microbiol. *3:* 290–297 (1949).

Anon. Japanese Commission: Report on the results obtained by the special committee for the investigation of infectious anemia among horses. Horse Administration Bureau, Tokyo Rept. No. 2 (1914).

Anon. Leading article. Myopathy and scrapie. Lancet *ii:* 767–768 (1956).

Anon. Leading article. Reovirus 3 and lymphoblastis. Lancet *i:* 965–966 (1966).

Anon. Leading article. Diseases caused by cytomegaloviruses. Brit. med. J. *1:* 72–73 (1968).

ARAKAWA, S.; KANEKO, T.; SEKI, T., and MUTO, S.: Experimental study on equine infectious anemia. Rep. 1. On the adaptation of the virus to mouse brain and others (in Japanese). Seitai no Kagaku *4:* 143–144 (1952).

ARAKAWA, S.; KANEKO, T.; SEKI, T., und MUTO, S.: Experimentelle Studien über den Virus der infektiösen Anämie der Pferde. 1. Mitteilung: Isolierung und Fixierung des Virus in weissen Mäusen. Wien. tierärztl. Mschr. *6:* 321–326 (1953).

Armstrong, C.: Studies on choriomeningitis and poliomyelitis. Harvey Lect. *36:* 39–65 (1940).

Armstrong, C.: Some recent research in the field of neurotropic viruses with especial reference to lymphocytic choriomeningitis and herpes simplex. Milit. Surg. *91:* 129–146 (1942).

Armstrong, C. and Dickens, P. F.: Benign lymphocytic choriomeningitis (acute aseptic meningitis). Publ. Hlth Rep., Wash. *50:* 831–842 (1935).

Armstrong, C. and Lillie, R. D.: Experimental lymphocytic choriomeningitis of monkeys and mice produced by a virus encountered in studies of the 1933 St. Louis encephalitis epidemic. Publ. Hlth Rep., Wash. *49:* 1019–1027 (1934).

Armstrong, C. and Sweet, L. K.: Lymphocytic choriomeningitis. Report of two cases, with recovery of the virus from gray mice (*Mus musculus*) trapped in the two infected households. Publ. Hlth Rep., Wash. *54:* 673–684 (1939).

Armstrong, C.; Wooley, J. G., and Onstott, R. H.: Distribution of lymphocytic choriomeningitis virus in the organs of experimentally inoculated monkeys. Publ. Hlth Rep., Wash. *51:* 298–303 (1936).

Armstrong, D.; Fortner, J. G.; Rowe, W. P., and Parker, J. C.: Meningitis due to lymphocytic choriomeningitis virus endemic in a hamster colony. J. amer. med. Ass. *209:* 265–267 (1969).

Bader, J. P.: The role of deoxyribonucleic acid in the synthesis of Rous sarcoma virus. Virology *22:* 462–468 (1964).

Bader, J. P.: The requirement of DNA synthesis in the growth of Rous sarcoma and Rous-associated viruses. Virology *26:* 253–261 (1965).

Baker, A. B.: Chronic lymphocytic choriomeningitis. J. Neuropath. exp. Neurol. *6:* 253–264 (1947).

Baker, F. D. and Hotchin, J.: Slow virus kidney disease of mice. Science *158:* 502–504 (1967).

Balozet, L.: Filtrabilité du virus de l'anémie infectieuse des équidés. Essai de détermination de la dimension des particules du virus. C. R. Acad. Sci. *209:* 703–707 (1939).

Bankier, J. C.: Equine infectious anemia. Attempted vaccination with crystal violet tissue vaccine. Canad. J. comp. Med. *9:* 197–199 (1945).

Baratawidjaja, R. K.; Morrissey, L. P., and Labzoffsky, N. A.: Demonstration of vaccinia, lymphocytic choriomeningitis and rabies viruses in the leucocytes of experimentally infected animals. Arch. ges. Virusforsch. *17:* 273–279 (1965).

Barker, L. F. and Ford, F. R.: Chronic arachnoiditis obliterating the spinal subarachnoid space. J. amer. med. Ass. *109:* 785–786 (1937).

Barlow, J. L.: The effect of alkylating agents on lymphocytic choriomeningitis infection in mice. N. Y. State Dep. Hlth, Ann. Rep. Div. Lab. Res., pp. 47–48 (1961).

Barlow, J. L.: Hyperreactivity to endotoxin in mice infected with lymphocytic choriomeningitis virus; in Bacterial endotoxins, pp. 448–454 (Quinn & Boden Co. Inc., New Jersey 1964).

Barlow, J. L. and Fairley, R. J.: Hyperreactivity to endotoxin in mice infected with lymphocytic choriomeningitis virus. N. Y. State Dep. Health, Ann. Rep. Div. Lab. Res., pp. 39–40 (1962).

BARLOW, J. L. and HOTCHIN, J.: The effect of certain drugs on lymphocytic cho-
    riomeningitis infection in mice. N. Y. State Dep. Health, Ann. Rep. Div. Lab.
    Res., pp. 22–23 (1960).
BARLOW, J. L. and HOTCHIN, J.: Induction of persistent tolerant infection with lym-
    phocytic choriomeningitis virus in adult mice by amethopterin treatment. N. Y.
    State Dep. Health, Ann. Rep. Div. Lab. Res., pp. 39 (1962).
BARLOW, J. L. and KELLER, E.: Effect of 5-Fluoro-2'-deoxyuridine on formation of
    lymphocytic choriomeningitis virus in continuous baby hamster kidney cells.
    N. Y. State Dep. Health, Ann. Rep. Div. Lab. Res., p. 51 (1964a).
BARLOW, J. L. and KELLER, E.: Propagation of lymphocytic choriomeningitis virus
    in tissue cell cultures. N. Y. State Dep. Health, Ann. Rep. Div. Lab. Res.,
    pp. 50–51 (1964b).
BARLOW, J. L. and KELLER E.: Studies of lymphocytic choriomeningitis virus in baby
    hamster kidney cells. N. Y. State Dep. Health, Ann. Rep. Div. Lab. Res., p. 61
    (1965).
BARLOW, J. L. and MUSTICO, T.: Noninfectious antigens associated with lymphocytic
    choriomeningitis virus infection. N. Y. State Dep. Health, Ann. Rep. Div. Lab.
    Res., p. 52 (1964).
BARLOW, J. L. and MUSTICO, T.: Noninfectious antigens associated with lymphocytic
    choriomeningitis infection. N. Y. State Dep. Health, Ann. Rep. Div. Lab. Res.,
    pp. 60–61 (1965).
BARLOW, J. and WIELAND, M. H.: Effect of low salt concentration on neutralizing
    antibody reactions for lymphocytic choriomeningitis virus. N. Y. State Dep.
    Health, Ann. Rep. Div. Lab. Res., p. 23 (1959).
BARLOW, J. L.: COHEN, S. M., and TRIANDAPHILLI, I.: The effect of 5-halogen-2'-
    deoxyuridine derivatives on the synthesis of lymphocytic choriomeningitis vi-
    rus. Fed. Proc. 24: 319 (1965a).
BARLOW, J. L.; COHEN, S. M.; TRIANDAPHILLI, I., and KELLER, E.: Identification of
    the nucleic acid of lymphocytic choriomeningitis virus. N. Y. State Dep.
    Health, Ann. Rep. Div. Lab. Res., pp. 59–60 (1965b).
BARON, S.; DU BUY, H. G.; BUCKLER, C. E., and JOHNSON, M. L.: Relationship of int-
    erferon production to virus growth in vivo. Proc. Soc. exp. Biol., N. Y. 117:
    338–341 (1964).
BARSKI, G. et YOUN, J. K.: Interférence entre la chorioméningite lymphocytaire et la
    leucémie de souris de Rauscher. C. R. Acad. Sci. 259: 4191–4194 (1964).
BASRUR, P. K. and KARSTAD, L.: Studies on viral plasmacytosis (Aleutian disease) of
    mink. VII. Infection of mink with DNA extracted from diseased spleens. Can-
    ad. J. comp. Med. 30: 295–300 (1966).
BASRUR, P. K.; GRAY, D. P., and KARSTAD, L.: Aleutian disease (plasmacytosis) of
    mink. III. Propagation of the virus in mink tissue cultures. Canad. J. comp.
    Med. 27: 301–306 (1963).
BAUBLIS, J. V. and BROWN, G. C.: Specific response of the immunoglobulins to ru-
    bella infection. Proc. Soc. exp. Biol., N. Y. 128: 206–210 (1968).
BAUM, S. G.; LEWIS, A. M.; ROWE, W. P., and HUEBNER, R. J.: Epidemic nonmenin-
    gitic lymphocytic-choriomeningitis-virus infection. An outbreak in a population
    of laboratory personnel. New Engl. J. Med. 274: 934–936 (1966).

BAYER, M. E.; BLUMBERG, B. S., and WERNER, B.: Particles associated with Australia antigen in the sera of patients with leukaemia, Down's syndrome and hepatitis. Nature, Lond. *218:* 1057–1059 (1968).

BECK, E. and DANIEL, P. M.: Kuru and scrapie compared: are they examples of system degeneration? NINDB Monograph No. 2. Slow, latent and temperate virus infections, pp. 85–93 (US Dept. of Health, Education and Welfare, Washington, D. C. 1965).

BECK, E.; DANIEL, P. M.; ALPERS, M.; GAJDUSEK, D. C., and GIBBS, C. J., jr.: Experimental 'kuru' in chimpanzees. A pathological report. Lancet *ii:* 1056–1059 (1966).

BELL, J. F.: Chronic rabies infection. Proc. Nat. Rabies Symp., National Communicable Disease Center, Atlanta, pp. 17–21 (US Dept. of Health, Education and Welfare, 1966).

BELL, T. M. and ROSS, M. G. R.: Persistent latent infection of human embryonic cells with reovirus type 3. Nature, Lond. *212:* 412–414 (1966).

BELL, T. M.; MASSIE, A.; ROSS, M. G. R.; SIMPSON, D. I. H., and GRIFFIN, E.: Further isolations of reovirus type 3 from cases of Burkitt's lymphoma. Brit. med. J. *1:* 1514–1517 (1966).

BELLANTI, J. A.; ARTENSTEIN, M. S.; OLSON, L. C.; BUESCHER, E. L.; LUHRS, C. E., and MILSTEAD, K. L.: Congenital rubella. Clinicopathologic, virologic, and immunologic studies. Amer. J. Dis. Child *110:* 464–472 (1965).

BELLER, K. und SCHWARZMAIER, E.: Untersuchungen über die ansteckende Blutarmut der Pferde. I. Zur Epidemiologie und Diagnostik der ansteckenden Blutarmut (Erfahrungen in Hessen über einen Zeitraum von 7 Jahren). Arch. Tierheilk. *76:* 24–38 (1940).

BENDA, R.: Passive immunoprophylaxis and immunotherapy of inhalation lymphocytic choriomeningitis in guinea pigs. J. Hyg. *8:* 243–251 (1964).

BENDA, R. and ČINÁTL, J.: Multiplication of lymphocytic choriomeningitis virus in bottle cell cultures. Experimental data for the preparation of highly infectious fluids. Acta Virol. *5:* 159–164 (1962).

BENDA, R. and ČINÁTL, J.: Active immunoprophylaxis of experimental inhalation lymphocytic choriomeningitis. J. Hyg. *8:* 252–261 (1964).

BENDA, R.; DANES, L., and FUCHSOVA, M.: Experimental inhalation infection of guinea pigs with the virus of lymphocytic choriomeningitis. J. Hyg. *8:* 87–99 (1964).

BENDA, R.; HRONOVSKY, V.; CĚRVA, L., and ČINÁTL, J.: Demonstration of lymphocytic choriomeningitis virus in cell cultures and mouse brain by the fluorescent antibody technique. Acta Virol. *9:* 347–351 (1965).

BENGTSON, I. A.: Cultivation of the virus of lymphocytic choriomeningitis in the developing chick embryo. Publ. Hlth Rep., Wash. *51:* 29–41 (1936).

BÉNION, A.: Traité complet de l'élevage et des maladies du mouton (in 4 parts), pp. 444–450 (Paris, Asselin 1874).

BENNETT, J. H.: Population and family studies on kuru. Eugen. Quart. *9:* 59–68 (1962a).

BENNETT, J. H.: Population studies in the kuru region of New Guinea. Oceania *33:* 24–46 (1962b).

BENNETT, J. H.; RHODES, F. A., and ROBSON, H. N.: A possible genetic basis for kuru. Amer. J. hum. Genet. *11:* 169–187 (1959).

BENSON, L.: Tissue culture experiments and plaque assay with lymphocytic choriomeningitis virus. N. Y. State Dep. Health, Ann. Rep. Div. Lab. Res., pp. 22–23 (1959).

BENSON, L.: The use of strain L mouse cells in an improved plaque assay of lymphocytic choriomeningitis virus. N. Y. State Dep. Health, Ann. Rep. Div. Lab. Res., pp. 23–24 (1960a).

BENSON, L.: Suppression of lymphocytic choriomeningitis virus production in Maitland-type tissue culture by antibody. N. Y. State Dep. Health, Ann. Rep. Div. Lab. Res., p. 22 (1960b).

BENSON, L. M.: Autointerference due to lymphocytic choriomeningitis virus in tissue culture. N. Y. State Dep. Health, Ann. Rep. Div. Lab. Res., pp. 46–47 (1961).

BENSON, L.: The effect of X-ray on the foot-pad response of mice injected with lymphocytic choriomeningitis virus. N. Y. State Dep. Health. Ann. Rep. Div. Lab. Res., p. 41 (1962a).

BENSON, L.: Effects of immune mouse lymphocytes on normal and virus infected mouse tissue culture. N. Y. State Dep. Health, Ann. Rep. Div. Lab. Res., pp. 41–42 (1962b).

BENSON, L. M. and HOTCHIN, J. E.: Cytopathogenicity and plaque formation with lymphocytic choriomeningitis virus. Proc. Soc. exp. Biol., N. Y. *103:* 623–625 (1960).

BENSON, L. M. and HOTCHIN, J.: Tumor production in mice by strain L tissue culture cells carrying lymphocytic choriomeningitis virus. N. Y. State Dep. Health, Ann. Rep. Div. Lab. Res., pp. 44–46 (1961).

BENSON, L. and HOTCHIN, J.: Antibody formation in persistent tolerant infection with lymphocytic choriomeningitis virus. Nature, Lond. *222:* 1045–1047 (1969).

BENSON, L. M.; WEIGAND, H., and HOTCHIN, J. E.: Relationship between blood lymphocyte counts and susceptibility to lymphocytic choriomeningitis after X-irradiation. N. Y. State Dep. Health, Ann. Rep. Div. Lab. Res., pp. 21–22 (1959).

BENSON, L.; MAGNUSSON, A., and HOTCHIN, J.: Long-term *in vitro* cultivation of lymphocytic choriomeningitis virus in tissue cultures. N. Y. State Dep. Health, Ann. Rep. Div. Lab. Res., pp. 21–22 (1960).

BENYESH-MELNICK, M.; DESSY, S. I., and FERNBACH, D. J.: Cytomegaloviruria in children with acute leukemia and in other children. Proc. Soc. exp. Biol., N. Y. *117:* 624–630 (1964).

BERMAN, P. H.; GILES, J. P., and KRUGMAN, S.: Correlation of measles and subacute sclerosing panencephalitis. Neurology, Minneap. *18:* 91–94 (1968).

BERNHARD, W.; KASTEN, F. H. et CHANY, C.: Étude cytochimique et ultrastructurale des cellules infectées par le virus K du rat et le virus H. C. R. Acad. Sci. *257:* 1566–1569 (1963).

BERTRAND, I.; CARRÉ, H. et LUCAM, F.: La tremblante du mouton. Rec. med. Vet. *113:* 540–561, 586–603 (1937).

BERTRAND, I.; CARRÉ, H. et LUCAM, F.: La tremblante du mouton (recherches histo-pathologiques). Ann. Anat. path. *14:* 565–586 (1937).

BESNOIT, M. M. et MOREL, C.: Note sur les lésions nerveuses de la tremblante du mouton. Rev. vet. Toulouse *23:* 397–400 (1898).

BEST, J. M.; BANATVALA, J. E., and MOORE, B. M.: Growth of rubella virus in human embryonic organ cultures. J. Hyg. *66:* 407–413 (1968).

BIGNAMI, A. and PALLADINI, G.: Experimentally produced cerebral status spongiosus and continuous pseudorhythmic electro-encephalographic discharges with a membrane-ATPase inhibitor in the rat. Nature, Lond. *209:* 413–414 (1966).

BIGOTEAU, M. L.: Sur la tremblante du mouton. Rev. gén. Med. Vét. *28:* 433–434 (1919).

BILLINGHAM, R. E.; BRENT, L., and MEDAWAR, P. B.: Quantitative studies on tissue transplantation immunity. III. Actively acquired tolerance. Philos. Trans. B. *239:* 357–414 (1956).

BIRDSONG, McL.; SMITH, D. E.; MITCHELL, F. N., and COREY, J. H., jr.: Generalized cytomegalic inclusion disease in newborn infants. J. amer. med. Ass. *162:* 1305–1308 (1956).

BLANC, G.: Pneumopathie du cobaye et chorioméningite lymphocytaire. Sem. Hôp., Paris *28:* 3805–3810 (1952).

BLANC, G. et BRUNEAU, J.: Comportement du virus de la chorioméningite chez la lapine en gestation. C. R. Acad. Sci. *233:* 1704–1705 (1951).

BLATTNER, R. J.: Parotitis, orchitis, and meningoencephalitis due to lymphocytic choriomeningitis virus. J. Pediat. *110:* 633–635 (1962).

BLATTNER, R. J.: Congenital rubella: Persistent infection of the brain and liver. J. Pediat. *68:* 997–999 (1966).

BLUMBERG, B. S.: Polymorphisms of the serum proteins and the development of iso-precipitins in transfused patients. Bull. N. Y. Acad. Med. *40:* 377–386 (1964).

BLUMBERG, B. S.: An inherited serum isoantigen in leukemia and Down's syndrome. J. clin. Invest. *45:* 988 (1966).

BLUMBERG, B. S. and MELARTIN, L.: Conjectures on inherited susceptibility to lepromatous leprosy. Int. J. Leprosy *34:* 60–64 (1966).

BLUMBERG, B. S. and RIDDELL, N. M.: Inherited antigenic differences in human serum beta-lipoproteins. A second antiserum. J. clin. Invest. *42:* 867–875 (1963).

BLUMBERG, B. S.; ALTER, H. J., and VISNICH, S.: A 'new' antigen in leukemia sera. J. amer. med. Ass. *191:* 541–546 (1965).

BLUMBERG, B. S.; MELARTIN, L.; GUINTO, R. A., and WERNER, B.: Family studies of a human serum isoantigen system (Australia antigen). Amer. J. hum. Genet. *18:* 594–608 (1966).

BLUMBERG, B. S.; GERSTLEY, B. J. S.; HUNGERFORD, D. A.; LONDON, W. T., and SUTNICK, A. I.: A serum antigen (Australia antigen) in Down's syndrome, leukemia and hepatitis. Ann. intern. Med. *66:* 924–931 (1967a).

BLUMBERG, B. S.; MELARTIN, L.; LECHAT, M., and GUINTO, R. S.: Association between lepromatous leprosy and Australia antigen. Lancet *ii:* 173–176 (1967b).

BLUMBERG, B. S.; SUTNICK, A. I., and LONDON, W. T.: Hepatitis and leukemia: their relation to Australia antigen. Bull. N. Y. Acad. Sci. *44:* 1566–1586 (1968).

BLUMBERG, B. S.; SUTNICK, A. I., and LONDON, W. T.: Australia antigen and hepatitis. J. amer. med. Ass. *207:* 1895–1896 (1969).

BOHIGIAN, G. M.; FOX, J., and COTLIER, E.: Immunofluorescent localization of rubella virus in the lens, retina and heart of congenital rubella-infected rats. Amer. J. Ophthal. *65:* 196–201 (1968).

BOREL, Y.; FAUCONNET, M., and MIESCHER, P. A.: Selective suppression of delayed hypersensitivity by the induction of immunologic tolerance. J. exp. Med. *123:* 585–598 (1966).

BOS, S. E.: Over alveolair-celltumoren (Thesis, Amsterdam 1951).

BOSANQUET, F. D.; DANIEL, P. M., and PARRY, H. B.: Myopathy in sheep. Its relationship to scrapie and to dermatomyositis and muscular dystrophy. Lancet *ii:* 737–746 (1956).

BOUÉ, A. and BOUÉ, J. G.: Effects of rubella infection on the division of human cells. Amer. J. Dis. Child *118:* 45–48 (1969).

BOULANGER, P.; BANNISTER, G. L.; RUCKERBAUER, G. M., and CORNER, A. H.: Equine infectious anemia: Preliminary investigation of the complement-fixation test for the demonstration of antibodies and antigen. Canad. J. comp. Med. *33:* 148–154 (1969).

BOUTEILLE, M.; FONTAINE, C.; VEDRENNE, C. et DELARUE, J.: Sur un cas d'encéphalite subaiguë à inclusions. Etude anatomoclinique et ultrastructurale. Rev. Neurol. *113:* 454–458 (1965).

BOXACA, M. C.; PARODI, A. S.; RUGIERO, H., and BLAY, R.: Experimental hemorrhagic fever in the guinea pig (Junin virus). Rev. Soc. Argent. Biol. *37:* 170–179 (1961).

BRASH, A. G.: Scrapie in imported sheep in New Zealand. New Zeald vet. J. *1:* 27–30 (1952).

BREESE, S. S., jr. and DE BOER, C. J.: Electron microscope observations of African swine fever virus in tissue culture cells. Virology *28:* 420–428 (1966).

BREESE, S. S., jr. and HESS, W. R.: Electron microscopy of African swine fever virus hemadsorption. J. Bact. *92:* 272–274 (1966).

BREESE, S. S., jr.; HOWATSON, A. F., and CHANY, C. H.: Isolation of virus-like particles associated with Kilham rat virus infection of tissue cultures. Virology *24:* 598–603 (1964).

British Medical Dictionary: MACNALTY (ed.) (Caxton Publishing Co. Ltd., London 1961).

BROTHERSTON, J. G.; VANTSIS, J. T.; MACKAY, J. M.K., and DRYSDALE, A.: Tissue culture studies on scrapie. Report of Scrapie Seminar, Washington, D. C., 1964, pp. 282–287 (US Dept. of Agriculture, ARS 91–53, Washington, D. C. 1966).

BROTHERSTON, J. G.; VANTSIS, J. T.; MACKAY, J. M. K., and DRYSDALE, A.: Tissue culture studies on scrapie. NINDB Monograph No. 2. Slow, latent and temperate virus infections, pp. 209–214 (US Dept. of Health, Education and Welfare, Washington, D. C. 1965).

BROTHERSTON, J. G.; RENWICK, C. C.; STAMP, J. T., and ZLOTNIK, I.: Spread of scrapie by contact to goats and sheep. J. comp. Path. *78:* 9–17 (1968).

BROWN, P.: Evolution of lymphocytic choriomengitis virus infection from neonatal inoculation through development of adult 'late onset disease' and glomerulonephritis. Arch. ges. Virusforsch. *24:* 220–230 (1968).

Brown, G. C.; Maassab, H. F.; Veronelli, J. A., and Francis, T. J., jr.: Rubella antibodies in human serum: Detection by the indirect fluorescent-antibody technique. Science *145:* 943–945 (1964).

Brown, G. C.; Maassab, H. F.; Veronelli, J. A., and Francis, T., jr.: Detection of rubella antibodies in human serum by the indirect fluorescent antibody technique. Arch. ges. Virusforsch. *16:* 459–463 (1965).

Brownlee, A.: Histo-pathological studies of scrapie, an obscure disease of sheep. Vet. J. *96:* 254–264 (1940).

Bruno-Lobo, G. G.; Bruno-Lobo, M.; Johnson, K. M.; Webb, P. A., and De Paola, D.: Pathogenesis of junin virus infection in the infant hamster; in Anais de Microbiologia, vol. 15, pp. 11–33 (Instituto de Microbiologia, Universidade do Federal, Rio De Janeiro 1968).

Brustad, T.: Molecular and cellular effects of fast charged particles. Radiat. Res. *15:* 139–158 (1961).

Buck, L. L. and Pfau, C. J.: Inhibition of lymphocytic choriomeningitis virus replication by actinomycin D and 6-azauridine. Virology *27:* 698–701 (1969).

Buckley, S. M. and Casals, J.: Lassa fever, a new virus disease of man from West Africa. III. Isolation and characterization of the virus. Amer. J. trop. Med. Hyg. *19:* 680–691 (1970).

Buko, L. and Kenyon, A. J.: Aleutian disease gammopathy of mink induced with an ultra-filtrable agent. Nature, Lond. *216:* 69–70 (1967).

Burger, D. and Hartsough, G. R.: Encephalopathy of mink. II. Experimental and natural transmission. J. infect. Dis. *115:* 393–399 (1965).

Burger, D. and Hartsough, G. R.: A 'scrapie'-like disease of mink. Report of Scrapie Seminar, Washington, D. C., 1964, pp. 225–227 (US Dept. of Agriculture, ARS 91–53, Washington, D. C. 1966).

Burger, D.; Gorham, J. R., and Leader, R. W.: Some physical and chemical characteristics of partially purified Aleutian disease virus. NINDB Monograph No. 2. Slow, latent and temperate virus infections, pp. 307–313 (US Dept. of Health, Education and Welfare, Washington, D. C. 1965).

Burnet, F. M. and Fenner, F.: The production of antibodies. Monograph of the Walter and Eliza Hall Institute. 2nd ed., 142 pp. (Macmillan and Co. Ltd., Melbourne 1949).

Butler, E. J. and Smith, W.: An attempt to separate the scrapie agent from brain tissue. Vet. Rec. *72:* 417–418 (1960).

Campbell, A. M.; Norman, R. M., and Sandry, R. J.: Subacute encephalitis in an adult associated with necrotizing myelitis and results of animal inoculation experiments. J. Neurol. Neurosurg. Psychiat. *26:* 439–446 (1963).

Camyre, K. P. and Pfau, C. J.: Biophysical and biochemical characterization of lymphocytic choriomeningitis virus. IV. Strain differences. J. Virol. *2:* 161–166 (1968).

Casals-Ariet, J. and Webster, L. T.: Characteristics of a strain of lymphocytic choriomeningitis virus encountered as a contaminant in tissue cultures of rabies virus. J. exp. Med. *71:* 147–154 (1940).

Caspary, E. A. and Sewell, F. M.: Synthesis of nuclear basic proteins in normal and scrapie-affected mice and rats. Biochem. J. *108:* 37P (1968).

CASSIRER, K.: Über die Traberkrankheit der Schafe. Virchows Arch. path. Anat. *153:* 89–110 (1898).

CEGLOWSKI, W. S. and FRIEDMAN, H.: Leukemia virus-induced depression of cellular and humoral antibody formation in mice. Bact. Proc. 90–91 (1967).

CHAN, G.; RANCOURT, M. W.; CEGLOWSKI, W. S., and FRIEDMAN, H.: Leukemia virus suppression of antibody-forming cells: Ultrastructure of infected spleens. Science *159:* 437–439 (1968).

CHANDLER, R. L.: Attempts to demonstrate antibodies in scrapie disease. Vet. Rec. *71:* 58–59 (1959).

CHANDLER, R. L.: Encephalopathy in mice produced with scrapie brain material. Lancet *i:* 1378–1379 (1961).

CHANDLER, R. L.: Encephalopathy in mice. Lancet *i:* 107–108 (1962).

CHANDLER, R. L.: Transmissible encephalopathy in mice inoculated with scrapie brain material J. gen. Microbiol. *31:* XIV (1963a).

CHANDLER, R. L.: Experimental scrapie in the mouse. Res. Vet. Sci. *4:* 276–285 (1963b).

CHANDLER, R. L.: A degenerative disease of the nervous system of mice, produced by inoculation with scrapie brain material. Proc. 17th World Vet. Congr., Hanover *2:* 1575–1579 (1963c).

CHANDLER, R. L.: An experimental mixed infection of mice with scrapie and an oncogenic virus. J. comp. Path. *75:* 323–326 (1965).

CHANDLER, R. L.: Cytopathology of scrapie in the rat: An electron microscopic study of thalamic and hippocampal areas. Res. Vet. Sci. *8:* 98–102 (1967a).

CHANDLER, R. L.: Electron microscopic and other observations on the ependyma and small cerebral blood vessels in mice and rats affected with scrapie. Res. Vet. Sci. *8:* 166–169 (1967b).

CHANDLER, R. L.: Ultrastructural pathology of scrapie in the mouse: An electron microscopic study of spinal cord and cerebellar areas. Brit. J. exp. Path. *49:* 52–59 (1968).

CHANDLER, R. L. and SMITH, K.: Electron microscopic observations on scrapie in the mouse, with reference to glucosaminidase activity. Res. Vet. Sci. *9:* 228–230 (1968).

CHANG, H. T.; CH'IU, F. H., and WANG, H. C.: Lymphocytic choriomeningitis; Report of a chronic case. Chin. med. J. *72:* 113–117 (1954).

CHAPMAN, I. and JIMENEZ, F. A.: Aleutian-mink disease in man. New Engl. J. Med. *269:* 1171–1174 (1963).

CHASTEL, CL.: Technique des plages et de l'inhibition des plages en cultures cellulaires pour l'identification du virus de la chorioméningite lymphocytaire. Ann. Inst. Pasteur *109:* 874–886 (1965).

CHAUVEAU, J.; MOULÉ, Y.; ROUILIER, L., and SCHNEEBELI, J.: Isolation of smooth vesicles and free ribosomes from rat liver microsomes. J. cell Biol. *12:* 17–29 (1962).

CHELLE, P.: Un cas de tremblante chez la chèvre. Bull. Acad. vet. Fr. *15:* 294–295 (1942).

CHEN, T. T.; WATANABE, I.; ZEMAN, W., and MEALY, J., jr.: Subacute sclerosing panencephalitis. Propagation of measles virus from brain biopsy in tissue culture. Science *163:* 1193–1194 (1969).

Chou, S. M.: Myxovirus-like structures in a case of human chronic polymyositis. Science *158:* 1453–1455 (1967).

Clark, H. F.: Suckling mouse cataract agent. J. infect. Dis. *114:* 476–487 (1964).

Clark, H. F.: The suckling mouse cataract agent (SMCA) in mice: Studies on viral growth in eyes and viscera and the immune response. Thesis (Ph. D.). State University of New York at Buffalo, Buffalo, N. Y. (1967).

Clark, H. F.: Rat cataract induced by suckling mouse cataract agent. Amer. J. Ophthal. *68:* 304–308 (1969).

Clark, H. F. and Karzon, D. T.: Suckling mouse cataract agent (SMCA) in mice. I. Factors affecting the incidence of cataracts and growth of virus in several strains of mice. J. Immunol. *101:* 776–781 (1968a).

Clark, H. F. and Karzon, D. T.: Suckling mouse cataract agent (SMCA) in mice. II. Transfer of protection to progeny of SMCA-infected dams. J. Immunol. *101:* 782–787 (1968b).

Clark, H. F. and Karzon, D. T.: Suckling mouse cataract agent (SMCA) in mice. III. The antigenic specificity of maternal protection against SMCA and the comparative ability of other viruses to replicate in the eye of the suckling mouse. J. Immunol. *101:* 890–895 (1968c).

Clark, H. F. and Karzon, D. T.: Growth curve studies of the suckling mouse cataract agent in individual compartments of the eye. Proc. Soc. exp. Biol., N. Y. *131:* 693–696 (1969).

Clarke, M. C.: The antibody response of scrapie-affected mice to immunization with sheep red blood cells. Res. Vet. Sci. *9:* 595–597 (1968).

Clarke, M. C. and Haig, D. A.: Attempts to demonstrate neutralizing antibodies in the sera of scrapie-affected animals. Vet. Rec. *78:* 647–649 (1966).

Clarke, M. C. and Haig, D. A.: Presence of the transmissible agent of scrapie in the serum of affected mice and rats. Vet. Rec. *80:* 504 (1967).

Clarke, M. C. and Haig, D. A.: Evidence for the multiplication of scrapie agent in cell culture. Nature, Lond. *225:* 100–101 (1970).

Coggeshall, L. T.: The transmission of lymphocytic choriomeningitis by mosquitoes. Science *89:* 515–516 (1939).

Coggins, L. and Heuschele, W. P.: Use of agar diffusion precipitation test in the diagnosis of African swine fever. Amer. J. Vet. Res. *27:* 485–488 (1966).

Cohen, S. M.; Triandaphilli, I. A.; Barlow, J. L., and Hotchin, J.: Immunofluorescent detection of antibody to lymphocytic choriomeningitis virus in man. J. Immunol. *96:* 777–784 (1966).

Colgrove, G. S.; Haelterman, E. O., and Coggins, L.: Pathogenesis of African swine fever in young pigs. Amer. J. vet. Res. *30:* 1343–1359 (1969).

Collins, D. N. and Hotchin, J.: Glomerulonephritis and glomerulosclerosis as a late manifestation of persistent tolerant infection of mice with lymphocytic choriomeningitis virus. N. Y. State Dep. Health, Ann. Rep. Div. Lab. Res., pp. 100–101 (1963).

Collins, D. N.; Weigand, H., and Hotchin, J.: The effects of pretreatment with X-rays on the pathogenesis of lymphocytic choriomeningitis in mice. II. The pathological histology. J. Immunol. *87:* 682–687 (1961).

COLMORE, J. P.: Severe infections with the virus of lymphocytic choriomeningitis. J. amer. med. Ass. *148:* 1199—1201 (1952).

CONNOLLY, J. H.: Additional data on measles virus antibody and antigen in subacute sclerosing panencephalitis. Neurology, Minneap. *18:* 87–90 (1968).

COOPER, L. Z. and KRUGMAN, S.: Diagnosis and management: Congenital rubella. Pediatrics *37:* 335–338 (1966).

COOPER, L. Z. and KRUGMAN, S.: Clinical manifestations of postnatal and congenital rubella. Arch. Ophthal., Chicago *77:* 434–439 (1967).

COTLIER, E.; FOX, J., and SMITH, M.: Rubella virus in the cataractous lens of congenital rubella syndrome. Amer. J. Ophthal. *62:* 233–235 (1966).

COTO, C. E.; REY, E., and PARODI, A. S.: Tacaribe virus infection of guinea pig. Virus distribution, appearance of antibodies and immunity against Junin virus infection. Arch. ges. Virusforsch. *20:* 81–86 (1967).

COUGHLIN, J. and WHITNEY, E.: Lymphocytic choriomeningitis virus latently infecting monkey kidney tissue cultures. N. Y. State Dep. Health, Ann. Rep. Div. Lab. Res., pp. 37–38 (1957).

COWAN, K. M.: Immunological studies on African swine fever virus. I. Elimination of the procomplementary activity of swine serum with formalin. J. Immunol. *86:* 465–470 (1961).

COWAN, K. M.: Immunologic studies on African swine fever virus. II. Enhancing effect of normal bovine serum on the complement-fixation reaction. Amer. J. vet. Res. *24:* 756–761 (1963).

CRAWFORD, L. V.: A minute virus of mice. Virology *29:* 605–612 (1966).

CREECH, G. T. and GOCHENOUR, W. S.: Chronic progressive pneumonia with particular reference to its etiology and transmission. J. agric. Res. *52:* 667–679 (1936).

CRISPENS, C. G.: On the epizootiology of the lactic dehydrogenase agent. J. nat. Cancer Inst. *32:* 497–505 (1964a).

CRISPENS, C. G.: Mouse plasma lactic dehydrogenase elevation: Evidence for two particles. Virology *24:* 501–502 (1964b).

CRISPENS, C. G.: Preliminary studies on in utero transmission of the lactic dehydrogenase agent. Anat. Rec. *149:* 511 (1964c).

CRISPENS, C. G.: On the transmission of the lactic dehydrogenase agent from mother to offspring. J. nat. Cancer Inst. *34:* 331–335 (1965a).

CRISPENS, C. G.: On the properties of the lactic dehydrogenase agent. J. nat. Cancer Inst. *35:* 975–979 (1965b).

CRISPENS, C. G.: Properties of lactic dehydrogenase elevating agents. Anat. Rec. *151:* 448–449 (1965c).

CRISPENS, C. G.: Effect of thymectomy on mice infected with the lactate dehydrogenase agent. J. nat. Cancer Inst. *36:* 81–87 (1966).

CRISPENS, C. G.: Lactate dehydrogenase virus and mouse embryos. Nature, Lond. *214:* 819 (1967).

CRISPENS, C. G. and REY, I. F.: Additional studies on the effects of neonatal thymectomy and lactate dehydrogenase virus infection on mice. Experimentia *23:* 681–683 (1967).

CUILLÉ, J. et CHELLE, P. L.: La maladie dite tremblante du mouton est-elle inoculable? C. R. Acad. Sci. *203:* 1552–1554 (1936).

Cuillé, J. et Chelle, P. L.: La tremblante du mouton est bien inoculable. C. R. Acad. Sci. *206:* 78–79 (1938a).

Cuillé, J. et Chelle, P. L.: La tremblante du mouton. Son étologie (recherches cliniques et experimentales). Rev. Path. comp. *38:* 1358–1372 (1938b).

Cuillé, J. et Chelle, P. L.: La tremblante du mouton est-elle déterminée par un virus filtrable? C. R. Acad. Sci. *206:* 1687–1688 (1938c).

Cuillé, J. and Chelle, P. L.: Investigations of scrapie in sheep. Vet. Med. *34:* 417–418 (1939a).

Cuillé, J. et Chelle, P. L.: Transmission expérimentale de la tremblante à la chèvre. C. R. Acad. Sci. *208:* 1058–1060 (1939b).

Cutie, T. and Sikora, E.: Effect of Evans blue on the foot pad reaction to lymphocytic choriomeningitis virus. N. Y. State Dep. Health, Ann. Rep. Div. Lab. Res., p. 52 (1964).

Cutting, W.; Furusawa, E.; Furusawa, S., and Woo, Y. K.: Antiviral activity of herbs on Columbia SK in mice, LCM, vaccinia and adeno Type 12 viruses *in vitro.* Proc. Soc. exp. Biol., N. Y. *120:* 330–333 (1965).

Dalldorf, G.: The simultaneous occurrence of the viruses of canine distemper and lymphocytic choriomeningitis. J. exp. Med. *70:* 19–27 (1939a).

Dalldorf, G.: Studies of the sparing effect of lymphocytic choriomeningitis on experimental poliomyelitis. I. Effect on the infectivity of monkey tissues. J. Immunol. *37:* 245–259 (1939b).

Dalldorf, G.: Lymphocytic choriomeningitis of dogs. Cornell Vet. *33:* 347–350 (1943).

Dalldorf, G.: Viruses and cancer. Med. Clin. N. Amer. *45:* 753–768 (1961).

Dalldorf, G. and Douglass, M.: Simultaneous distemper and lymphocytic choriomeningitis in dog spleen and the sparing effect on poliomyelitis. Proc. Soc. exp. Biol., N. Y. *39:* 294–297 (1938).

Dalldorf, G.; Jungeblut, C. W. und Umphlet, M. D.: Multiple Fälle von Choriomeningitis in einer Wohnung, in welcher infizierte Mäuse festgestellt wurden. Wien med. Wschr. *96:* 473–474 (1946).

Dalton, A. J.; Kilham, L., and Zeigel, R. F.: A comparison of polyoma, 'K', and Kilham rat viruses with the electron microscope. Virology *20:* 391–398 (1963).

Dalton, A. J.; Rowe, W. P.; Smith, G. H.; Wilsnack, R. E., and Pugh, W. E.: Morphological and cytochemical studies on lymphocytic choriomeningitis virus. J. Virol. *2:* 1465–1478 (1968).

Dammann, P. T.: Zur Ätiologie der Traberkrankheit. Thierärztl. Umsch. 255 (1869).

Daneš, L.; Benda, R., i Fuchsová, M.: Experimentălnĭ inhalačni nakaza opic druhŭ *Macacus cynomolgus* a *Macacus rhesus* virem lymfocitarni choriomeningitidy (Kmenem WE). Bratsil. Lek. Listy *73:* 71–79 (1963).

Darcel, C. le Q.; Merriman, M.; Beauregard, M.; Avery, R. J., and Kasting, R.: Scrapie. I. Transmission and pathogenesis. Canad. J. comp. Med. *27:* 81–84 (1963).

David-Ferreira, J. F.; David-Ferreira, K. L.; Gibbs, C. J., jr., and Morris, J. A.: Scrapie in mice: Ultrastructural observations in the cerebral cortex. Proc. Soc. exp. Biol., N. Y. *127:* 313–320 (1968).

De Boer, C. J.: Antibody studies in animals infected with African swine fever virus (ASFV). Abstract. Fed. Proc. *26:* 7130 (1967a).

De Boer, C. J.: Studies to determine neutralizing antibody in sera from animals recovered from African swine fever and laboratory animals inoculated with African virus with adjuvants. Arch. ges. Virusforsch. *20:* 164–179 (1967b).

De Boer, C. J.; Hess, W. R., and Dardiri, A. H.: Studies to determine the presence of neutralizing antibody in sera and kidneys from swine recovered from African swine fever. Arch. ges. Virusforsch. *27:* 44–54 (1969).

DeBruyn, W. M.: A lymphopenia-causing agent, probably a virus, found in mice after injection with tumor tissue and with cell-free filtrates of lymphosarcoma T 86157 (MB). Cancer Res. *9:* 395–397 (1949).

Deibel, R.; Osterhout, G., and Quinlan, L.: Propagation of lymphocytic choriomeningitis virus in chick embryo fibroblast cells. N. Y. State Dep. Health, Ann. Rep. Div. Lab. Res., p. 50 (1964).

Deinhardt, F.; Holmes, A. W.; Capps, R. B., and Popper, H.: Studies on the transmission of human viral hepatitis to marmoset monkeys. I. Transmission of disease, serial passages, and description of liver lesions. J. exp. Med. *125:* 673–688 (1967).

DeKock, G.; Robbinson, E. M., and Keppel, J. J. G.: Swine fever in South Africa. Onderstepoort J. vet. Sci. *14:* 31–93 (1940).

Dent, P. B.; Olson, G. B.; Good, R. A.; Rawls, W. E., and South, M. A.: Rubella-virus/leucocyte interaction and its role in the pathogenesis of the congenital rubella syndrome. Lancet *i:* 291–293 (1968).

Desmond, M. M.; Wilson, G. S.; Melnick, J. L.; Singer, D. B.; Zion, T. E.; Rudolph, A. J.; Pineda, R. G.; Ziai, M., and Blattner, R. J.: Congenital rubella encephalitis. J. Pediat. *71:* 311–331 (1967).

Desmyter, J.; Rawls, W. E.; Melnick, J. L.; Yow, M. D., and Barrett, F. F.: Interferon in congenital rubella: response to live attenuated measles vaccine. J. Immunol. *99:* 771–777 (1967).

De-Thé G. and Notkins, A. L.: Ultrastructure of the lactic dehydrogenase virus (LDV) and cell-virus relationships. Virology *26:* 512–516 (1965).

DeTray, D. E.: Persistence of viremia and immunity in African swine fever. Amer. J. vet. Res. *18:* 811–816 (1957).

DeTray, D. E.: African swine fever. Adv. vet. Sci. *8:* 299–333 (1963).

DeTray, D. E. and Scott, G. R.: Blood changes in swine with African swine fever. Amer. J. vet. Res. *18:* 484–490 (1957).

DeTray, D. E.; Zaphiro, D., and Hay, D.: The incidence of African swine fever in wart hogs in Kenya – A preliminary report. J. amer. vet. med. Ass. *138:* 78–80 (1961).

Devries, M. J.; Putten, L. M.; Van Halner, H., et Bekkum, D. W.: Lésions suggérant une réactivité auto-immune chez des souris atteintes de la 'runt disease' après thymectomie néonatale. Rev. franç. et. clin. biol. *9:* 381–397 (1964).

Dick, G.; McAlister, J. J.; McKeown, F., and Campbell, A. M. G.: Multiple sclerosis and scrapie. J. Neurol. Neurosurg. Psychiat. *28:* 560–562 (1965).

Dickinson, A. G. and Fraser, H.: Genetical control of the concentration of ME7 scrapie agent in mouse spleen. J. comp. Path. *79:* 363–366 (1969a).

DICKINSON, A. G. and FRASER, H.: Modification of the pathogenesis of scrapie in mice by treatment of the agent. Nature, Lond. *222:* 892–893 (1969b).

DICKINSON, A. G. and MACKAY, J. M. K.: Genetical control of the incubation period in mice of the neurological disease, scrapie. Heredity *19:* 279–288 (1964).

DICKINSON, A. G. and MEIKLE, V. M. H.: A comparison of some biological characteristics of the mouse-passaged scrapie agents, 22A and ME7. Genet. Res. *13:* 213–225 (1969).

DICKINSON, A. G.; MACKAY, J. M. K., and ZLOTNIK, I.: Transmission by contact of scrapie in mice. J. comp. Path. *74:* 250–254 (1964).

DICKINSON, A. G.; YOUNG, G. B.; STAMP, J. T., and RENWICK, C. C.: The distribution of scrapie in sheep of different ages. Report of Scrapie Seminar, Washington, D. C., 1964, pp. 207–213 (US Dept. of Agriculture, ARS 91–53, Washington, D. C. 1996a).

DICKINSON, A. G.; YOUNG, G. B., and RENWICK, C. C.: Scrapie: Experiments involving maternal transmission in sheep. Report of Scrapie Seminar, Washington, D. C., 1964, pp. 244–248 (US Dept. of Agriculture, ARS 91–53, Washington, D. C. 1966b).

DICKINSON, A. G.; STAMP, J. T.; RENWICK, C. C., and SMITH, W.: Genetical control of susceptibility to experimental challenge with scrapie in Cheviot sheep. Report of Scrapie Seminar, Washington, D. C., 1964, pp. 249–250 (US Dept. of Agriculture, ARS 91–53, Washington, D. C. 1966c).

DICKINSON, A. G.; MACKAY, J. M. K., and ZLOTNIK, I.: Transmission by contact of scrapie in mice. Report of Scrapie Seminar, Washington, D. C., 1964, pp. 259–163 (US Dept. of Agriculture, ARS 91–53, Washington, D. C. 1966d).

DICKINSON, A. G.; YOUNG, G. B.; STAMP, J. T., and RENWICK, C. C.: Scrapie in Suffolk sheep. A genetical investigation using experimental matings. Report of Scrapie Seminar, Washington, D. C., 1964, pp. 228–244 (US Dept. of Agriculture, ARS 91–53, Washington, D. C. 1966e).

DICKINSON, A. G.; STAMP, J. T.; RENWICK, C. C., and RENNIE, J. C.: Some factors controlling the incidence of scrapie in Cheviot sheep injected with a Cheviot-passaged scrapie agent. J. comp. Path. *78:* 313–321 (1968a).

DICKINSON, A. G.; MEIKLE, V. M. H., and FRASER, H.: Identification of a gene which controls the incubation period of some strains of scrapie agent in mice. J. comp. Path. *78:* 293–299 (1968b).

DIOSI, P.; BABUSCEAC, L.; NEVINGLOVSCHI, O., and STOICANESCU, A.: Duration of cytomegaloviruria in nursery children. Path. Microbiol. *29:* 513–518 (1966).

DIOSI, P.; BABUSCEAC, L., and DAVID, C.: Recovery of cytomegalovirus from the submaxillary glands of ground squirrels. Arch. ges. Virusforsch. *20:* 383–386 (1967).

DITCHFIELD, J.: Equine infectious anemia. A review of the disease and diagnostic tests. Canad. vet. J. *8:* 273–278 (1967).

DITCHFIELD, W. J. B.; WADDELL, G. H.; SAURINO, V. R., and TEIGLAND, M. B.: A preliminary evaluation of serologic tests for equine infectious anemia. J. amer. vet. med. Ass. *151:* 1840–1846 (1967).

DIXON, M. and WEBB, E. C.: Enzymes, 2nd ed. (Academic Press, New York 1964).

DMOCHOWSKI, L.; RECHER, L.; TANAKA, T.; YUMOTO, T.; SYKES, J. A., and YOUNG, L.: Studies on the biologic relationship of some murine leukemia viruses. Cancer Res. *26:* 382–394 (1966).

DOBBERSTEIN, J.: Kritische Betrachtungen zur Pathogenese der ansteckenden Blutarmut des Pferdes. Berl. Münch. tierärztl. Wschr. *50:* 192–196 (1934).

DOLESCHALL, F. VON und PAUL, B.: Zur Frage der Meningitis serosa epidemica. Gehäuftes Auftreten in Debrecen Mai bis August 1935. Dtsch. Arch. klin. Med. *178:* 341–352 (1936).

DOWNS, W. G.; ANDERSON, C. R.; SPENCE, L.; AITKEN, T. H. G., and GREENHALL, A. H.: Tacaribe virus, a new agent isolated from *Artibeus* bats and mosquitoes in Trinidad, West Indies. Amer. J. trop. Med. Hyg. *12:* 640–646 (1963).

DRAPER, G. J.: 'Epidemics' caused by a late-manifesting gene. Application to scrapie. Heredity *18:* 165–171 (1963).

DRAPER, G. J. and PARRY, H. B.: Scrapie in sheep: The hereditary component in high incidence environment. Nature, Lond. *195:* 670–672 (1962).

DREESMAN, G. R. and BENYESH-MELNICK, M.: Spectrum of human cytomegalovirus complement-fixing antigens. J. Immunol. *99:* 1106–1114 (1967).

DREGUSS, M. N.: Hemagglutination of chicken cells by serum of horses infected with the virus of infectious anemia. Vet. ext. Quart. Univ. Pa. *116:* 3–13 (1949).

DREGUSS, M. N. and LOMBARD, L. S.: Experimental studies in equine infectious anemia (Oxford University Press, London 1954).

DUBUY, H. and JOHNSON, M. L.: Studies on the *in vivo* and *in vitro* multiplication of the LDH virus of mice. J. exp. Med. *123:* 985–998 (1966).

DUBUY, H. G. and JOHNSON, M. L.: Further studies on the *in vitro* replication of lactic dehydrogenase virus in peritoneal macrophage cultures. Proc. Soc. exp. Biol., N. Y. *128:* 1210–1214 (1968).

DUDGEON, J. A.: Rubella. Clinical aspects of prenatal and postnatal infection. Publ. Hlth, Lond. *81:* 268–279 (1967a).

DUDGEON, J. A.: Rubella; in Modern trends in medical virology, vol. 1., 110–140 (Butterworths, London 1967b).

DUDGEON, J. A.; BUTLER, N. R., and PLOTKIN, S. A.: Further serological studies on the rubella syndrome. Brit. med. J. *ii:* 155–160 (1964).

DUNGAL, N.; GILASON, G., and TAYLOR, E. L.: Epizootic adenomatosis in the lungs of sheep. Comparisons with Jaagsiekte, verminous pneumonia and progressive pneumonia. J. comp. Path. *51:* 46–68 (1938).

DURAN-REYNALS, F.; JUNGHERR, E.; CUBA-CAPARÓ, A.; RAFFERTY, K. A., jr., and HELMBOLDT, C.: The pulmonary adenomatosis complex in sheep. Ann. N. Y. Acad. Sci. *70:* 726–742 (1958).

EAGLE, H.; HABEL, K.; ROWE, W. P., and HUEBNER, R. J.: Viral susceptibility of a human carcinoma cell (strain KB). Proc. Soc. exp. Biol., N. Y. *91:* 361–364 (1956).

EAST, J.; PARROTT, D. M. V., and SEAMER, J.: The ability of mice thymectomized at birth to survive infection with lymphocytic choriomeningitis virus. Virology *22:* 160–162 (1964).

EGGERS, H. J.: Quantitative investigations on the complement-fixation reaction and lymphocytic choriomeningitis. Arch. ges. Virusforsch. *8:* 221–229 (1958).

EKLUND, C. M.; HADLOW, W. J., and KENNEDY, R. C.: Some properties of the scrapie agent and its behavior in mice. Proc. Soc. exp. Biol., N. Y. *112:* 974–979 (1963).

EKLUND, C. M.; KENNEDY, R. C., and HADLOW, W. J.: Pathogenesis of scrapie virus infection in the mouse. NINDB Monograph No. 2. Slow, latent and temperate virus infections. pp. 207–208 (US Dept. of Health, Education and Welfare, Washington, D. C. 1965).

EKLUND, C. M.; KENNEDY, R. C., and HADLOW, W. J.: Evolution of scrapie virus infection in mice. Report of Scrapie Seminar, Washington, D. C., 1964, pp. 288–291 (US Dept. of Agriculture, ARS 91–53, Washington, D. C. 1966).

EKLUND, C. M.; KENNEDY, R. C., and HADLOW, W. J.: Pathogenesis of scrapie virus infection in the mouse. J. infect. Dis. *117:* 15–22 (1967).

EKLUND, C. M.; HADLOW, W. J.; KENNEDY, R. C.; BOYLE, C. C., and JACKSON, T. A.: Aleutian disease of mink: Properties of the etiologic agent and the host responses. J. infect. Dis. *118:* 510–526 (1968).

ELIZAN, T. S.; FABIYI, A., and SEVER, J. L.: Study of rubella virus as a teratogen in experimental animals: A short review. J. Mount Sinai Hosp. N. Y. *36:* 108–112 (1969).

ELI-ZEIN, A.; MYERS, W. L., and SEGRE, D.: Behavior of equine infectious anemia virus in cell culture and development of a diagnostic test for the disease. J. infect. Dis. *118:* 473–480 (1968).

EVANS, R. and RILEY, V.: Circulating interferon in mice infected with the lactate dehydrogenase-elevating virus. J. gen. Virol. *3:* 449–452 (1968).

EVANS, R. and SALAMAN, M. H.: Studies on the mechanism of action of Riley virus. III. Replication of Riley's plasma enzyme-elevating virus *in vitro*. J. exp. Med. *122:* 993–1002 (1965).

FARMER, T. W. and JANEWAY, C. A.: Infections with the virus of lymphocytic choriomeningitis. Medicine *21:* 1–63 (1942).

FEDOROV, Iu. V.; IGOLKIN, N. I., and TYUSHNYAKOVA, M. K.: Some data on fleas, virus-carriers in foci of tick-borne encephalitis and lymphocytic choriomeningitis. Meditsinskaia parazitologiia i parazitarnye bolezni (Moskva) *28:* 149–152 (1959).

FELDMAN, R. A.: Cytomegaloviruses in stored urine specimens. A quantitative study. J. Pediat. *73:* 611–614 (1968).

FERM, V. H. and KILHAM, L.: Congenital anomalies induced in hamster embryo with H-1 virus. Science *145:* 510–511 (1964).

FERM, V. H. and KILHAM, L.: Histopathologic basis of the teratogenic effects of H-1 virus on hamster embryos. J. Embryol. exp. Morph. *13:* 151–158 (1965a).

FERM, V. H. and KILHAM, L.: Skeletal studies of virus-induced dwarfism. Growth *29:* 7–16 (1965b).

FERNANDES, M. V.; WIKTOR, T. J., and KOPROWSKI, H.: Mechanism of the cytopathic effect of rabies virus in tissue culture. Virology *21:* 128–131 (1963).

Fernandes, M. V.; Wiktor, T. J., and Koprowski, H.: Endosymbiotic relationship between animal viruses and host cells. A study of rabies virus in tissue culture. J. exp. Med. *120:* 1099–1116 (1964).

Field, E. J.: Transmission experiments with multiple sclerosis. An interim report. Brit. med. J. *ii:* 564–565 (1966).

Field, E. J.: Invasion of the mouse nervous system by scrapie agent. Brit. J. exp. Path. *48:* 662–664 (1967).

Field, E. J.: Transmission of kuru to mice. Lancet *i:* 981–982 (1968).

Field, E. J. and Raine, C. S.: An electron microscopic study of scrapie in the mouse. Acta neuropath. *4:* 200–211 (1964).

Field, E. J. and Raine, C. S.: Observations on 'dense-body' structure in nerve cells with special reference to scrapie. Res. Vet. Sci. *7:* 292–295 (1966).

Field, E. J. and Windsor, G. D.: Cultural characters of scrapie mouse brain. Res. Vet. Sci. *6:* 130–132 (1965).

Field, E. J.; Miller, H., and Russell, D. S.: Observations on glial inclusion bodies in a case of acute disseminated sclerosis. J. clin. Path. *15:* 278–284 (1962).

Field, E. J.; Caspary, E. A., and Windsor, G. D.: Sodium and potassium in scrapie brain. Res. Vet. Sci. *7:* 72–73 (1966).

Field, E. J.; Raine, C. S., and Joyce, G.: Scrapie in the rat: an electron-microscope study. I. Amyloid bodies and deposits. Acta neuropath. *8:* 47–56 (1967).

Findlay, G. M. and Stern, R. O.: Pathological changes due to infection with the virus of lymphocytic choriomeningitis. J. Path. Bact. *43:* 327–338 (1936).

Findlay, G. M.; Alcock, N. S., and Stern, R. O.: The virus aetiology of one form of lymphocytic meningitis. Lancet *i:* 650–654 (1936).

Findlay, G. M.; Kleinberger, E.; Maccallum, F. O., and Mackenzie, R. D.: Rolling disease. New syndrome in mice associated with a pleuropneumonia-like organism. Lancet *ii:* 1511–1513 (1938).

Fitzsimmons, W. M. and Pattison, I. H.: Unsuccessful attempts to transmit scrapie by nematode parasites. Res. Vet. Sci. *9:* 281–283 (1968).

Földes, P.; Szeri, I.; Bános, Z.; Anderlik, P., and Balázs, M.: LCM infection of mice thymectomized in newborn age. Acta microbiol. hung. *11:* 277–282 (1964).

Fortner, J.: Über das Dauervirusträgertum bei ansteckender Blutarmut der Einhufer. Dtsch. tierärztl. Wschr. *52:* 265–266 (1944).

Fortner, J. et Ulbrich, F.: Etat actuel de nos expériences sur la transmission de l'anémie infectieuse des équinés à des petits animaux d'expérience. Bull. off. int. Epizoot. *42:* 737–742 (1952).

Foster, K. M. and Jack, I.: Isolation of cytomegalovirus from the blood leucocytes of a patient with post-transfusion mononucleosis. Austr. Ann. Med. *14:* 135–140 (1968).

Fowler, M. and Robertson, E. G.: Observations on kuru. III. Pathological features in five cases. Austr. Ann. Med. *8:* 16–26 (1959).

Frame, J. D.; Baldwin, J. M., jr.; Gocke, D. J., and Traup, J. M.: Lassa fever, a new virus disease of man from West Africa. I. Clinical description and pathological findings. Amer. J. trop. Med. Hyg. *19:* 670–676 (1970).

Frantsi, C.: Reproduction of the Riley virus in cell culture and its interaction with the Friend leukemia virus. M. Sc. Thesis, University of Guelph, Guelph, Ontario, Canada (1968).

Frantsi, C. and Gregory, K. F.: Reproduction of the lactate dehydrogenase-elevating (Riley) virus in mouse embryonic liver cell cultures. Virology *37:* 145–148 (1969).

Fraser, H.: The occurrence of nerve fibre degeneration in brains of mice inoculated with scrapie. Res. vet. Sci. *10:* 338–341 (1969).

Fraser, H. and Dickinson, A. G.: Distribution of experimentally induced scrapie lesions in the brain. Nature, Lond. *216:* 1310–1311 (1967).

Fraser, H. and Dickinson, A. G.: The sequential development of the brain lesions of scrapie in three strains of mice. J. comp. Path. *78:* 301–311 (1968).

Friedmann, J. C.: L'anémie infectieuse des équinés. Nouv. Rev. franç. Hémat. *4:* 421–442 (1964).

Furusawa, E. and Cutting, W.: Antiviral activity of higher plants on lymphocytic choriomeningitis *in vitro* and *in vivo*. Proc. Soc. exp. Biol., N. Y. *122:* 280–282 (1966).

Furusawa, E.; Cutting, W., and Furst, A.: Inhibitory effect of antiviral compounds on Columbia SK, LCM, vaccinia and adeno type 12 viruses *in vitro*. Chemotherapie *8:* 95–105 (1964).

Furusawa, E.; Ramanathan, S.; Furusawa, S.; Woo, Y. K., and Cutting, W.: Antiviral activity of higher plants and propionin on lymphocytic choriomeningitis infection. Proc. Soc. exp. Biol., N. Y. *125:* 234–239 (1967).

Furusawa, E.; Furusawa, S.; Kroposki, M., and Cutting, W.: Activity of *Sambucus sieboldiana* on Columbia SK and LCM virus infection in mice. Proc. soc. Exp. Biol., N. Y. *128:* 1196–1199 (1968).

Gajdusek, D. C.: Kuru. Trans. roy. Soc. trop. Med. Hyg. *57:* 151–169 (1963).

Gajdusek D. C.: A kuru research laboratory at the Awande kuru center; in: Annual Report of the Lutheran Missions in New Guinea, Lae, Territory of New Guinea (1967).

Gajdusek, D. C.: Kuru and experimental kuru in chimpanzees. Presented at the 13th Sci. Session of the Inst. for Poliomyelitis and Virus Encephalitides, Acad. of Med. Sci., USSR, Moscow, June 27–30, 1967. Issued in modified form as a Document of the Meeting of Investigators on the Genetics of Primitive Groups (Wld. Hlth Org., Geneva, July 3–7, 1967a).

Gajdusek, D. C.: Discussion on kuru, scrapie and the experimental kuru-like syndrome in chimpanzees; in: Current topics in microbiology, vol. 40, pp. 59–63 (Springer, New York 1967b).

Gajdusek, D. C. and Alpers, M. C.: Kuru in childhood: Disappearance of the disease in the younger age group. J. Pediat. *69:* 886–887 (1966).

Gajdusek, D. C. and Gibbs, C. J.: Attempts to demonstrate a transmissible agent in kuru, amyotrophic lateral sclerosis, and other sub-acute and chronic nervous system degenerations of man. Nature, Lond. *204:* 257–259 (1964).

Gajdusek, D. C. and Zigas, V.: Kuru. Clinical, pathological and epidemiological study of an acute progressive degenerative disease of the central nervous system among natives of the Eastern Highlands of New Guinea. Amer. J. Med. *26:* *442–469 (1959).*

GAJDUSEK, D. C.; GIBBS, C. J., and ALPERS, M.: Experimental transmission of a kuru-like syndrome to chimpanzees. Nature, Lond. *209:* 794–796 (1966).

GAJDUSEK, D. C.; GIBBS, C. J., jr., and ALPERS, M.: Transmission and passage of experimental 'kuru' to chimpanzees. Science *155:* 212–214 (1967).

GAJDUSEK D. C.; GIBBS, C. J., jr.; ASHER, D. M., and DAVID, E.: Transmission of experimental kuru to the spider monkey (*Ateles geoffreyi).* Science *162:* 693–694 (1968).

GALLAGHER, N. D. and GOULSTON, S. J. M.: Persistent acute viral hepatitis. Brit. med. J. *i:* 906–908 (1962).

GARDINER, A. C.: Gel diffusion reactions of tissues and sera from scrapie-affected animals. Res. Vet. Sci. *7:* 190–195 (1965).

GARDINER, A. C. and MARUCCI, A. A.: Immunological responsiveness of scrapie infected mice. J. comp. Path. *79:* 233–235 (1969).

GEORGII, A.; LENZ, I., and ZOBEL, H.: Penetration of the placental barrier by the lactate dehydrogenase-elevating virus (Riley) and its behavior in mouse embryo cultures following infection *in utero.* Proc. Soc. exp. Biol., N. Y. *117:* 322–326 (1964).

GIBBONS, R. A. and HUNTER, G. D.: Nature of the scrapie agent. Nature, Lond. *215:* 1041–1043 (1967a).

GIBBONS, R. A. and HUNTER, G. D.: A consideration of the nature of the scrapie agent – a membrane hypothesis. Biochem. J. *105:* 7P (1967b).

GIBBS, C. J., jr.: Search for infectious etiology in chronic and subacute degenerative disease of the central nervous system; in: Current topics in microbiology, vol. 40, pp. 44–58 (Springer, New York 1967).

GIBBS, C. J. and GAJDUSEK, D. C.: General considerations of slow virus infections. Int. Symp. on Rabies, France 1965; Series immunobiol. Standard vol. 1, pp. 131–146 (Karger, Basel/New York 1966).

GIBBS, C. J. and GAJDUSEK, D. C.: The epidemiology of slow virus infection. Trans. 32nd North American Wildlife and Natural Resources Conference, pp. 396–404 (Wildlife Management Institute, Washington 1967).

GIBBS, C. J., jr. and GAJDUSEK, D. C.: Infection as the etiology of spongiform encephalopathy (Creutzfeldt-Jakob disease). Science *165:* 1023–1025 (1969).

GIBBS, C. J., jr.; GAJDUSEK, D. C., and MORRIS, J. A.: Viral characteristics of the scrapie agent in mice. NINDB Monograph No. 2. Slow, latent and temperate virus infections, pp. 195–202 (US Dept. of Health, Education and Welfare, Washington, D. C. 1965).

GIBBS, C. J., jr.; GAJDUSEK, D. C., and MORRIS, J. A.: Further observations in mice following inoculation of scrapie goat and sheep brain material. Report of Scrapie Seminar, Washington, D. C., 1964, pp. 292–298 (US Dept. of Agriculture, ARS 91–53, Washington, D. C. 1966).

GIBBS, C. J.; GAJDUSEK, D. C.; ASHER, D. M.; ALPERS, M. P.; BECK, E.; DANIEL, P. M., and MATTHEWS, W. B.: Creutzfeldt-Jakob disease (spongiform encephalopathy): Transmission to the chimpanzee. Scienc*e 161:* 388–389 (1968).

GILES, J. P.; MCCOLLUM, R. W.; BERNDSON, L. W., jr., and KRUGMAN, S.: Viral hepatitis. Relation of Australia/SH antigen to the Willowbrook MS-2 strain. New Engl. J. Med. *281:* 119–122 (1969).

GINOZA, W.: Radiosensitive molecular weight of single stranded virus nucleic acids. Nature, Lond. *199:* 453–456 (1963).

GLASGOW, L. A.; HANSHAW, J. B.; MERIGAN, T. C., and PETRALLI, J. K.: Interferon and cytomegalovirus *in vivo* and *in vitro*. Proc. Soc. exp. Biol., N. Y. *125:* 843–849 (1967).

GLASSE, R. M.: The spread of kuru among the Fore: A preliminary report. Mimeographed manuscript. Dept. of Publ. Hlth., Territory of Papua and New Guinea (1962).

GLASSE, R. M.: Cannibalism in the kuru region. Mimeographed manuscript. Dept. of Publ. Hlth., Territory of Papua and New Guinea (1963).

GLATZEL, H.: Zur Frage der gutartigen lymphocytären Meningitis. Klin. Wschr. *17:* 1360–1362 (1938).

GLEDHILL, A. W.: Fatal effect of some bacterial toxins on mice preinfected with mouse hepatitis virus (MHVI). J. gen. Microbiol. *18:* xvii (1958).

GLEDHILL, A. W.: Protective effect of anti-lymphocytic serum on murine lymphocytic choriomeningitis. Nature, Lond. *214:* 178–179 (1967).

GLEDHILL, A. W. and NIVEN, J. S. F.: The toxicity of some bacterial filtrates for mice pre-infected with *Eperythrozoon coccoides*. Brit. J. exp. Path. *38:* 284–290 (1957).

GLEDHILL, A. W. and SEAMER, J.: The effect of *Eperythrozoon coccoides* upon lymphocytic choriomeningitis in mice. N. Y. State Dep. Health, Ann. Rep. Div. Lab. Res., p. 21 (1960).

GLEDHILL, A. W.; SEAMER, J., and HOTCHIN, J.: The relationship between mouse hepatitis and lymphocytic choriomeningitis viruses. N. Y. State Dep. Health, Ann. Rep. Div. Lab. Res., p. 24 (1960).

GOCKE, D. J. and KAVEY, N. B.: Hepatitis antigen. Correlation with disease and infectivity of blood donor. Lancet *i:* 1055–1059 (1969).

GOLDBERG, S. A.; BRODIE, M., and STANLEY, D.: Effect of X-ray on experimental encephalitis in mice inoculated with St. Louis strain. Proc. Soc. exp. Biol., N. Y. *32:* 587–590 (1935).

GORDON, W. S.: Advances in veterinary research. Vet. Rec. *58:* 516–525 (1946).

GORDON, W. S.: Discussion of paper by PALMER. Vet. Rec. *69:* 1324 (1957).

GORDON, W. S.: Variation in susceptibility of sheep to scrapie and genetic implications. Report of Scrapie Seminar, Washington, D. C., 1964, pp. 53–68 (US Dept. of Agriculture, ARS 91–53, Washington, D. C. 1966a).

GORDON, W. S.: Transmission of scrapie and evidence of spread of infection in sheep at pasture. Report of Scrapie Seminar, Washington, D. C., 1964, pp. 8–18 (US Dept. of Agriculture, ARS 91–53, Washington, D. C. 1966b).

GORDON, W. S.: Review of work on scrapie at Compton, England, 1952–1964. Report of Scrapie Seminar, Washington, D. C., 1964, pp. 19–40 (US Dept. of Agriculture, ARS 91–53, Washington, D. C. 1966c).

GORDON, W. S.; BROWNLEE, A., and WILSON, D. R.: Studies in louping-ill, tick-borne fever and scrapie. Proc. 3rd int. Congr. Microbiol., New York, 1939, pp. 362–363 (Waverly Press. Inc., 1940).

GORDON, D. A.; FRANKLIN, A. E., and KARSTAD, L.: Viral plasmacytosis (Aleutian disease) of mink resembling human collagen disease. Canad. med. Ass. J. *96:* 1245–1251 (1967).

GORHAM, J. R.; LEADER, R. W., and HENSON, J. B.: Neutralizing ability of hypergammaglobulinemic serum on the Aleutian disease virus of mink. Abstract. Fed. Proc. *22:* 265 (1963).

GORHAM, J. R.; LEADER, R. W., and HENSON, J. B.: The experimental transmission of a virus causing hypergammaglobulinemia in mink: Sources and modes of infection. J. infect. Dis. *114:* 341–345 (1964).

GORHAM, J. R.; LEADER, R. W.; PADGETT, G. A.; BURGER, D., and HENSON, J. B.: Some observations on the natural occurrence of Aleution disease. NINDB Monograph No. 2. Slow, latent and temperate virus infections. pp. 279–285 (US Dept. of Health, Education and Welfare, Washington, D. C. 1965).

GORHAM, J. R.; HENSON, J. B.; PADGETT, G. A., and McGUIRE, T. C.: Aleutian disease; in: Infectious diseases of wild mammals (Iowa State College Press, in press).

GREIG, J. R.: Scrapie. Observations on the transmission of the disease by mediate contact. Vet. J. *96:* 203–206 (1940a).

GREIG, J. R.: Scrapie. Trans. highl. agric. soc. Scot. *52:* 71–90 (1940b).

GREIG, J. R.: Scrapie in sheep. J. comp. Path. *60:* 263–266 (1950).

GREŠIKOVÁ, M. and CASALS, J.: A simple method of preparing a complement-fixing antigen for lymphocytic choriomeningitis virus. Acta Virol. *7:* 380 (1963).

GRESSER, I. and PATTISON, I. H.: An attempt to modify scrapie in mice by the administration of interferon. J. gen. Virol. *3:* 295–297 (1968).

GRIFFITH, J. S.: Self-replication and scrapie. Nature, Lond. *215:* 1043–1044 (1967).

GRIFFITH, J. F. and KATZ, S. L.: Subacute sclerosing panencephalitis, laboratory findings in 6 cases. Neurology, Minneap. *18:* 98–100 (1968).

GRUN, R.: Über benigne fieberhafte lymphocytäre Meningitis unbekannter Ätiologie. Dtsch. Arch. klin. Med. *172:* 429–442 (1932).

GUDNADÓTTIR, M.: Experiments with maedi, a chronic progressive virus disease affecting the lungs of sheep in Iceland. Unio Nordica Contra Cancrum, Symposium on Virus and Cancer, Stockholm, 1964, pp. 49–58 (Swedish Cancer Soc., Stockholm 1965).

GUDNADÓTTIR, M.: Host-virus interaction in maedi-infected sheep. Lung tumours in animals, June 24–29, Perugia, Italy. Division of Cancer Research, Univ. of Perugia, pp. 381–391 (1966).

GUDNADÓTTIR, M. and KRISTINSDÓTTIR, K.: Complement-fixing antibodies in sera of sheep affected with visna and maedi. J. Immunol. *98:* 663–667 (1967).

GUDNADÓTTIR, M. and PÁLSSON, P. A.: Successful transmission of visna by intrapulmonary inoculation. J. infect. Dis. *115:* 217–225 (1965).

GUDNADÓTTIR, M. and PÁLSSON, P. A.: Host-virus interaction in visna infected sheep. J. Immunol. *95:* 1116–1120 (1966).

GUDNADÓTTIR, M. and PÁLSSON, P. A.: Transmission of maedi by inoculation of a virus grown in tissue culture from maedi-affected lungs. J. infect. Dis. *117:* 1–6 (1967).

GUDNADÓTTIR, M.; HELGADÓTTIR, H.; BJARNASON, O., and JÓNSDÓTTIR, K.: Virus isolated from the brain of a patient with multiple sclerosis. Exp. Neurol. *9:* 85–95 (1964).

GUDNADÓTTIR, M.; GÌSLASON, G., and PÁLSSON P. A.: Studies on natural cases of maedi in search for diagnostic laboratory methods. Res. Vet. Sci. *9:* 65–67 (1968).

GUNTHER, A.: Über akute 'aseptische' Meningitis. Jb. Kinderh. phys. Erzieh. *128:* 127–154 (1930).

GUSTAFSON, D. P. and KANITZ, C. L.: *In vitro* studies of scrapie virus. Abstract. Fed. Proc. *24:* 248 (1965a).

GUSTAFSON, D. P. and KANITZ, C. L.: Evidence of the presence of scrapie in cell cultures of brain. NINDB Monograph No. 2. Slow, latent and temperate virus infections, pp. 221–236 (US Dept. of Health, Education and Welfare, Washington, D. C. 1965b).

GUSTAFSON, D. P. and KANITZ, C. L.: Long-term cell cultures from the brain of a sheep affected with scrapie. Report of Scrapie Seminar, Washington, D. C., 1964, pp. 69–92 (US Dept. of Agriculture, ARS 91–53, Washington, D. C. 1966).

HAAS, V. H.: Studies on the natural history of the virus of lymphocytic choriomeningitis in mice. Publ. Hlth. Rep., Wash. *56:* 285–292 (1941).

HAAS, V. H.: Some relationships between lymphocytic choriomeningitis (LCM) virus and mice. J. infect. Dis. *94:* 187–198 (1954).

HAAS, V. H.: Serial passage of a lymphocytic tumor and choriomeningitis virus in immune mice. J. nat. Cancer Inst. *25:* 75–83 (1960).

HAAS, V. H. and STEWART, S. E.: Sparing effect of amethopterin and guanazolo in mice with the virus of lymphocytic choriomeningitis. Virology *2:* 511–516 (1956).

HAAS, V. H.; BRIGGS, G. M., and STEWART, S. E.: Inapparent lymphocytic choriomeningitis infection in folic acid-deficient mice. Science *126:* 405–406 (1957a).

HAAS, V. H.; STEWART, S. E., and BRIGGS, G. M.: Folic acid deficiency and the sparing of mice infected with the virus of lymphocytic choriomeningitis. Virology *3:* 15–21 (1957b).

HADLOW, W. J.: Myopathies of livestock. Lab. Invest. *8:* 1478–1498 (1959a).

HADLOW, W. J.: Scrapie and kuru. Lancet *ii:* 289–290 (1959b).

HADLOW, W. J.: The pathology of experimental scrapie in the dairy goat. Res. Vet. Sci. *2:* 289–314 (1961).

HADLOW, W. J. and KARSTAD, L.: Transmissible encephalopathy of mink in Ontario. Canad. vet. J. *9:* 193–196 (1968).

HAIG, D. A. and CLARKE, M. C.: Observations on the agent of scrapie. NINDB Monograph No. 2. Slow, latent and temperate virus infections, pp. 215–219 (US Dept. of Health, Education und Welfare, Washington, D. C. 1965).

HAIG, D. A. and PATTISON, I. H.: *In vitro* growth of pieces of brain from scrapie-affected mice. J. Path. Bact. 93: 724–727 (1967).

HAIG, D. A.; CLARKE, M. C.; BLUM, E., and ALPER, T.: Further studies on the inactivation of the scrapie agent by ultraviolet light. J. gen. Virol. *5:* 455–457 (1969).

HAMBIDGE, K. M.; SHAFFER, D.; MARSHALL, W. C., and HAYES, K.: Congenital rubella: Report of two cases with generalized infection. Brit. med. J. *1:* 650–652 (1966).

HAMPERS, C. L.; KOLKER, P., and HAGER, E. B.: Isolation and characterization of antibodies and other immunologically reactive substances from rejecting renal allografts. J. Immunol. *99:* 514–525 (1967).

HANCOCK, M. P.; HUNTLEY, C. C., and SEVER, J. L.: Congenital rubella syndrome with immunoglobulin disorder. J. Pediat. *72:* 636–645 (1968).

HANOAKA, M.; SUZUKI, S., and HOTCHIN, J.: Destruction of thymus dependent lymphocytes by lymphocytic choriomeningitis virus. Science *163:* 1216–1219 (1969).

HANSHAW, J. B.: Cytomegaloviruses; in: Monographs in virology, vol. 3, pp. 1–23 (Springer, New York 1968).

HANSHAW, J. B.; STEINFELD, H. J., and WHITE, C. J.: Fluorescent-antibody test for cytomegalovirus macroglobulin. New Engl. J. Med. *279:* 566–570 (1968).

HARDING, J. D. J.; DONE, J. T., and DARBYSHIRE, J. H.: Congenital tremors in piglets and their relation to swine fever. Vet. Rec. *79:* 388–390 (1966).

HARNDEN, D. G.; ELSDALE, T. R.; YOUNG, D. E., and ROSS, A.: The isolation of cytomegalovirus from peripheral blood. Blood *30:* 120–125 (1967).

HARTER, D. H. and CHOPPIN, P. W.: Plaque assay of visna virus using a secondary cellular overlay as an indicator. Virology *31:* 176–178 (1967a).

HARTER, D. H. and CHOPPIN, P. W.: Cell-fusing activity of visna virus particles. Virology *31:* 279–288 (1967b).

HARTER, D. H. and TELLEZ-NAGEL, I.: Attempts to isolate SSPE agents in cell culture. Neurology, Minneap. *18:* 133–137 (1968).

HARTER, D. H.; HSU, K. C., and ROSE, H. M.: Immuno-fluorescence and cytochemical studies of visna virus in cell culture. J. Virol. *1:* 1265–1270 (1967).

HARTER, D. H.; HSU, K. C., and ROSE, H. M.: Multiplication of visna virus in bovine and porcine cell lines. Proc. Soc. exp. Biol., N. Y. *129:* 295–300 (1968).

HARTLEY, E. G.: Action of disinfectants on experimental mouse scrapie. Nature, Lond. *213:* 1135 (1967).

HARTSOUGH, G. R. and BURGER, D.: Encephalopathy of mink. I. Epizootiologic and clinical observations. J. infect. Dis. *115:* 387–392 (1965).

HARTSOUGH, G. R. and GORHAM, J. R.: Aleutian disease in mink. Nat. Fur News *28:* 10–11 (1956).

HASHIMI, A.; CARRUTHERS, M. M.; WOLF, P., and LERNER, A. M.: Congenital infections with reovirus. J. exp. Med. *124:* 33–46 (1966).

HASSAN, S. A. and COCHRAN, K. W.: Teratogenicity of reo and poliovirus in mice. Abstract. Bact. Proc., p. 115 (1966).

HAYES, G. S. and HARTMAN, T. L.: Lymphocytic choriomeningitis; report of laboratory infection. Bull. Johns Hopk. Hosp. *73:* 275–286 (1943).

HEINE, U.; BEARD, D., and BEARD, J. W.: Ultracytochemical studies on aberrant structures in avian virus tumor cells. Cancer Res. *28:* 585–594 (1968).

HEITZMAN, R. J.: Nucleotide-sugar enzymes in scrapie. Lancet *i:* 427 (1968).

HEITZMAN, R. J. and CORP, C. R.: Behaviour in emergence and open-field tests of normal and scrapie mice. Res. Vet. Sci. *9:* 600–601 (1968).

HELMBOLDT, C. F. and JUNGHERR, E. L.: The pathology of Aleutian disease in mink. Amer. J. vet. Res. *19:* 212–222 (1958).

HELYER, B. J. and HOWIE, J. B.: Spontaneous auto-immune disease in NZB/BL mice. Brit. J. Haemat. *9:* 119–131 (1963).

HENSON, J. B.; LEADER, R. W., and GORHAM, J. R.: Hypergammaglobulinemia in mink. Proc. Soc. exp. Biol., N. Y. *107:* 919–920 (1961).

HENSON, J. B.; GORHAM, J. R.; LEADER, R. W., and WAGNER, B. M.: Experimental hypergammaglobulinemia in mink. J. exp. Med. *116:* 357–364 (1962).

HENSON, J. B.; GORHAM, J. R., and LEADER, R. W.: Hypergammaglobulinemia in mink initiated by a cell-free filtrate. Nature, Lond. *197:* 206–207 (1963a).

HENSON, J. B.; GORHAM, J. R., and LEADER, R. W.: The familial occurrence of hypergammaglobulinemia in mink. Texas Rep. Biol. Med. *21:* 37–42 (1963b).

HENSON, J. B.; LEADER, R. W.; GORHAM, J. R., and PADGETT, G. A.: The sequential development of lesions in spontaneous Aleutian disease of mink. Path. vet. *3:* 289–314 (1966).

HENSON, J. B.; GORHAM, J. R., and TAKAKA, Y.: Renal glomerular ultrastructure in mink affected by Aleutian disease. Lab. Invest. *17:* 123–139 (1967a).

HENSON, J. B.; McGUIRE, T. C.; KOBAYASHI, K., and GORHAM, J. R.: The diagnosis of equine infectious anemia using the complement-fixation test, siderocyte counts, hepatic biopsies, and serum protein alterations. J. amer. vet. med. Ass. *151:* 1830–1839 (1967b).

HENSON, J. B.; GORHAM, J. R.; TANAKA, Y., and PADGETT, G. A.: The sequential development of ultrastructural lesions in the glomeruli of mink with experimental Aleutian disease. Lab. Invest. *19:* 153–162 (1968).

HENSON, J. B.; GORHAM, J. R.; PADGETT, G. A., and DAVIS, W. C.: Pathogenesis of the glomerular lesions in Aleutian disease of mink. Arch. Path. *87:* 21–28 (1969).

HERNDON, R. M. and RUBINSTEIN, L. J.: Light and electron microscopy observations on the development of viral particles in the inclusions of Dawson's encephalitis (subacute sclerosing panencephalitis). Neurology, Minneap. *18:* 8–20 (1968).

HERSEY, D. F. and SHAW, E. D.: Viral agents in hepatitis. A review. Lab. Invest. *19:* 558–572 (1968).

HEUSCHELE, W. P.: Studies on the pathogenesis of African swine fever. I. Quantitative studies on the sequential development of virus in pig tissues. Arch. ges. Virusforsch. *21:* 349–356 (1967).

HEUSCHELE, W. P.; COGGINS, L., and STONE, S. S.: Fluorescent antibody studies on African swine fever virus. Amer. J. vet. Res. *27:* 477–484 (1966).

HEYL, J. T.; ALLEN, H. F., and CHEEVER, F. S.: Quantitative assay of neutralizing antibody content of pools of gamma globulin from different sections of the United States against the viruses of herpes simplex, lymphocytic choriomeningitis and epidemic keratoconjunctivitis. J. Immunol. *60:* 37–45 (1948).

HIGASHI, O.: Congenital gigantism of peroxidase granules: the first case ever reported of qualitative abnormality of peroxidase. Tohoku J. exp. Med. *59:* 315–332 (1954).

HIRSCH, M. S. and MURPHY, F. A.: The effect of anti-lymphocyte serum on lymphocytic choriomeningitis (LCM) virus infection in mice. Abstract. Fed. Proc. *26:* 481 (1967).

HIRSCH, M. S. and MURPHY, F. A.: Effects of anti-lymphoid sera on viral infections. Lancet *ii:* 37–40 (1968).

HIRSCH, M. S.; MURPHY, F. A.; RUSSE, H. P., and HICKLIN, M. D.: Effects of anti-thymocyte serum on lymphocytic choriomeningitis (LCM) virus infection in mice. Proc. Soc. exp. Biol., N. Y. *125:* 980–983 (1967).

HIRSCH, M. S.; MURPHY, F. A., and HICKLIN, M. D.: Immunopathology of lymphocytic choriomeningitis virus infection of newborn mice. Antithymocyte serum effects on glomerulonephritis and wasting disease. J. exp. Med. *127:* 757–766 (1968).

HOLMAN, H. H. and PATTISON, I. H.: Further evidence on the significance of vacuolated nerve cells in the medulla oblongata of sheep affected with scrapie. J. comp. Path. *53:* 231–236 (1943).

HOLTERMANN, O. A. and MAJDE, J. A.: Skin grafting between lymphocytic choriomeningitis virus-infected and noninfected inbred mice. Abstract. Bact. Proc., p. 199 (1969a).

HOLTERMANN, O. A. and MAJDE, J. A.: Rejection of skin grafts from mice chronically infected with lymphocytic choriomeningitis virus by non-infected syngeneic recipients. Nature, Lond. *223:* 624 (1969b).

HORSTMANN, D. M.; BANATVALA, J. E.; RIORDAN, J. T.; PAYNE, M. C.; WHITTEMORE, R.; OPTON, E. M., and FLOREY, C. de Ve.: Maternal rubella and the rubella syndrome in infants. Amer. J. Dis. Child. *110:* 408–415 (1965).

HORTA-BARBOSA, L.; FUCCILLO, D. A., and SEVER, J. L.: Subacute sclerosing panencephalitis: Isolation of measles virus from a brain biopsy. Nature, Lond. *221:* 974 (1969).

HOTCHIN, J. E.: The cultivation of Novikoff rat hepatoma cells *in vitro.* Cancer Res. *17:* 682–687 (1957).

HOTCHIN, J.: Some aspects of induced latent infection of mice with the virus of lymphocytic choriomeningitis; in: Symposium on latency and masking in viral and rickettsial infections, pp. 59–65 (Burgess Co., Minneapolis 1958).

HOTCHIN, J.: Discussion of 'specific immunity as a factor in the ecology of animal viruses;' in: Perspectives in virology, p. 182 (John Wiley & Sons, Inc., New York 1959).

HOTCHIN, J. E.: The role of immunological tolerance in neonatal infection of mice with lymphocytic choriomeningitis virus. Quart. Rev. Pediat. *16:* 97–101 (1961).

HOTCHIN, J.: The biology of lymphocytic choriomeningitis infection: Virus-induced immune disease. Cold Spr. Harb. Symp. quant. Biol. *27:* 479–499 (1962a).

HOTCHIN, J.: The foot pad reaction of mice to lymphocytic choriomeningitis virus. Virology *17:* 214–215 (1962b).

HOTCHIN, J.: Chronic disease following lymphocytic choriomeningitis virus inoculation and possible mechanisms of slow virus pathogenesis. NINDB Monograph No. 2. Slow, latent and temperate virus infections, pp. 341–359 (US Dept. of Health, Education and Welfare, Washington, D. C. 1965).

HOTCHIN, J.: Kuru as a persisting tolerated infection. Lancet *ii:* 28–31 (1966).

HOTCHIN, J.: Immune and autoimmune reactions in the pathogenesis of slow virus disease. Curr. Topics Microbiol. *40:* 33–43 (1967).

HOTCHIN, J.: Lymphocytic choriomeningitis as a model of persistent virus infection.

Proc. 1st int. Congr. for Virology, Helsinki 1968, pp. 109–112 (Karger, Basel/ New York 1969).

HOTCHIN, J.: A concept of persistent virus infection. Proc. of the 3rd int. Symp. on medical and applied virology: Viruses affecting man and animals (1970a).

HOTCHIN, J.: Virus-induced autoimmunity and the aging process. Proc. of a Symp. on tolerance, autoimmunity and molecular aging, in press (1970b).

HOTCHIN, J. and BENSON, L. M.: Mouse-weight measurements as an index of virus disease. N. Y. State Dep. Health, Ann. Rep. Div. Lab. Res., pp. 42–43 (1961).

HOTCHIN, J. and BENSON, L.: The pathogenesis of lymphocytic choriomeningitis in mice: The effects of different inoculation routes and the footpad response. J. Immunol. *91:* 460–468 (1963).

HOTCHIN, J. and BENSON L.: Differences between surface and cytoplasmic antigens in LCM virus infected cells (to be published).

HOTCHIN, J. E. and CINITS, M.: Lymphocytic choriomeningitis infection of mice as a model for the study of latent virus infection. Canad. J. Microbiol. *4:* 149–163 (1958).

HOTCHIN, J. and COLLINS, D. N.: Glomerulonephritis and late onset disease of mice following neonatal virus infection. Nature, Lond. *203:* 1357–1359 (1964).

HOTCHIN, J. and SIKORA, E.: Protection against the lethal effect of lymphocytic choriomeningitis virus in mice by neonatal thymectomy. Nature, Lond. *202:* 214–215 (1964).

HOTCHIN, J. E. and WEIGAND, H.: Relationship between age at inoculation and outcome of infection of mice with lymphocytic choriomeningitis virus. N. Y. State Dep. Health, Ann. Rep. Div. Lab. Res., p. 21 (1959).

HOTCHIN, J. and WEIGAND, H.: Studies of lymphocytic choriomeningitis in mice. I. The relationship between age at inoculation and outcome of infection. J. Immunol. *86:* 392–400 (1961a).

HOTCHIN, J. and WEIGAND, H.: The effects of pretreatment with X-rays on the pathogenesis of lymphocytic choriomeningitis in mice. I. Host survival, virus multiplication and leukocytosis. J. Immunol. *87:* 675–681 (1961b).

HOTCHIN, J. E.; COHEN, S. M.; RUSKA, H., and RUSKA, C.: Electron microscopical aspects of hemadsorption in tissue cultures infected with influenza virus. Virology *6:* 689–701 (1958).

HOTCHIN, J.; BENSON, L. M., and SEAMER, J.: Factors affecting the induction of persistent tolerant infection of newborn mice with lymphocytic choriomeningitis. Virology *18:* 71–78 (1962).

HOTCHIN, J.; BENSON, L., and SIKORA, E.: Detection of neutralizing antibody to lymphocytic choriomeningitis virus in mice. J. Immunol. *102:* 1128–1135 (1969).

HOTCHIN, J.; BENSON, L., and GARDNER, J.: Mother-infant interaction in lymphocytic choriomeningitis virus infection of the newborn mouse: The effect of maternal health on mortality of offspring. Pediat. Res. *4:* 193–199 (1970).

HOURRIGAN, J. L.: Scrapie in the United States and the scrapie eradication program. Report of Scrapie Seminar, Washington, D. C., 1964, pp. 340–360 (US Dept. of Agriculture, ARS 91–53, Washington, D. C. 1966).

HOWARD, M. E.: Infection with the virus of choriomeningitis in man. Yale J. Biol. Med. *13:* 161–180 (1940).

HOWARD, R. J.; NOTKINS, A. L., and MERGENHAGEN, S. E.: Inhibition of cellular immune reactions in mice infected with lactic dehydrogenase virus. Nature, Lond. *221:* 873–874 (1969).

HOWITT, B. F.: Complement fixation test differentiating 3 strains of equine encephalomyelitic virus and the virus of lymphocytic choriomeningitis. Proc. Soc. exp. Biol., N. Y. *35:* 526–528 (1937a).

HOWITT, B. F.: The complement fixation reaction in experimental equine encephalomyelitis, lymphocytic choriomeningitis, and the St. Louis type of encephalitis. J. Immunol. *33:* 235–250 (1937b).

HUMMELER, K. and KOPROWSKI, H.: Investigating the rabies virus. Nature, Lond. *221:* 418–421 (1969).

HUMPHREYS, S. R.; VENDETTI, J. M.; MANTEL, N., and GOLDIN, A.: Observations on a leukemic cell variant in mice. J. nat. Cancer Inst. *17:* 447–457 (1956).

HUNT, J. W.; TILL, J. E., and WILLIAMS, J. F.: Radiation damage and free radical production in irradiated ribonuclease. Radiat. Res. *17:* 703–711 (1962).

HUNTER, G. D.: Progress toward the isolation and characterization of the scrapie agent. NINDB Monograph No. 2. Slow, latent and temperate virus infections, pp. 259–262 (US Dept. of Health, Education and Welfare, Washington, D. C. 1965).

HUNTER, G. D. and MILLSON, G. C.: Studies on the heat stability and chromatographic behaviour of the scrapie agent. J. gen. Microbiol. *37:* 251–258 (1964a).

HUNTER, G. D. and MILLSON, G. C.: Further experiments on the comparative potency of tissue extracts from mice infected with scrapie. Res. Vet. Sci. *5:* 149–153 (1964b).

HUNTER, G. D. and MILLSON, G. C.: Distribution and activation of lysosomal enzyme activities in subcellular components of normal and scrapie-affected mouse brain. J. Neurochem. *13:* 375–383 (1966).

HUNTER, G. D. and MILLSON, G. C.: Attempts to release the scrapie agent from tissue debris. J. comp. Path. *77:* 301–307 (1967).

HUNTER, G. D.; MILLSON, G. C., and CHANDLER, R. L.: Observations on the comparative infectivity of cellular fractions derived from homogenates of mouse-scrapie brain. Res. Vet. Sci. *4:* 543–549 (1963).

HUNTER, G. D.; MILLSON, G. C., and MEEK, C.: The intracellular location of the agent of mouse scrapie. J. gen. Microbiol. *34:* 319–325 (1964).

HUNTER, G. D.; MILLSON, G. C., and VOCKINS, M. D.: Lysosomal enzymes and scrapie. Biochem. J. *102:* 43P–44P (1967a).

HUNTER, G. D.; MILLSON, G. C., and GIBBONS, R. A.: Some new information concerning the stability of the scrapie agent. Biochem. J. *105:* 7P (1967b).

HYSLOP, N. St. G.: Equine infectious anaemia (swamp fever). A review. Vet. Rec. *78:* 858–864 (1966).

INGALLS, T. H.; PLOTKIN, S. A.; MEYER, H. M. jr., and PARKMAN, P. D.: Rubella: Epidemiology, virology, and immunology. Amer. J. med. Sci. *253:* 349–373 (1967).

ISACSON, P.: Myxoviruses and autoimmunity. Progr. Allergy vol. 10, pp. 256–292 (Karger, Basel/New York 1967).

ISHII, S.: On the existence of virus in semen and the possibility of infection by the copulation in the horse affected with infectious anemia. Jap. J. appl. vet. Med. *11:* 647–652 (1938).

ISHII, S.: Equine infectious anaemia or swamp fever. Adv. vet. Sci. *8:* 263–298 (1963).

ISHII, S.; AKAI, M., and YONEDA, T.: On the virus of equine infectious anemia. II. Is found the virus in the blood of colt born from the horse affected with infectious anemia and in the milk secreted from diseased horse. J. jap. soc. anim. Hyg. *8:* 119–142 (1940).

ISHITANI, R.: Research in Japan on control of equine infectious anemia. Proc. of 1st int. Conf. on Equine Infectious Diseases, Italy, pp. 1–21 (1966).

JABBOUR, J. T.; GARCIA, J. H.; LEMMI, H.; RAGLAND, J.; DUENAS, D. A., and SEVER, J. L.: Subacute sclerosing panencephalitis. A multidisciplinary study of eight cases. J. amer. med. Ass. *207:* 2248–2254 (1969).

JACK, I. and GRUTZNER, J.: Cellular viraemia in babies infected with rubella virus before birth. Brit. med. J. *1:* 289–292 (1969).

JACK, I. and MCAULIFFE, K. C.: Sero-epidemiological study of cytomegalovirus infections in Melbourne children and some adults. Med. J. Austr. *1:* 206–209 (1968).

JACK, I.; TODD, H., and TURNER, E. K.: Isolation of human cytomegalovirus from the circulating leucocytes of a leukaemic patient. Med. J. Austr. *1:* 210–213 (1968).

JENSON, A. B.; RABIN, E. R.; BENTINCK, D. C., and RAPP, F.: Reovirus viremia in newborn mice. An electron microscopic, immunofluorescent and virus assay study. Amer. J. Path. *49:* 1171–1183 (1966).

JOCHHEIM, K. A.; SCHEID, W.; LIEDTKE, G.; HANSEN, I. und STAUSBERG, G.: Komplementbindende Antikörper gegen den Virus der lymphozytären Choriomeningitis im Serum von Versuchstieren und Beobachtungen zur Immunität. Arch. ges. Virusforsch. *7:* 143–162 (1957).

JOHNSON, R. H.: Feline panleucopaenia virus. II. Some features of the cytopathic effects in feline kidney monolayers. Res. Vet. Sci. *6:* 472–481 (1965).

JOHNSON, K. M.; WIEBENGA, N. H.; MACKENZIE, R. B.; KUNS, M. L.; TAURASO, N. M.; SHELOKOV, A.; WEBB, P. A.; JUSTINES, G., and BEYE, H. K.: Virus isolations from human cases of hemorrhagic fever in Bolivia. Proc. Soc. exp. Biol., N. Y. *118:* 113–118 (1965a).

JOHNSON, K. M.; MACKENZIE, R. B.; WEBB, P. A., and KUNS, M. L.: Chronic infection of rodents by Machupo virus. Science *150:* 1618–1619 (1965b).

JOHNSON, K. M.; KUNS, M. L.; MACKENZIE, R. B.; WEBB, P. A., and YUNKER, C. E.: Isolation of Machupo virus from wild rodent *Calomys callosus.* Amer. J. trop. Med. *15:* 103–106 (1966).

JOHNSON, R. H.; MARGOLIS, G., and KILHAM, L.: Identity of feline ataxis virus with feline panleucopenia virus. Nature, Lond. *214:* 175–177 (1967).

JOSKE, R. A.; LEAK, P. J.; PAPADIMITRIOU, J. M.; STANLEY, N. F., and WALTERS, M. N. I.: Murine infection with reovirus: IV. Late chronic disease and the induction of lymphoma after reovirus type 3 infection. Brit. J. exp. Path. *47:* 337–346 (1966).

Joske, R. A.; Stanley, N. F., and Walters, M. N. I.: Experimental viral induction of autoimmune liver disease. Proc. 3rd Wld. Congr. Gastroenterology; Recent Advances in Gastroenterology vol. 3, pp. 233–235 (1967).

Jungeblut, C. W. and Kodza, H.: Interference between lymphocytic choriomeningitis virus and the leukemia-transmitting agent of leukemia L_2C in guinea pigs. Arch. ges. Virusforsch. *12:* 552–560 (1963).

Justines, G. and Johnson, K. M.: Immune tolerance in *Calomys callosus* infected with Machupo virus. Nature, Lond. *222:* 1090–1091 (1969).

Kajima, M. and Majde, J.: LCM virus as a carrier of non-viral cellular components. Naturwissenschaften, in press.

Kakulas, B. A.; Lecours, A. R., and Gajdusek, D. C.: Further observations on the pathology of kuru (A study of the two cerebra in serial section). J. Neuropath. exp. Neurol. *26:* 85–97 (1967).

Kaplan, M. M.: Epidemiology of rabies. Nature, Lond. *221:* 421–452 (1969).

Karasaki, S.: Size and ultrastructure of the H-viruses as determined with the use of specific antibodies. J. Ultrastruct. Res. *16:* 109–122 (1966).

Karmody, C. S.: Subclinical maternal rubella and congenital deafness. New Engl. J. Med. *278:* 809–814 (1968).

Karstad, L.: Viral plasmacytosis (Aleutian disease) in mink. V. The occurrence of hyalin glomerular lesions and fibrinoid arteritis in experimental infection. Canad. J. comp. Med. *29:* 66–74 (1965).

Karstad, L.: Aleutian disease. A slowly progressive viral infection of mink; in: Current tropics in microbiology and immunology, vol. 40, pp. 9–21 (Springer, New York 1967).

Karstad, L. and Pridham, T. J.: Aleutian disease of mink. Evidence of its viral etiology. Canad. J. comp. Med. *26:* 97–102 (1962).

Karstad, L.; Pridham, T. J., and Gray, D. P.: Aleutian disease (plasmacytosis) of mink. II. Responses of mink to formalin-treated diseased tissues and to subsequent challenge with virulent inoculum. Canad. J. comp. Med. *27:* 124–128 (1963).

Kasting, R. and Darcel, C. LeQ.: Comparisons by paper chromatography of extracts of brain, urine and plasma from normal and scrapie sheep. Res. Vet. Sci. *4:* 518–525 (1963).

Kay, H. E. M.; Peppercorn, M. E.; Porterfield, J. S.; McCarthy, K., and Taylor-Robinson, C. H.: Congenital rubella infection of a human embryo. Brit. med. J. *ii:* 166–167 (1964).

Keast, D. and Stanley, N. F.: Studies on a murine lymphoma induced by reovirus type 3: Some general aspects of the lymphoma 2731/L. Proc. Soc. exp. Biol., N. Y. *122:* 1091–1098 (1966).

Keast, D.; Stanley, N. F., and Phillips, P. A.: The association of murine lymphoma with reovirus type 3 infection: The development of neoplasia in an animal suffering from chronic reovirus 3 disease. Proc. Soc. exp. Biol., N. Y. *128:* 1033–1038 (1968).

Kennedy, R. C.; Eklund, C. M.; Lopez, C., and Hadlow, W. J.: Isolation of a virus from the lungs of Montana sheep affected with progressive pneumonia. Virology *35:* 483–484 (1968).

KENRICK, K. G.; SLINN, R. F.; DORMAN, D. C., and MENSER, M. A.: Immunoglobulins and rubella-virus antibodies in adults with congenital rubella. Lancet *i:* 548–551 (1968).

KENYON, A. J.: Enhancement of Aleutian disease plasmacytosis by immunoglobulins from infected mink. NINDB Monograph No. 2. Slow, latent and temperate virus infections. pp. 321–328 (US Dept. of Health, Education and Welfare, Washington, D. C. 1965).

KENYON, A. J.: Immunologic deficiency in Aleutian disease of mink. Amer. J. vet. Res. *27:* 1780–1782 (1966).

KENYON, A. J. and WILLIAMS, R. C.: Lymphatic leukaemia associated with dysproteinaemia in ferrets. Nature, Lond. *214:* 1022–1024 (1967).

KENYON, A. J.; HELMBOLDT, C. F., and NIELSEN, S. W.: Experimental transmission of Aleutian disease with urine. Amer. J. vet. Res. *24:* 1066–1067 (1963a).

KENYON, A. J.; TRAUTWEIN, G., and HELMBOLDT, C. F.: Characterization of blood serum proteins from mink with Aleutian disease. Amer. J. vet. Res. *24:* 168–173 (1963b).

KENYON, A. J.; WILLIAMS, R. C. jr., and HOWARD, E. B.: Monoclonal γ-globulins in ferrets with lymphoproliferative lesions. Proc. Soc. exp. Biol., N. Y. *123:* 510–513 (1966a).

KENYON, A. J.; MAGNANO, T.; HELMBOLDT, C. F., and BUKO, L.: Aleutian disease in the ferret. J. amer. vet. med. Ass. *149:* 920–923 (1966b).

KENYON, A. J.; HOWARD, E., and BUKO, L.: Hypergammaglobulinemia in ferrets with lymphoproliferative lesions (Aleutian disease). Amer. J. vet. Res. *28:* 1167–1172 (1967).

KENYON, A. J.; WILLIAMS, R. C., and HOWARD, E. B.: Alpha$_2$-macroglobulinemia with associated renal amyloidosis in mink. Amer. J. vet. Res. *29:* 1453–1462 (1968).

KILHAM, L.: Mongolism associated with rat virus (RV) infection in hamsters. Virology *13:* 141–142 (1961).

KILHAM, L.: Viruses of laboratory and wild rats; in: National Cancer Institute Monograph No. 20, pp. 117–135 (US Dept. of Health, Education and Welfare, Maryland 1966).

KILHAM, L. and MARGOLIS, G.: Cerebellar ataxia in hamsters inoculated with rat virus. Science *143:* 1047–1048 (1964).

KILHAM, L. and MARGOLIS, G.: Viral etiology of spontaneous ataxia of cats. Amer. J. Path. *48:* 991–1011 (1966a).

KILHAM, L. and MARGOLIS, G.: Spontaneous hepatitis and cerebellar 'hypoplasia' in suckling rats due to congenital infections with rat virus. Amer. J. Path. *49:* 457–475 (1966b).

KILHAM, L. and MOLONEY, J. B.: Association of rat virus and Moloney leukemia virus in tissues of inoculated rats. J. nat. Cancer Inst. *32:* 523–531 (1964).

KILHAM, L. and OLIVIER, L. J.: A latent virus of rats isolated in tissue culture. Virology *7:* 428–437 (1959).

KILHAM, L.; MARGOLIS, G., and COLBY, E. D.: Congenital infections of cats and ferrets by feline panleukopenia virus manifested by cerebellar hypoplasia. Lab. Invest. *17:* 465–480 (1967).

KIMBERLIN, R. H.: RNA metabolism in the brains of mice clinically affected with scrapie. J. comp. Path. *78:* 237–241 (1968).

KIMBERLIN, R. H. and ANGER, H. S.: Further observations on the synthesis of DNA in scrapie-affected mouse by using radioautographic techniques. Biochem. J. *107:* 32P (1968).

KIMBERLIN, R. H. and HUNTER, G. D.: DNA synthesis in the brains of scrapie-affected mice. Biochem. J. *96:* 64P (1965).

KIMBERLIN, R. H. and HUNTER, G. D.: DNA synthesis in scrapie-affected mouse brain. J. gen. Virol. *1:* 115–124 (1967).

KIMBERLIN, R. H. and MILLSON, G. C.: Some biochemical aspects of mouse scrapie. J. comp. Path. *77:* 359–366 (1967).

KINDIG, D.; SPARGO, B., and KIRSTEN, W. H.: Glomerular response in Aleutian disease of mink. Lab. Invest. *16:* 436–443 (1967).

KLATZO, I.; GAJDUSEK, D. C., and ZIGAS, V.: Pathology of kuru. Lab. Invest. *8:* 799–847 (1959).

KLEMOLA, E.; KAARIÄINEN, L.; VON ESSEN, R.; HALTIA, K.; KOIVUNIEMI, A., and VON BONSDORFF, C. H.: Further studies on cytomegalovirus mononucleosis in previously healthy individuals. Acta med. scand. *182:* 311–322 (1967).

KOBAYASHI, K.: Studies on the cultivation of equine infectious anemia virus *in vitro.* I. Serial cultivation on the virus in the culture of various horse tissues. Virus (Osaka) *2:* 177–189 (1961a).

KOBAYASHI, K.: Studies on the cultivation of equine infectious anemia. II. Propagation of the virus in horse bone-marrow cell culture. Virus (Osaka) *2:* 189–201 (1961b).

KOBAYASHI, K.: Studies on the cultivation of equine infectious anemia virus *in vitro.* III. Propagation of the virus in horse leucocyte culture. Virus (Osaka) *2:* 249–256 (1961c).

KOBAYASHI, K.: Studies on the cultivation of equine infectious anemia *in vitro.* I. Propagation of the virus in horse leucocyte culture. Jap. J. vet. Sci. *24:* 376 (1962).

KOBAYASHI, K.; HENSON, J. B., and GORHAM, J. R.: Viral neutralizing antibodies in equine infectious anemia. Abstract. Fed. Proc. *28:* 429 (1969).

DeKOCK, G.: Are lesions of Jaagiekte in sheep of nature of neoplasm. Union S. Africa, Dir. Vet. Serv., 15th Ann. Rep., 611–641 (1929).

KOENS, H.: De 'Zwoegers' op Texel. Thesis, Univ. Utrecht, 1943.

KOFENDER, M.; CHASON, J. L., and LERNER, A. M.: Persistence of reovirus in the eyes of neonatally infected mice. Amer. J. Ophthal. *64:* 312–313 (1967).

KOLTAY, M.; VIRÁG, I.; BÁNOS, Z.; ANDERLIK, P., and SZERI, I.: Interaction of graft-versus-host reaction and lymphocytic choriomeningitis infection in mice. Experientia *24:* 63–65 (1968).

KOMROWER, G. M.; WILLIAMS, B. L., and STONES, P. B.: Lymphocytic choriomeningitis in the newborn. Probable transplacental infection. Lancet *i:* 697–69 (1955).

KONO, Y. and KOBAYASHI, K.: Complement fixation test of equine infectious anemia. II. Relation between CF antibody response and the disease. Nat. Inst. anim. hlth. Quart (Tokyo) *6:* 204–207 (1966).

KOPROWSKI, H.; WIKTOR, T. J., and KAPLAN, M. M.: Enhancement of rabies virus infection by lymphocytic choriomeningitis virus. Virology *28:* 754–756 (1966).

KORONES, S. B.; AINGER, L. E.; MONIF, R. G.; ROANE, J.; SEVER, J. L., and FUSTE, F.: Congenital rubella syndrome: New clinical aspects with recovery of virus from affected infants. J. Pediat. *67:* 166–181 (1965).

KREIS, B.: La maladie d'Armstrong: Chorio-méningite lymphocytaire, une nouvelle entité morbide? 160 p. (Thesis for Doctor of Med.) (Baillière et Fils, Paris 1937).

KRITZLER, R. A.; TERNER, J. Y.; LINDENBAUM, J.; MAGIDSON, J.; WILLIAMS, R.; PRESIG, R., and PHILLIPS, G. B.: Chediak-Higashi syndrome. Cytologic and serum lipid observations in a case and family. Amer. J. Med. *36:* 583–594 (1964).

KRUGMAN, R. D. and GOODHEART, C. R.: Human cytomegalovirus. Thermal inactivation. Virology *23:* 290–291 (1964).

KUNDIN, W. D.; LIU, C., and GIGSTAD, J.: Reovirus infection in suckling mice: Immunofluorescent and infectivity studies. J. Immunol. *97:* 393–401 (1966).

KUNS, M. L.: Epidemiology of Machupo virus infection. II. Ecological and control studies of hemorrhagic fever. Amer. J. trop. Med. Hyg. *14:* 813–816 (1965).

KÜPPER, B.; BLOEDHORN, H.; ACKERMANN, R. und SCHEID, W.: Über die Verbreitung des Virus der lymphozytären Choriomeningitis unter den Mäusen in Westdeutschland. Zbl. Bakt. Parasitenk. Infek. Hyg. *195:* 1–11 (1964).

KUTTNER, A. G.: The problem of the significance of the inclusion bodies found in the salivary glands of infants, and the occurrence of inclusion bodies in the submaxillary glands of hamsters, white mice, and wild rats (Peiping). J. exp. Med. *60:* 773–792 (1934).

LAMBERT, H. P.; STERN, H., and WELLSTEED, A. J.: Congenital rubella syndrome. Lancet *ii:* 826–827 (1965).

LANDAUER, T. K.; KILHAM, L., and BUCHTEL, H. A.: Behavioral characteristics associated with the rat virus-induced 'hamster mongolism' syndrome. J. psychiat. Res. *5:* 95–106 (1967).

LANG, D. J.: The association of indirect inguinal hernia with congenital cytomegalic inclusion disease. Pediatrics *38:* 913–916 (1966).

LANG, D. J. and NOREN, B.: Cytomegaloviremia following congenital infection. J. Pediat. *73:* 812–819 (1968).

LARSEN, J. H.: On the induction of immunological tolerance to LCM virus in the adult mouse. 15th Scand. Congr. Path. Microbiol., pp. 60–61 (1967).

LARSEN, J. H.: Studies on immunological tolerance to LCM virus. 9. Induction of immunological tolerance to the virus in the adult mouse. Acta path. microbiol. scand. *73:* 106–114 (1968).

LARSEN, J. H.: Development of humoral and cell-mediated immunity to lymphocytic choriomeningitis virus in the mouse. J. Immunol. *102:* 941–946 (1969a).

LARSEN, J. H.: On the induction of immunological tolerance to a self-reproducing antigen. Immunology, Lond. *16:* 15–23 (1969b).

LARSEN, J. H. and VOLKERT, M.: Studies on immunological tolerance to LCM virus. 7. Adoptive immunization of virus carrier mice by grafts of normal syngeneic lymphoid cells. Acta path. microbiol. scand. *70:* 95–106 (1967).

LAW, L. W. and DUNN, T. B.: Effects of a filtrable self-propagating contaminant on a transplantable acute lymphoid leukemia in mice. J. nat. Cancer Inst. *11:* 1037–1053 (1951).

LEA, D. E.: Actions of radiation on living cells, chapt. 3 (Cambridge University Press, New York 1946).

LEADER, R. W.: Mink disease. New Engl. J. Med. *270:* 373 (1964).

LEADER, R. W.; GORHAM, J. R.; HENSON, J. B., and BURGER, D.: Pathogenesis of Aleutian disease of mink. NINDB Monograph No. 2. Slow, latent and temperate virus infections, pp. 287–295 (US Dept. of Health, Education and Welfare, Washington, D. C. 1965).

LEHMANN-GRUBE, F.: Lymphocytic choriomeningitis in the mouse. I. Growth in the brain. Arch. ges. Virusforsch. *14:* 344–350 (1964a).

LEHMANN-GRUBE, F.: Lymphocytic choriomeningitis in the mouse. II. Establishment of carrier colonies. Arch. ges. Virusforsch. *14:* 351–357 (1964b).

LEHMANN-GRUBE, F.: A carrier state of lymphocytic choriomeningitis virus in L cell cultures. Nature, Lond. *213:* 770–773 (1967).

LEHMANN-GRUBE, F.: Untersuchungen über das Virus der lymphozytären Choriomeningitis. I. Stabilisierung des Virus. Arch. ges. Virusforsch. *23:* 202–217 (1968).

LEHMANN-GRUBE, F. and HESSE, R.: A new method for the titration of lymphocytic choriomeningitis viruses. Arch. ges. Virusforsch. *20:* 256–259 (1967).

LEHMANN-GRUBE, F.; ACKERMANN, R.; JOCHHEIM, K. A.; LIEDTKE, G. und SCHEID, W.: Über die Technik der Neutralisation des Virus der lymphozytären Choriomeningitis in der Maus. Arch. ges. Virusforsch. *9:* 64–72 (1959).

LEICHENGER, H.; MILZER, A., and LACK, H.: Recurrent lymphocytic choriomeningitis treated with sulfanilamide: Isolation of virus. J. amer. med. Ass. *115:* 436–440 (1940).

LEIFER, E.; GOCKE, D. J., and BOURNE, H.: Lassa fever, a new virus disease of man from West Africa. II. Report of a laboratory-acquired infection treated with plasma from a person recently recovered from the disease. Amer. J. trop. Med. Hyg. *19:* 677–679 (1970).

LENNETTE, E. H.; MAGOFFIN, R. L., and FREEMAN, J. M.: Immunologic evidence of measles virus as an etiologic agent in subacute sclerosing panencephalitis. Neurology, Minneap. *18:* 21–29 (1968).

LÉPINE, P. et SAUTTER, V.: Contamination de laboratoire avec le virus de la chorioméningite lymphocytaire. Ann. Inst. Pasteur *61:* 519–526 (1938).

LÉPINE, P.; MOLLARET, P. et KREIS, B. Réceptivité de l'homme au virus murin de la chorioméningitis lymphocytaire: Reproduction expérimentale de la méningite lymphocytaire bénigne. Compt. rend. Acad. sci. *204:* 1846–1848 (1937).

LERNER, A. M.: Concentration and purification of viruses with special reference to reoviruses. Bact. Rev. *28:* 391–396 (1964).

LERNER, E. M. II and HAAS, V. H.: Histopathology of lymphocytic choriomeningitis in mice spared by amethopterin. Proc. Soc. exp. Biol., N. Y. *98:* 395–399 (1958).

LEVENE, C. and BLUMBERG, B. S.: Additional specificities of Australia antigen and the possible identification of hepatitis carriers. Nature, Lond. *221:* 195–196 (1969).

LEVEY, R. H.; TRAININ, N.; LAW, L. W.; BLACK, P. H., and ROWE, W. P.: Lymphocytic choriomeningitis infection in neonatally thymectomized mice bearing diffusion chambers containing thymus. Science *142:* 483–485 (1963).

LEVY, H. B. and HAAS, V. H.: Alteration of the course of lymphocytic choriomeningitis in mice by certain antimetabolites. Virology *5:* 401–407 (1958).

LEVY, J. A.; HENLE, G.; HENLE, W., and ZAJAC, B. A.: Effect of reovirus type 3 on cultured Burkitt's tumour cells. Nature, Lond. *220:* 607–608 (1968).

LEWIS, J. M. and UTZ, J. P.: Orchitis, parotitis and meningoencephalitis due to lymphocytic choriomeningitis virus. New Engl. J. Med. *265:* 776–780 (1961).

LEWIS, A. M., jr.; ROWE, W. P.; TURNER, H. C., and HUEBNER, R. J.: Lymphocytic choriomeningitis virus in hamster tumor: Spread to hamster and humans. Science *150:* 363–364 (1965).

LILLIE, R. D.: Histopathologic reaction to the virus of lymphocytic choriomeningitis in the chick embryo. Publ. Hlth Rep., Wash. *51:* 41–42 (1936a).

LILLIE, R. D.: Pathologic histology of lymphocytic choriomeningitis in monkeys. Publ. Hlth Rep., Wash *51:* 303–310 (1936b).

LILLIE, R. D. and ARMSTRONG, C.: Pathologic reaction to the virus of lymphocytic choriomeningitis in guinea pigs. Publ. Hlth Rep., Wash. *59:* 1391–1405 (1944).

LILLIE, R. D. and ARMSTRONG, C.: Pathology of lymphocytic choriomeningitis in mice. Arch. Path. *40:* 141–152 (1945).

LINDQUIST, J. M.; PLOTKIN, S. A.; SHAW, L.; GILDEN, R. V., and WILLIAMS, M. L.: Congenital rubella syndrome as a systemic infection. Studies of affected infants born in Philadelphia, USA. Brit. med. J. *2:* 1401–1406 (1965).

LONDON, W. T.; FUCCILLO, D. A., and SEVER, J. L.: Congenital rubella in rabbits. Abstract Bact. Proc. 201 (1969).

LOVE, R.; FERNANDES, M. V., and KOPROWSKI, H.: Cytochemistry of inclusion bodies in tissue culture cells infected with rabies virus. Proc. Soc. exp. Biol., N. Y. *116:* 560–563 (1964).

LUCAM, F.: La 'bouhite' ou 'lymphomatose pulmonaire maligne du Mouton'. Rec. Méd. vét. *118:* 273–285 (1942).

LÜHRS, E.: Die ansteckende Blutarmut der Pferde. Z. Veterinärk. *31:* 369–490 (1919).

LÜHRS, E.: Ist das Wechselfieber der Pferde auf den Menschen übertragbar? Z. Veterinärk. *32:* 89–95 (1920).

LUNDSTEDT, C.: Interaction between antigenically different cells. Virus-induced cytotoxicity by immune lymphoid cells *in vitro*. Acta path. microbiol. scand. *75:* 139–152 (1969).

LUNDSTEDT, C. and VOLKERT, M.: Studies on immunological tolerance to LCM virus. 8. Induction of tolerance to the virus in adult mice treated with anti-lymphocytic serum. Acta path. microbiol. scand. *71:* 471–480 (1967).

LUTZNER, M. A.; TIERNEY, J. H., and BENDITT, E. P.: Giant granules and widespread cytoplasmic inclusions in a genetic syndrome of Aleutian mink. Lab. Invest. *14:* 2063–2079 (1966).

LYON, R. A.: Period of antibody development to lymphocytic choriomeningitis in mice. Publ. Hlth Rep., Wash. *55:* 2178–2180 (1940).

MACCALLUM, F. O. and FINDLAY, G. M.: Lymphocytic choriomeningitis. Isolation of the virus from the nasopharynx. Lancet *i:* 1370–1373 (1939).

MACCALLUM, F. O. and FINDLAY, G. M.: The cultivation of lymphocytic choriomeningitis in tissue culture. Brit. J. exp. Path. *21:* 110–116 (1940).

MACCALLUM, F. O.; FINDLAY, G. M., and SCOTT, T. M.: Pseudo-lymphocytic choriomeningitis. Brit. J. exp. Path. *20:* 260–269 (1939).

MACCALLUM, F. O.; SCOTT, T. F. M.; DALLDORF, G., and GIFFORD, R.: Pseudo-lymphocytic choriomeningitis: A correction. Brit. J. exp. Path. *38:* 120–121 (1957).

MACHELLA, T. E.; WEINBERGER, L. M., and LIPPINCOTT, S. W.: Lymphocytic choriomeningitis. Report of a fatal case with autopsy findings. Amer. J. med. Sci. *197:* 617–625 (1939).

MACKAY, J. M. K.: Detection of the scrapie agent in tissues of normal mice. Nature, Lond. *219:* 182–183 (1968).

MACKAY, J. M. K. and SMITH, W.: A case of scrapie in an uninoculated goat – a natural occurrence or a contact infection? Vet. Rec. *73:* 394–395 (1961).

MACKAY, J. M. K.; SMITH, W., and STAMP, J. T.: Experimental scrapie: Some recent work. Vet. Rec. *72:* 1002–1014 (1960).

MACKENZIE, A. and WILSON, A. M.: Accumulations of fat in the brains of mice affected with scrapie. Res. Vet. Sci. *7:* 45–54 (1966).

MACKENZIE, R. B.; WEBB, P. A., and JOHNSON K. M.: Detection of complement-fixing antibody after Bolivian hemorrhagic fever, employing Machupo, Junin and Tacaribe virus antigen. Amer. J. trop. med. Hyg. *14:* 1079–1084 (1965).

MACKENZIE, A.; MILLSON, G. C., and WILSON, A. M.: Glycosidase histochemistry in normal and scrapie mice, rats, sheep and goats. J. comp. Path. *78:* 43–52 (1968a).

MACKENZIE, A.; WILSON, A. M., and DENNIS, P. F.: Further observations on histochemical changes in scrapie mouse brain. Comparison with experimental viral encephalitides. J. comp. Path. *78:* 489–498 (1968b).

MAES, R.; VAHERI, A.; SEDWICK, D., and PLOTKIN, S.: Synthesis of virus and macromolecules by rubella-infected cells. Nature, Lond. *210:* 384–385 (1966).

MAHY, B. W. J.; ROWSON, K. E. K.; PARR, C. W., and SALAMAN, M. H.: Studies on the mechanism of action of Riley virus. J. exp. Med. *122:* 967–981 (1965).

MAHY, B. W. J.; ROWSON, K. E. K., and PARR, C. W.: Studies on the mechanism of action of Riley virus. IV. The reticuloendothelial system and impaired plasma enzyme clearance in infected mice. J. exp. Med. *125:* 277–288 (1967).

MALHERBE, H. and HARWIN, R.: Seven viruses isolated from the vervet monkey. Brit. J. exp. Path. *38:* 539–541 (1957).

MALMQUIST, W. A.: Serologic and immunologic studies with African swine fever virus. Amer. J. vet. Res. *24:* 450–459 (1963).

MALMQUIST, W. A. and HAY, D.: Hemadsorption and cytopathic effect produced by African swine fever virus in swine bone marrow and buffy coat cultures. Amer. J. vet. Res. *21:* 104–108 (1960).

MARAMOROSH, K.: Biological transmission of disease agents, vol. 1, p. 104 (Academic Press, New York 1962).

MARGOLIS, G. and KILHAM, L.: Rat virus, an agent with an affinity for the dividing cell. NINDB Monograph No. 2. Slow, latent and temperate virus infections. pp. 361–367 (US Dept. of Health, Education and Welfare, Washington, D. C. 1965).

MARGOLIS, G. and KILHAM, L.: Virus-induced cerebellar hypoplasia; in Infections of the nervous system, vol. 44, pp. 113–146 (Williams & Wilkins Co., Baltimore 1968a).

MARGOLIS, G. and KILHAM, L.: In pursuit of an ataxic hamster, or virus-induced cerebellar hypoplasia; in: The central nervous system. International Academy of Pathology Monograph No. 9, pp. 157–183 (Williams & Wilkins Co., Baltimore 1968b).

MARGOLIS, G.; KILHAM, L., and DAVENPORT, J.: A model for virus induced reproductive failure. Theory, observations and speculations. Proc. of the Conf. on comparative aspects of reproductive failure (Springer, New York 1967).

MARGOLIS, G.; KILHAM, L., and RUFFOLO, P. R.: Rat virus hepatitis, an experimental model of neonatal hepatitis. Exp. molec. Path. 8: 1–20 (1968).

MARKHAM, F. S.: A study of the submaxillary gland virus of the guinea pig. Amer. J. Path. 14: 311–322 (1938).

MARSH, H.: Infectious diseases of sheep; in Adv. vet. Sci, vol. 4, pp. 163–209 (Academic Press, New York 1958).

MARTIN, L. A.: L'incubation et la premier accès thermique au cours de l'anémie infectieuse expérimentales des équidés. Ann. Inst. Pasteur 62: 595–615 (1939).

MATHEWS, J. D.: The changing face of kuru. An analysis of pedigrees collected by R. M. GLASSE and SHIRLEY GLASSE and of recent census data. Lancet i: 1138–1141 (1965).

MATHEWS, J. D.; GLASSE, R., and LINDENBAUM, S.: Kuru and cannibalism. Lancet ii: 449–452 (1968).

MATSUO, Y. and SPENCER, H. J.: Studies on the infectivity of rat virus (RV) in BALB/c mice. Proc. Soc. exp. Biol., N. Y. 130: 294–299 (1969).

MAURER, F. D.: Lymphocytic choriomeningitis. Lab. Anim. Care 14: 415–419 (1964).

MAURER, F. D.; GRIESMER, R. A., and JONES, T. C.: The pathology of African swine fever – A comparison with hog cholera. Amer. J. vet. Res. 19: 517–539 (1958).

MAYOR, H. D. and MELNICK, J. L.: Small deoxyribonucleic acid-containing virus (Picodnavirus group). Nature, Lond. 210: 331–332 (1966).

McALLISTER, R. M.; FILBERT, J. E., and GOODHEART, C. R.: Human cytomegalovirus. Studies on the mechanism of viral cytopathology and inclusion body formation. Proc. Soc. exp. Biol., N. Y. 124: 932–937 (1967).

McCARTHY, K. and TAYLOR-ROBINSON, C. H.: Rubella. Brit. med. Bull. 23: 185–191 (1967).

McCOLLUM, R. W.: The size of serum hepatitis virus. Proc. Soc. exp. Biol., N. Y. 81: 157–160 (1952).

McCRACKEN, G. H., jr., and SHINEFIELD, H. R.: Immunoglobulin concentrations in newborn infants with congenital cytomegalic inclusion disease. Pediatrics 36: 933–937 (1965).

McDANIEL, H. A. and MOREHOUSE, L. G.: The diagnosis of scrapie. Report of Scrapie Seminar, Washington, D. C., 1964, pp. 41–52 (US Dept. of Agriculture, ARS 91–53, Washington, D. C. 1966).

McFadyean, J.: Scrapie. J. comp. Path. *31:* 102–131 (1918a).

McFadyean, J.: Sarcosporidiosis as the cause of scrapie. J. comp. Path. *31:* 290–299 (1918b).

McGiven, A. R. and Hicks, J. D.: The development of renal lesions in NZB/NZW mice. Immunohistological studies. Brit. J. exp. Path. *68:* 302–304 (1967).

McGowan, J. P.: Investigation into the disease of sheep called scrapie. Bull. Edinburgh and East. of Scot. Coll. Agric. (1914).

McGowan, J. P.: Scrapie. J. comp. Path. *31:* 278–290 (1918).

McKay, D. G.; Phillips, L. L.; Kaplan, H., and Henson, J. B.: Chronic intravascular coagulation in Aleutian disease of mink. Amer. J. Path. *50:* 899–911 (1967).

Medearis, D. N., jr.: Mouse cytomegalovirus infection. II. Observations during prolonged infections. Amer. J. Hyg. *80:* 103–112 (1964a).

Medearis, D. N., jr.: Mouse cytomegalovirus infection. III. Attempts to produce intrauterine infections. Amer. J. Hyg. *80:* 113–120 (1964b).

Medearis, D. N., jr.: Observations concerning human cytomegalovirus infection and disease. Bull. Johns. Hopk. Hosp. *114:* 181–211 (1964c).

Melnick, J. L. and Parks, W. P.: Hepatitis virus studies in marmosets. Proc. 8th Inter. Congr. Trop. Med. and Malaria, Tehran, 1968, p. 827.

Mendes, A. M. and Daskalos, A. M.: Studies on the lapinization of swine fever virus in Angola. Bull. epizoot. Dis. Afr. *3:* 9–14 (1955).

Menser, M. A.; Dods, L., and Harley, J. D.: A twenty-five year follow-up of congenital rubella. Lancet *ii:* 1347–1350 (1967a).

Menser, M. A.; Harley, J. D.; Hertzberg, R.; Dorman, D. C., and Murphy, A. M.: Persistence of virus in lens for three years after prenatal rubella. Lancet *ii:* 387–388 (1967b).

Menser, M. A.; Robertson, S. E. J.; Dorman, D. C.; Gillespie, A. M., and Murphy, A. M.: Renal lesions in congenital rubella. Pediatrics *40:* 901–904 (1967c).

Merchant, I. A.: Lymphocytic choriomeningitis virus; in: Veterinary bacteriology and virology, 6th ed., pp. 787–792 (1961).

Mergenhagen, S. E.; Notkins, A. L., and Dougherty, S. F.: Adjuvanticity of lactic dehydrogenase virus. Influence of virus infection on the establishment of immunologic tolerance to a protein antigen in adult mice. J. Immunol. *99:* 576–581 (1967).

Miller, J. F. and Howard, J. G.: Some similarities between the neonatal thymectomy syndrome and graft-versus-host disease. J. Reticuloendothel. Soc. *1:* 369–392 (1964).

Millman, I.; Zavatone, V.; Gerstley, B. J. S., and Blumberg, B. S.: Australian antigen detected in the nuclei of liver cells of patients with viral hepatitis by the fluorescent antibody technique. Nature, Lond. *222:* 181–184 (1969).

Millson, G. C.: Lysosomal enzymes in normal and scrapie mouse brain. J. Neurochem. *12:* 461–468 (1965).

Millson, G. C. and Hunter, G. D.: Protein synthesis in normal and scrapie mouse brain. J. Neurochem. *15:* 447–453 (1968).

Millson, G. C.; West, L. C., and Dew, S. M.: Biochemical and haematological observations on the blood and cerebrospinal fluid of clinically healthy and scrapie-affected goats. J. comp. Path. *70:* 194–198 (1960).

Milzer, A.: Studies on the transmission of lymphocytic choriomeningitis virus by arthropods. J. infect. Dis. *70:* 152–172 (1942).

Milzer, A. and Levinson, S. O.: Laboratory infection with the virus of lymphocytic choriomeningitis. J. amer. med. Ass. *120:* 27–30 (1942).

Milzer, A. and Levinson, S. O.: Production of potent inactivated vaccines with ultraviolet irradiation. V. Active and passive immunization with lymphocytic choriomeningitis vaccine. J. Bact. *51:* 622 (1946).

Milzer, A. and Levinson, S. O.: Active immunization of mice with ultraviolet inactivated lymphocytic choriomeningitis virus vaccine and results of immune serum therapy. J. infect. Dis. *85:* 251–255 (1949).

Mims, C. A.: Immunofluorescence study of the carrier state and mechanism of vertical transmission in lymphocytic choriomeningitis virus infection in mice. J. Path. Bact. *91:* 395–402 (1966).

Mims, C. A. and Subrahmanyan, T. P.: Immunofluorescence study of the mechanism of resistance to superinfection in mice carrying the lymphocytic choriomeningitis virus. J. Path. Bact. *91:* 403–415 (1966).

Mims, C. A. and Wainwright, S.: The immunodepressive action of lymphocytic choriomeningitis virus in mice. J. Immunol. *101:* 717–724 (1968).

Miura, S.; Kuchii, T.; Shionoya, K., and Ueda, S.: Experimental studies on the simple inactivation of infectious anemia virus presented in the horse serum. I. Results from experiment I–III. Jap. J. vet. Sci. *9:* 87–102 (1947).

Miura, S.; Sato, G., and Miyamae, T.: Further observations on the transmission of equine infectious anemia virus of sheep. Jap. J. vet. Res. *3:* 136–139 (1955).

Möhlmann, H.: Über vier durch Wechselpassage Pferde-Schaf-Pferd experimentell erzeugte Fälle der stummen Form der infektiösen Anämie. Arch. exp. Vet. Med. *10:* 709–712 (1956).

Möhlmann, H. und Gralheer, H.: Grössenbestimmung des Virus der infektiösen Anämie der Einhufer durch Ultrafiltration. Arch. exp. Vet. Med. *8:* 199–203 (1954).

Molomut, N. and Padnos, M.: Inhibition of transplantable and spontaneous murine tumors by the M-P virus. Nature, Lond. *208:* 948–950 (1965).

Molomut, N.; Padnos, M.; Gross, L., and Satory, V.: Inhibition of a transplantable murine leukemia by a lymphocytopenic virus. Nature, Lond. *204:* 1003–1004 (1964).

Molomut, N.; Padnos, M., and Smith, L. W.: A lymphocytopenic filterable agent derived from tissue cell cultures of murine carcinoma. J. nat. Cancer Inst. *34:* 403–413 (1965).

Monif, G. R. G. and Sever, J. L.: Chronic infection of the central nervous system with rubella virus. Neurology, Minneap. *16:* 111–112 (1966).

MONTGOMERY, R. E.: On a form of swine fever occurring in British East Africa (Kenya colony). J. comp. Path. *34:* 159–191 (1921).

MONTGOMERY, J. R.; SOUTH, M. A.; RAWLS, W. E.; MELNICK, J. L.; OLSON, G. B.; DENT, P. F., and GOOD, R. A.: Viral inhibition of lymphocyte response to phytohemagglutinin. Science *157:* 1068–1070 (1967).

MOORE, R. W.; LIVINGSTONE, C. W., and REDMOND, H. E.: Equine infectious anemia. I. Preparation and preliminary investigation of a precipitinogen for equine infectious anema (EIA). Sth West. vet. J. *19:* 187–191 (1966).

MORRIS, J. A. and GAJDUSEK, D. C.: Encephalopathy in mice following inoculation of scrapie sheep brain. Nature, Lond. *197:* 1084–1086 (1963).

MORRIS, J. A.; GAJDUSEK, D. C., and GIBBS, C. J., jr.: Spread of scrapie from inoculated to uninoculated mice. Proc. Soc. exp. Biol., N. Y. *120:* 108–110 (1965).

MOULD, D. L. and DAWSON, A. McL.: Free and esterified cholesterol in the cerebrospinal fluid of goats affected with experimental scrapie. Res. Vet. Sci. *6:* 274–279 (1965).

MOULD, D. L. and DAWSON, A. McL.: Unsuccessful studies in the dialysis of the mouse scrapie agent. J. comp. Path. *78:* 115–120 (1968).

MOULD, D. L. and SLATER, J. S.: An investigation into the nature of the causal agent of sheep scrapie and some observations on the biochemistry of the disease. Report of Scrapie Seminar, Washington, D. C., 1964, pp. 270–281 (US Dept. of Agriculture, ARS 91–53, Washington, D. C. 1966).

MOULD, D. L. and SMITH, W.: The causal agent of scrapie. I. Extraction of the agent from infected sheep tissue. J. comp. Path. *72:* 97–105 (1962a).

MOULD, D. L. and SMITH, W.: The causal agent of scrapie. II. Extraction of the agent from infected goat tissue. J. comp. Path. *72:* 106–112 (1962b).

MOULD, D. L.; SMITH, W., and DAWSON, A. McL.: The elution of scrapie brain tissue through calcium phosphate columns. Biochem. J. *91:* 13P (1964).

MOULD, D. L.; DAWSON, A. McL., and SMITH, W.: Scrapie in mice. The stability of the agent to various suspending media, pH and solvent extraction. Res. Vet. Sci. *6:* 151–154 (1965a).

MOULD, D. L.; SMITH, W., and DAWSON, A. McL.: Centrifugation studies on the infectivities of cellular fractions derived from mouse brain infected with scrapie ('Suffolk strain'). J. gen. Microbiol. *40:* 71–79 (1965b).

MOULD, D. L.; DAWSON, A. McL., and SMITH, W.: Determination of the dosage-response curve of mice inoculated with scrapie. J. comp. Path. *77:* 387–391 (1967a).

MOULD, D. L.; DAWSON, A. McL.; SLATER, J. S., and ZLOTNIK, I.: Relationships between chemical changes and histological damage in the brains of scrapie affected mice. J. comp. Path. *77:* 393–403 (1967b).

MOULTON, J. and COGGINS, L.: Synthesis and cytopathogenesis of African swine fever virus in porcine cell cultures. Amer. J. vet. Res. *29:* 219–232 (1968a).

MOULTON, J. and COGGINS, L.: Comparison of lesions in acute and chronic African swine fever. Cornell Vet. *58:* 364–388 (1968b).

MOULTON, J. E. and PALMER, A. C.: Attempts to demonstrate the transmissible agent of scrapie in experimentally infected goats by means of fluorescent antibody. Cornell Vet. *49:* 349–359 (1959).

MURPHY, A. M.; REID, R. R.; POLLARD, I.; GILLESPIE, A. M.; DORMAN, D. C.; MENSER, M. A.; HARLEY, J. D., and HERTZBERG, R.: Rubella cataracts. Further clinical and virologic observations. Amer. J. Ophthal. *64:* 1109–1119 (1967).

MURPHY, F. A.; WEBB, P. A.; JOHNSON, K. M., and WHITFIELD, S. G.: Morphological comparison of machupo with lymphocytic choriomeningitis virus: Basis for a new taxonomic group. J. Virology *4:* 535–541 (1969).

MYERS, W. L.; SEGRE, D., and EL-ZEIN, A.: Equine infectious anemia: Reports of progress in research. J. amer. vet. med. Ass. *155:* 352–354 (1969).

NADEL, E. and HAAS, V. H.: Inhibitory effect of virus of lymphocytic choriomeningitis on course of leukemia in guinea pigs. Fed. Proc. *14:* 414–415 (1955).

NADEL, E. M. and HAAS, V. H.: Effect of the virus of lymphocytic choriomeningitis on the course of leukemia in guinea pigs and mice. J. nat. Cancer Inst. *17:* 221–231 (1956).

NAEYE, R. L.: Cytomegalic inclusion disease. The fetal disorder. Amer. J. clin. Path. *47:* 738–744 (1967).

NAEYE, R. L. and BLANC, W.: Pathogenesis of congenital rubella. J. amer. med. Ass. *194:* 1277–1283 (1965).

NEUMANN, M.; GAJDUSEK, D. C., and ZIGAS, V.: Neuropathologic findings in exotic neurologic disorders among natives of the highlands of New Guinea. J. Neuropath. exp. Neurol. *23:* 486–507 (1964).

NIKOLITSCH, M.: Der Weg des neurotropen Virus, dargestellt in Modellversuchen an Tollwut und lymphozytärer Choriomeningitis. Zbl. Bakt. Parasitkde (I. Abt.). *175:* 1–10 (1959).

NOTKINS, A. L.: Recovery of an infectious ribonucleic acid from the lactic dehydrogenase agent by treatment with ether. Virology *22:* 563–567 (1964).

NOTKINS, A. L.: Lactic dehydrogenase virus. Bact. Rev. *29:* 143–160 (1965).

NOTKINS, A. L. and SCHEELE, C.: Studies on the transmission and the excretion of the lactic dehydrogenase agent. J. exp. Med. *118:* 7–12 (1963).

NOTKINS, A. L. and SCHEELE, C.: Impaired clearance of enzymes in mice infected with the lactic dehydrogenase agent. J. nat. Cancer Inst. *33:* 741–749 (1964).

NOTKINS, A. L. and SHOCHAT, S. J.: Studies of the multiplication and the properties of the lactic dehydrogenase agent. J. exp. Med. *117:* 735–747 (1963).

NOTKINS, A. L.; MERGENHAGEN, S. E.; RIZZO, A. A.; SCHEELE, C., and WALDMANN, T. A.: Elevated γ globulin and increased antibody production in mice infected with lactic dehydrogenase virus. J. exp. Med. *123:* 347–364 (1966a).

NOTKINS, A. L.; MAHAR, S.; SCHEELE, C., and GOFFMAN, J.: Infectious virus-antibody complex in the blood of chronically infected mice. J. exp. Med. *124:* 81–97 (1966b).

NOTKINS, A. L.; MERGENHAGEN, S. E.; RIZZO, A. A.; SCHEELE, C., and WALDMANN, T. A.: Lactic dehydrogenase virus (LDV) as an immunologic adjuvant. Abstract. Proc. amer. Ass. Cancer Res. *7:* 53 (1966c).

NOTKINS, A. L.; MAGE, M.; ASHE, W. K., and MAHAR, S.: Neutralization of sensitized lactic dehydrogenase virus by anti-γ globulin. J. Immunol. *100:* 314–320 (1968).

NUSBAUM, S. R.: The challenge of field diagnosis and control of equine infectious anemia. J. amer. vet. med. Ass. *151:* 1847–1851 (1967).

OBEL, A. L.: Studies on a disease in mink with systemic proliferation of the plasma cells. Amer. J. vet. Res. *20:* 384–393 (1959).

OKADA, S. and FLETCHER, G. L.: Radiation inactivation of deoxyribonuclease in the dry and hydrated states. Radiat. Res. *13:* 92–98 (1960).

OLDSTONE, M. B. A. and DIXON, F. J.: Lymphocytic choriomeningitis: Production of antibody by 'tolerant' infected mice. Science *158:* 1193–1195 (1967).

OLDSTONE, M. B. A. and DIXON, F. J.: Susceptibility of different mouse strains to lymphocytic choriomeningitis virus. J. Immunol. *100:* 355–357 (1968a).

OLDSTONE, M. B. A. and DIXON, F. J.: Direct immunofluorescent tissue culture assay for lymphocytic choriomeningitis virus. J. Immunol. *100:* 1135–1138 (1968b).

OLDSTONE, M. B. A. and DIXON, F. J.: Pathogenesis of chronic disease associated with persistent lymphocytic choriomeningitis viral infection. I. Relationship of antibody production to disease in neonatally infected mice. J. exp. Med. *129:* 483–505 (1969).

OLDSTONE, M. B. A.; HABEL, K., and DIXON, F. J.: The pathogenesis of cellular injury associated with persistent LCM viral infection. Abstract Fed. Proc. *28:* 429 (1969).

OLMSTED, E.; PRASAD, S.; SHEFFER, J.; CLARK, H. F., and KARZON, D. T.: Ocular lesions induced in C57 mice by the suckling mouse cataract agent (SMCA). Invest. Ophthal. *5:* 413–420 (1966).

OLSON, G. B.; SOUTH, M. A., and GOOD, R. A.: Phytohemagglutinin unresponsiveness of lymphocytes from babies with congenital rubella. Nature, Lond. *214:* 695–696 (1967).

OLSON, G. B.; DENT, P. B.; RAWLS, W. E.; SOUTH, M. A.; MONTGOMERY, J. R.; MELNICK, J. L., and GOOD, R. A.: Abnormalities of *in vitro* lymphocyte responses during rubella virus infections. J. exp. Med. *128:* 47–68 (1968).

O'REILLY, K. J.; PATERSON, J. S., and HARRISS, S. T.: The persistence in kittens of maternal antibody to feline infectious enteritis (panleucopenia). Vet. Rec. *84:* 376–378 (1969).

OSBORN, J. E.; BLAZKOVEC, A. A., and WALKER, D. L.: Immunosuppression during acute murine cytomegalovirus infection. J. Immunol. *100:* 835–844 (1968).

PADGETT, G. A.; GORHAM, J. R., and HENSON, J. B.: Epizootiologic studies of Aleutian disease. I. Transplacental transmission of the virus. J. infect. Dis. *117:* 35–38 (1967).

PADGETT, G. A.; REIQUAN, C. W.; HENSON, J. B., and GORHAM, J. R.: Comparative studies of susceptibility to infection in the Chediak-Higashi syndrome. J. Path. Bact. *95:* 509–522 (1968).

PADNOS, M.; HOFER, R. J., and FERRIS, P.: Characteristics of a murine hemagglutinin induced by the M-P virus. Proc. Soc. exp. Biol., N. Y. *128:* 546–550 (1968).

Page, A. R.; Berendes, H.; Warner, J., and Good, R. A.: The Chediak-Higashi syndrome. Blood *20:* 330–343 (1962).

Palmer, A. C.: Studies in scrapie. Vet. Rec. *69:* 1318–1324 (1957).

Palmer, A. C.: Attempt to transmit scrapie by injection of semen from an affected ram. Vet. Rec. *71:* 664 (1959a).

Palmer, A. C.: Scrapie, a review of the literature. Vet. Rev. Annot. *5:* 1–15 (1959b).

Pálsson, P. A.; Pattison, I. H., and Field, E. J.: Transmission experiments with multiple sclerosis. NINDB Monograph No. 2. Slow, latent and temperate virus infections. pp. 49–54 (US Dept. of Health, Education and Welfare, Washington, D. C. 1965).

Papadimitriou, J. M.: Electron microscopic findings of a murine lymphoma associated with reovirus type 3 infection. Proc. Soc. exp. Biol., N. Y. *121:* 93–96 (1966).

Parikh, G. C.: Cytological changes by lymphocytic choriomeningitis virus in the human amnion cells. Jap. J. Microbiol. *5:* 129–132 (1961).

Parkman, P. D.; Phillips, P. E., and Meyer, H. M., jr.: Experimental rubella virus infection in pregnant monkeys. Amer. J. Dis. Child. *110:* 390–394 (1965).

Parodi, A. S.; Coto, C. E.; Boxaca, M.; Lajmanovich, S., and González, S.: Characteristics of Junin virus. Etiological agent of Argentine hemorrhagic fever. Arch. ges. Virusforsch. *19:* 393–402 (1966).

Parry, H. B.: Scrapie and related myopathies in sheep. Preliminary observation on their investigation and attempted control by a voluntary health scheme. Vet. Rec. *69:* 43–55 (1957).

Parry, H. B.: Scrapie: A transmissible hereditary disease of sheep. Nature, Lond. *185:* 441–443 (1960).

Parry, H. B.: Scrapie: A transmissible and hereditary disease of sheep. Heredity *17:* 75–105 (1962).

Parry, H. B.: The hereditary mechanism in the causation of natural scrapie in sheep. IV. The possible relationships of the transmissible scrapie agent (provirus) to the genetical component. Report of Scrapie Seminar, Washington, D. C., 1964, pp. 168–171 (US Dept. of Agriculture, ARS 91–53, Washington, D. C. 1966).

Patrick, M. H. and Rupert, C. S.: The effects of host-cell reactivation on assay of U. V.-irradiated *Haemophilus influenzae* transforming DNA. Photochem. Photobiol. *6:* 1–20 (1967).

Pattison, I. H.: The spread of scrapie by contact between affected and healthy sheep, goats or mice. Vet. Rec. *76:* 333–336 (1964).

Pattison, I. H.: Experiments with scrapie with special reference to the nature of the agent and the pathology of the disease. NINDB Monograph No. 2. Slow, latent and temperate virus infections, pp. 249–257 (US Dept. of Health, Education and Welfare, Washington, D. C. 1965a).

Pattison, I. H.: Resistance of the scrapie agent to formalin. J. comp. Path. *75:* 159–164 (1965b).

Pattison, I. H.: Scrapie in the welsh mountain breed of sheep and its experimental transmission to goats. Vet. Rec. *77:* 1388–1390 (1965c).

PATTISON, I. H.: The relative susceptibility of sheep, goats and mice to two types of the goat scrapie agent. Res. Vet. Sci. *7:* 207–212 (1966).

PATTISON, I. H.: Scrapie; in POOL The veterinary annal, p. 83 (Wright, Bristol (1968).

PATTISON, I. H. and JONES, K. M.: The possible nature of the transmissible agent of scrapie. Vet. Rec. *80:* 2–9 (1967a).

PATTISON, I. H. and JONES, K. M.: The astrocytic reaction in experimental scrapie in the rat. Res. Vet. Sci. *8:* 160–165 (1967b).

PATTISON, I. H. and JONES, K. M.: Detection of the scrapie agent in tissues of normal mice and in tumours of tumour-bearing but otherwise normal mice. Nature, Lond. *218:* 102–104 (1968).

PATTISON, I. H. and MILLSON, G. C.: Further observations on the experimental production of scrapie in goats and sheep. J. comp. Path. *70:* 182–193 (1960).

PATTISON, I. H. and MILLSON, G. C.: Scrapie produced experimentally in goats with special reference to the clinical syndrome. J. comp. Path. *71:* 101–108 (1961a).

PATTISON, I. H. and MILLSON, G. C.: Experimental transmission of scrapie to goats and sheep by the oral route. J. comp. Path. *71:* 171–176 (1961b).

PATTISON, I. H. and MILLSON, G. C.: Further experimental observations on scrapie. J. comp. Path. *71:* 350–359 (1961c).

PATTISON, I. H. and MILLSON, G. C.: Distribution of the scrapie agent in the tissues of experimentally inoculated goats. J. comp. Path. *72:* 233–244 (1962).

PATTISON, I. H. and SANSOM, B. F.: Dialysis of the scrapie agent. Res. Vet. Sci. *5:* 340–347 (1964).

PATTISON, I. H. and SMITH, K.: Experimental scrapie in goats: a modification of incubation period and clinical response following pretreatment with normal goat brain. Nature, Lond. *200:* 1342–1343 (1963).

PATTISON, I. H.; GORDON, W. S., and MILLSON, G. C.: Experimental production of scrapie in goats. J. comp. Path. *69:* 300-312 (1959).

PATTISON, I. H.; MILLSON, G. C., and SMITH, K.: An examination of the action of the whole blood, blood cells or serum on the goat scrapie agent. Res. Vet. Sci. *5:* 116–121 (1964).

PEDERSEN, I. R.: Methanol precipitation of lymphocytic choriomeningitis virus. Acta path. microbiol. scand. *67:* 514–522 (1966).

PEDERSEN, I. R. and VOLKERT, M.: Multiplication of lymphocytic choriomeningitis virus in suspension cultures of Earle's strain L cells. Acta path. microbiol. scand. *67:* 523–536 (1966).

PERIER, O. et VANDERHAEGHEN, J. J.: Indications étiologiques apportées par la microscope électronique dans certaines encéphalites humaines. Rev. neurol. *115:* 250–254 (1966).

PERRIN, T. L. and STEINHAUS, E. A.: Pathologic reaction in guinea pigs to the Humphreys' virus strain. Publ. Hlth Rep., Wash. *59:* 1603–1609 (1944).

PETERS, J. T.: L'anémia infectieuse du cheval chez l'homme. Presse méd. *10:* 105–106 (1924).

PETERS, J. T.: Trifur equorum infection in man. New Engl. J. Med. *251:* 1022–1023 (1954).

PETTE, E.; MANNWEILER, K., and PALACIOS, O.: A contribution to the problem of granuloma encephalomyelitis of viral origin. Dtsch. Z. Nervenheilk. *182:* 635–651 (1961).

PFAU, C. J.: Biophysical and biochemical characterization of lymphocytic choriomeningitis virus. I. Density gradient studies. Acta path. microbiol. scand. *63:* 188–197 (1965a).

PFAU, C. J.: Biophysical and biochemical characterization of lymphocytic choriomeningitis virus. 2. Partial purification by differential centrifugation and fluorocarbon techniques. Acta path. microbiol. scand. *63:* 198–205 (1965b).

PFAU, C. J.: Stabilization of the virus of lymphocytic choriomeningitis. Proc. 9th int. Congr. for Microbiol., Moscow 1966, p. 468.

PFAU, C. J. and CAMYRE, K. P.: Biophysical and biochemical characterization of lymphocytic choriomeningitis virus. III. Thermal and ultrasonic sensitivity. Arch. ges. Virusforsch. *20:* 430–437 (1967).

PFAU, C. J. and CAMYRE, K. P.: Inhibition of lymphocytic choriomeningitis virus multiplication by 2-(a-Hydroxybenzyl) benzimidazole. Virology *35:* 375–380 (1968).

PFAU, C. J.; PEDERSEN, I. R., and VOLKERT, M.: Inability of nucleic acid analogues to inhibit the synthesis of lymphocytic choriomeningitis virus. Acta path. microbiol. scand. *63:* 181–187 (1965).

PHILLIPS, L. L. and HENSON, J. B.: Coagulation changes in Aleutian mink disease. Abstract Fed. Proc. *25:* 620 (1966).

PHILLIPS, L. L. and HENSON, J. B.; YOW, M. D.; BAYATPOUR, M., and BURKHARDT, M.: Persistence of virus in infants with congenital rubella and in normal infants with a history of maternal rubella. J. amer. med. Ass. *193:* 1027–1029 (1965).

PHILLIPS, C. A.; RAWLS, W. E.; MELNICK, J. L., and YOW, M. D.: Viral studies of a congenital rubella epidemic. Health Lab. Sci. *3:* 118–123 (1966).

PHILLIPS, L. L.; KAPLAN, H. S.; PADGETT, G. A., and GORHAM, J. R.: Comparative studies on the Chediak-Higashi syndrome. Coagulation and fibrinolytic mechanisms of mink and cattle. Amer. J. vet. clin. Path. *1:* 1–6 (1967).

PLACIDI, L. et VERGE, J.: Essai de transmission au singe du virus de l'anémia infectieuse des équidés (maladie de Vallée et Carré). C. R. Acad. Sci. *237:* 1041–1043 (1953).

PLAGEMANN, P. G. W. and SWIM, H. E.: Studies of the plasma lactic dehydrogenase-elevating virus (PLDEV) of mice. Abstract Amer. Ass. Cancer Res. *4:* 53 (1963a).

PLAGEMANN, P. G. W. and SWIM, H. E.: Studies of virus associated with metabolic disease in mice. VIII. Internat. Congr. Microbiol., 1962, p. 91 (Toronto Press, Toronto 1963b).

PLAGEMANN, P. G. W. and SWIM, H. E.: Propagation of lactic dehydrogenase-elevating virus in cell culture. Proc. Soc. exp. Biol., N. Y. *121:* 1147–1152 (1966).

PLOTKIN, S. A.; DUDGEON, J. A., and RAMSAY, A. M.: Laboratory studies on rubella and the rubella syndrome. Brit. med. J. *ii:* 1296–1299 (1963).

PLOTKIN, S. A.; KLAUS, R. M., and WHITELY, J. P.: Hypogammaglobulinemia in an infant with congenital rubella syndrome; failure of Z-adamantanamine to stop virus excretion. J. Pediat. *69:* 1085–1091 (1966).

PLOWRIGHT, W.; PARKER, J., and STAPLE, R. F.: The growth of a virulent strain of African swine fever virus in domestic pigs. J. Hyg. *66:* 117–134 (1968).

PLUMMER, P. J. G.: Scrapie – A disease of sheep. A review of the literature. Canad. J. comp. Med. *10:* 49–54 (1946).

POLLARD, M.; KAJIMA, M., and SHARON, N.: LCM virus-induced immunopathology in congenitally infected gnotobiotic mice; in: Perspectives in virology, vol. 6, pp. 193–209 (Academic Press, New York 1968a).

POLLARD, M.; SHARON, N., and TEAH, B. A.: Congenital lymphocytic choriomeningitis virus infection in gnotobiotic mice. Proc. Soc. exp. Biol., N. Y. *127:* 755–761 (1968b).

POLLIKOFF, R. and SIGEL, M. M.: Factors influencing the neutralization of lymphocytic choriomeningitis virus. Bact. Proc., p. 105 (1952).

PORTELLA, O. B.: Hemadsorption and related studies on the hamster osteolytic viruses. Arch. ges. Virusforsch. *14:* 277–305 (1963).

PORTER, D. D. and LARSEN, A. E.: Aleutian disease of mink: Infectious virus-antibody complexes in the serum. Proc. Soc. exp. Biol., N. Y. *26:* 680–682 (1967).

PORTER, D. D.; DIXON, F. J., and LARSEN, A. E.: Metabolism and function of gamma globulin in Aleutian disease of mink. J. exp. Med. *121:* 889–900 (1965).

PORTER, D. D.; PORTER, H. G., and DEERHAKE, B. B.: Immunofluorescence assay for antigens and antibody in lactic dehydrogenase virus infection of mice. J. Immunol. *102:* 431–436 (1969a).

PORTER, D. D.; LARSEN, A. E., and PORTER, H. G.: The pathogenesis of Aleutian disease of mink. I. *In vivo* viral replication and the host antibody response to viral antigen. J. exp. Med. *130:* 575–593 (1969b).

POTTER, M. and HAAS, V. H.: Relationships between lymphocytic choriomeningitis virus, amethopterin, and an amethopterin-resistant lymphocytic neoplasm in mice. J. nat. Cancer Inst. *22:* 801–809 (1959).

PRICE, W. H.: Chronic disease and virus persistence in mice inoculated with Kyasanur Forest disease virus. Virology *29:* 679–681 (1966).

PRICK, J. J. G.: Virus meningitis. I. Clinical part. Antonie Van Leeuwenhoek *11:* 177–185 (1946).

PRINCE, A. M.: An antigen detected in the blood during the incubation period of serum hepatitis. Proc. nat. Acad. Sci., Wash. *60:* 814–821 (1968a).

PRINCE, A. M.: Relation of Australia and SH antigens. Lancet *ii:* 462–463 (1968b).

RASMUSSEN, A. F., jr.: The laboratory diagnosis of lymphocytic choriomeningitis and mumps. Presented at the Rocky Mountain Conf. on Poliomyelitis, Denver, Colorado, 1946, pp. 45–51.

RAWLS, W. E.: Congenital rubella: The significance of virus persistence. Progr. med. Virol., vol. 10, pp. 238–285 (Karger, Basel/New York 1968).

RAWLS, W. E. and MELNICK, J. L.: Rubella virus carrier cultures derived from congenitally infected infants. J. exp. Med. *123:* 795–816 (1966).

RAWLS, W. E.; PHILLIPS, C. A.; MELNICK, J. L., and DESMOND, M. M.: Persistent virus infection in congenital rubella. Arch. Ophthal., Chicago *77:* 430–433 (1967).

RAWLS, W. E.; DESMYTER, J., and MELNICK, J. L.: Virus carrier cells and virus free cells in fetal rubella. Proc. Soc. exp. Biol., N. Y. *129:* 477–483 (1968).

RECHER, L.; TANAKA, T.; SYKES, J. A.; YUMOTO, T.; SEMAN, G.; YOUNG, L., and DMOCHOWSKI, L.: Further studies on the biological relationship of murine leukemia viruses and on kidney lesions of mice with leukemia induced by these viruses. Nat. Cancer Inst. Monograph 22, pp. 459–479 (1966).

ŘEHÁČEK, J.: Cultivation of different viruses in tick tissue cultures. Acta Virol. 9: 332–337 (1965).

REID, R. R.; MURPHY, A. M.; GILLESPIE, A. M.; DORMAN, D. C.; MENSER, M. A.; HERTZBERG, R., and HARLEY, J. D.: Preliminary communication. Isolation ot rubella virus from congenital cataracts removed at operation. Med. J. Austr. i: 540–542 (1966).

REISS-GUTFREUND, R. J.: Antagonisme entre un virus de chorioméningite lymphocytaire (CML) et Rickettsia prowazeki. Ann. Inst. Pasteur 102: 227–231 (1962).

REMEZOV, P. I.: The influence of general X-irradiation and cooling on the course of certain neurotropic virus infections in white mice. Probl. Virol. 4: 58–61

REMEZOV, P. I. and TOPLENINOVA, K. A.: Detection of the virus of lymphocytic choriomeningitis by means of the indirect method of fluorescing antibodies. Vop. Paikhiat. Nevropat. 7: 113–120 (1961).

RENWICK, C. C. and ZLOTNIK, I.: The transmission of scrapie to mice by intracerebral inoculations of brain from an apparently normal lamb. Vet. Rec. 77: 984–985 (1965).

RESSANG, A. A.; DEBOER, G. F., and WIJN, G. C.: The lung in Zwoegerziekte. Path. vet. 5: 353–369 (1968).

RESSANG, A. A.; STAM, F. C., and DEBOER, G. F.: A meningo-leucoencephalomyelitis resembling visna in Dutch Zwoeger sheep. Path. vet. 3: 401–411 (1966).

RHIM, J. S.; JORDAN, L. E., and MAYOR, H. D.: Cytochemical, fluorescent antibody and electron microscopic studies on the growth of reovirus (ECHO 10) in tissue culture. Virology 17: 342–355 (1962).

RHODES, A. J. and CHAPMAN, M.: Some observations on interference between neurotropic viruses. Canad. J. Res. 27: 341–348 (1949).

RHODES, A. J. and CHAPMAN, M.: Further observations on interference between lymphocytic choriomeningitis and MM viruses. Canad. J. Res. 28: 245–255 (1950).

RIFKIND, D.: Cytomegalovirus infection after renal transplantation. Arch. intern. Med. 116: 554–558 (1965).

RILEY, V.: Enzymatic determination of transmissible replicating factors associated with mouse tumors. Ann. N. Y. Acad. Sci. 100: 762–789 (1963a).

RILEY, V.: Synergistic glycolytic activity associated with transmissible agents and neoplastic growth; in: Control mechanism in respiration and fermentation, pp. 211–241 (Ronald, New York 1963b).

RILEY, V.: Transmissible agents and anemia of mouse cancer. N. Y. St. J. Med. 63: 1523–1531 (1963c).

RILEY, V.: Synergism between a lactate dehydrogenase-elevating virus and Eperythrozoon coccoides. Science 146: 921–923 (1964).

RILEY, V.: Spontaneous mammary tumors: Decrease of incidence in mice infected with an enzyme-elevating virus. Science 153: 1657–1658 (1966).

RILEY, V.: Lactate dehydrogenase in the normal and malignant state in mice and the influence of a benign enzyme-elevating virus; in: Methods in cancer research, vol. IV, pp. 493–618 (Academic Press, New York 1968).

RILEY, V.; HUERTO, E.; LILLY, F.; BARDELL, D.; LOVELESS, J. D., and FITZMAURICE, M. A.: Some characteristics of virus-like entities associated with thirty varieties of experimental tumors. Abstract Proc. amer. Ass. Cancer Res. *3:* 261 (1961).

RILEY, V.; LOVELESS, J. D., and FITZMAURICE, M. A.: Comparison of a lactate dehydrogenase elevating virus-like agent and Eperythrozoon coccoides. Proc. Soc. exp. Biol., N. Y. *116:* 486–490 (1964).

RILEY, V.; LOVELESS, J. D.; FITZMAURICE, M. A., and SILER, W. M.: Mechanism of lactate dehydrogenase (LDH) elevation in virus-infected hosts. Life Sci. *4:* 487–507 (1965).

RILEY, V.; FITZMAURICE, M. A., and LOVELESS, J. D.: Decrease in 'spontaneous' mammary tumor incidence in mice infected with the LDH-elevating virus. Abstract Proc. amer. Ass. Cancer Res. *7:* 59 (1966).

ROCH, M.: Encore la méningite lymphocytaire bénigne: La forme meningée de l'encéphalite epidémique. Rev. méd. Suisse rom. *51:* 1–18 (1931).

ROGER, F.: Étude sur le pouvoir pathogène du virus de la chorioméningite lymphocytaire. I. Réactivité dermique chez le lapin. Ann. Inst. Pasteur *103:* 639–656 (1962).

ROGER, F.: Études sur le pouvoir pathogène expérimental du virus de la chorioméningite lymphocytaire. II. Inoculation dans le derme du cobaye. Ann. Inst. Pasteur *104:* 274–283 (1963a).

ROGER, F.: Études sur le pouvoir pathogène expérimental du virus de la chorioméningite lymphocytaire. III. Une réaction inflammatoire directement visible chez la souris oedème viral du membre inférieur. Ann. Inst. Pasteur *104:* 347–360 (1963b).

ROGER, F. and HOTCHIN, J.: Local reactivity to lymphocytic choriomeningitis virus in the mouse; its development as a new diagnostic test. N. Y. State Dep. Health, Ann. Rep. Div. Lab. Res., pp. 43–44 (1961).

ROGER, F. et ROGER, A.: Études sur le pouvoir pathogène expérimental du virus de la chorioméningite lymphocytaire. IV. Niveau de mortalité des souris après inoculation sous-cutanée plantaire. Ann. Inst. Pasteur *105:* 476–485 (1963a).

ROGER, F. et ROGER, A.: Études sur le pouvoir pathogène expérimental du virus de la chorioméningite lymphocytaire. V. Distribution de la mortalité des souris au cours des réactions locales. Ann. Inst. Pasteur *105:* 612–623 (1963b).

ROGER, F. et ROGER, A.: Titrage local du virus de la chorioméningite lymphocytaire chez la souris. I. Position du problème. Méthodes. Traitement 'en tout ou rien'. Ann. Inst. Pasteur *106:* 439–448 (1964a).

ROGER, F. et ROGER, A.: Études sur le pouvoir pathogène expérimental du virus de la chorioméningite lymphocytaire. VI. Mortalité des souris selon le mode d'inoculation et selon la dose. Ann. Inst. Pasteur *106:* 588–601 (1964b).

ROGER, F. et ROGER, A.: Titrage local du virus de la chorioméningite lymphocytaire chez la souris. II. Étude quantitative par la méthode des courbes de latence. Ann. Inst. Pasteur *106:* 738–751 (1964c).

ROGER, F. et ROGER, A.: Titrage local du virus de la chorioméningite lymphocytaire chez la souris. III. Liaison entre la durée ou l'étendue de la réaction locale et la concentration de virus inoculée. Implications théoretiques et practiques. Ann. Inst. Pasteur *106:* 878–893 (1964d).

ROGER, F. et ROGER, A.: Trois modalités d'action des anticorps en immunologie virale. I. Le 'masquage' des virus par les anticorps. Influence du récepteur sur les résultats apparents des réactions de séro-neutralisation. Ann. Inst. Pasteur *108:* 166–179 (1965).

ROGERS, N. G.: The effect of merthiolate on the infectivity of certain viruses. J. lab. clin. Med. *38:* 483–485 (1951).

RORKE, L. B.; FABIYI, A.; ELIZAN, T. S., and SEVER, J. L.: Experimental cerebrovascular lesions in congenital and neonatal rubella-virus infections of ferrets. Lancet *ii:* 153–154 (1968).

ROSS, C. A. C.; LENMAN, J. A. R., and RUTTER, C.: Infective agents and multiple sclerosis. Brit. med. J. *1:* 226–229 (1965).

ROWE, W. P.: Studies on pathogenesis and immunity in lymphocytic choriomeningitis infection of the mouse. Res. Rep. Naval Med. Res. Inst., Bethesda, Md. *12:* 167–220 (1954).

ROWE W. P.: Protective effect of pre-irradiation on lymphocytic choriomeningitis infection in mice. Proc. Soc. exp. Biol., N. Y. *92:* 194–198 (1956).

ROWE, W. P.; HARTLEY, J. W.; CRAMBLETT, H. G., and MASTROTA, F. M.: Detection of human salivary gland virus in mouth and urine of children. Amer. J. Hyg. *67:* 57–65 (1958).

ROWE, W. P.; BLACK, P. H., and LEVEY, R. H.: Protective effect of neonatal thymectomy on mouse LCM infection. Proc. Soc. exp. Biol., N. Y. *114:* 248–251 (1963).

ROWE, W. P.; MURPHY, F. A.; BERGOLD, G. H.; CASALS, J.; HOTCHIN, J.; JOHNSON, K. M.; LEHMANN-GRUBE, F.; MIMS, C. A.; TRAUB, E., and WEBB, P. A.: Arenoviruses: Proposed name for newly defined virus group. J. Virol. *5:* 651–652 (1970).

ROWSON, K. E. K.; MAHY, B. W., and SALAMAN, M. H.: Size estimation by filtration of the enzyme-elevating virus of Riley. Life Sci. *7:* 479–485 (1963).

ROWSON, K. E. K.; MAHY, B. W. J., and BENDINELLI, M.: Riley virus neutralizing activity in the plasma of infected mice with persistent viraemia. Virology *28:* 775–778 (1966).

RUBIN, H. and TEMIN, H. M.: A radiological study of cell-virus interaction in the Rous sarcoma. Virology *7:* 75–79 (1959).

RUBIN, H.; CORNELIUS, A., and FANSHIER, L.: The pattern of congenital transmission of an avian leukosis virus. Proc. nat. Acad. Sci., Wash. *47:* 1058–1069 (1961).

RUBIN, H.; FANSHIER, L.; CORNELIUS, A., and HUGHES, W. F.: Tolerance and immunity in chickens after congenital and contact infection with an avian leukosis virus. Virology *17:* 143–156 (1962).

RUDOLPH, A. J.; YOW, M. D.; PHILLIPS, A.; DESMOND, M. M.; BLATTNER, R. J., and MELNICK, J. L.: Transplacental rubella infection in newly born infants. J. amer. med. Ass. *191:* 843–845 (1965).

RUFFOLO, P. R.; MARGOLIS, G., and KILHAM, L.: The induction of hepatitis by prior partial hepatectomy in resistant adult rats injected with H-1 virus. Light and electron microscopy and virologic studies. Amer. J. Path. *49:* 795–824 (1966).

RUSSELL, J. D.; BENNETT, J. M., and HANCOCK, B. B.: The etiology and diagnosis of Aleutian disease in mink. Lab. Anim. Care *13:* 784–789 (1963).

SABIN, A. B.: Reoviruses. Science *130:* 1387–1389 (1959).

SAISON, R. and KARSTAD, L.: Evidence of an auto-immune reaction in viral plasmacytosis (Aleutian disease) of mink as demonstrated by the Coombs test. Proc. 11th Congr. int. Soc. Blood Transf., Sydney 1966; Bibl. haemat. No. 29, Part 2, pp. 486–494 (Karger, Basel/New York 1968).

SAISON, R.; KARSTAD, L., and PRIDHAM, T. J.: Viral plasmacytosis (Aleutian disease) in mink: VI. The development of positive Coombs tests in experimental infections. Canad. J. comp. Med. *30:* 151–156 (1966).

SARAIVA, L. G.; AZEVEDO, M.; CORREA, J. M.; CARVALHO, G., and PROSPERO, J. D.: Anomalous panleukocytic granulation. Blood *14:* 1112 (1959).

SATO, S.: On the fate of the colt born from anemia infected horse. Jap. J. ass. cent. vet. Med. *41:* 431–454 (1928).

SAUNDERS, M.; CHAMBERS, M. E.; KNOWLES, M., and CASPARY, E. A.: Cellular and humoral responses to measles in subacute sclerosing panencephalitis. Lancet *i:* 72–74 (1969).

SAURINO, V. R.; WADDELL, G. H.; FLYNN, J. H., and TEIGLAND, M. B.: Immunodiagnostic relations of three clinical types of equine infectious anemia. J. amer. vet. med. Ass. *149:* 1416–1422 (1966).

SAVAGE, R. D. and FIELD, E. J.: Brain damage and emotional behavior. The effects of scrapie on the emotional responses of mice. Anim. Behav. *13:* 443–446 (1965).

SCHEID, W.: Das Virus der lymphozytären Choriomeningitis und seine Bedeutung für die Neurologie. Fortschr. Neurol. Psychiat. *25:* 73–99 (1957).

SCHEID, W.; JOCHHEIM, K. A., und MOHR, W.: Laboratoriumsinfektionen mit dem Virus der lymphozytären Choriomeningitis. Dtsch. Arch. klin. Med. *203:* 88–109 (1956).

SCHEID, W.; JOCHHEIM, K. A. und STAMMLER, K. A.: Tödlicher Verlauf einer Infektion mit dem Virus der lymphozytären Choriomeningitis. Dtsch. Z. Nervenheilk. *174:* 123–139 (1956).

SCHEID, W.; ACKERMANN, R.; BLOEDHORN, N., and KÜPPER, B.: Distribution of the virus of lymphocytic choriomeningitis in Western Germany. German med. Mthl. *9:* 157–161 (1964).

SCHELL, K.; HUEBNER, R. J., and TURNER, H. C.: Concentration of complementfixing viral antigens. Proc. Soc. exp. Biol., N. Y. *121:* 41–46 (1966).

SCHERMER, S.: Die histologischen Veränderungen bei der infektiösen Anämie des Pferdes und ihr Vergleich mit denen bei experimentellen Anämien. Arch. Tierheilk. *55:* 121–145 (1926).

SCHIFF, G. M. and SEVER, J. L.: Rubella: Recent laboratory and clinical advances. Progr. med. Virol. vol. 8, pp. 30–61 (Karger, Basel/New York 1966).

SCHLEIFSTEIN, J. and COLLINS, D. N.: The pathology of lymphocytic choriomeningitis in nonirradiated and radiated mice. N. Y. State Dep. Health, Ann. Rep. Div. Lab. Res., p. 22 (1959).

SCHMUÑIS, G.; WEISSENBACHER, M., and PARODI, A. S.: Tolerance to Junin virus in thymectomized mice. Arch. ges. Virusforsch. *21:* 200–204 (1967).

SCHNEIDER, H.: Über epidemische akute 'Meningitis serosa'. Wien Klin. Wschr. *44:* 350–352 (1931).

SCHOOLEY, J. C.; KELLY, L. S.; DOBSON, E. L.; FINNEY, C. R.; HAVENS, V. W., and CANTOR, L. N.: Reticuloendothelial activity in neonatally thymectomized mice and irradiated mice thymectomized in adult life. J. Reticuloendothel. Soc. *2:* 396–405 (1965).

SCOTT, G. R.: The virus of African swine fever and its transmission. Bull. Off. int. Epiz. *63:* 645–677 (1965a).

SCOTT, G. R.: Prevention, control and eradication of African swine fever. Bull. Off. int. Epiz. *63:* 751–764 (1965b).

SCOTT, J. W.: The experimental transmission of swamp fever (infectious anemia) by means of secretions. Wyoming Agric. exp. station Bull No. 138, p. 17 (1924).

SCOTT, T. F. M. and ELFORD, W. J.: The size of the virus of lymphocytic choriomeningitis as determined by ultrafiltration and ultracentrifugation. Brit. J. exp. Path. *20:* 182–188 (1939).

SEAMER, J.: Mouse macrophages as host cells for murine viruses. Arch. ges Virusforsch. *17:* 654–663 (1965a).

SEAMER, J.: The growth, reproduction and mortality of mice made immunologically tolerant to lymphocytic choriomeningitis virus by congenital infection. Arch. ges. Virusforsch. *15:* 169–177 (1965b).

SEAMER, J. and GLEDHILL, A. W.: Role of the central nervous system in fatal murine lymphocytic choriomeningitis (Brief report). Arch. ges. Virusforsch. *17:* 664–668 (1965).

SEAMER, J. and HOTCHIN, J.: The effect of subcutaneous inoculation upon subsequent intracerebral challenge with lymphocytic choriomeningitis virus. N. Y. State Dep. Health, Ann. Rep. Div. Lab. Res., p. 20 (1960).

SEAMER, J.; GLEDHILL, A. W.; BARLOW, J. L., and HOTCHIN, J.: Effect of *Eperythrozoon coccoides* upon lymphocytic choriomeningitis in mice. J. Immunol. *86:* 512–515 (1961).

SEAMER, J.; BARLOW, J. L.; GLEDHILL, A. W., and HOTCHIN, J.: Increased susceptibility of mice to lymphocytic choriomeningitis virus after peripheral inoculation. Virology *21:* 309–316 (1963).

SEDWICK, W. D. and WIKTOR, T. J.: Reproducible plaquing system for rabies, lymphocytic choriomeningitis and other ribonucleic acid viruses in BHK-21/13S agarose suspensions. J. Virology *1:* 1224–1226 (1967).

SEIFERT, G. und OEHME, J. L.: Pathologie und Klinik der Cytomegalie (Thieme, Leipzig 1957).

SELZER, G.: Virus isolation, inclusion bodies, and chromosomes in a rubella-infected human embryo. Lancet *ii:* 336–337 (1963).

SETLOW, J. K. and DUGGAN, D. E.: The resistance of *Micrococcus radiodurans* to ultraviolet radiation. I. Ultraviolet-induced lesions in the cell's DNA. Biochem. biophys. Acta *87:* 664–668 (1964).

SEVER, J. L. and ZEMAN, W.: Serological studies of measles and subacute sclerosing panencephalitis. Neurology, Minneap. *18:* 95–97 (1968).

SEYDERHELM, R.: Über die perniciöse Anämie der Pferde. Beitrag zur vergleichenden Pathologie der Blutkrankheiten. Beitr. path. Anat. *58:* 285–318 (1914).

SHAUGHNESSY, H. J. and MILZER, A.: Experimental infection of Dermacentor andersoni Stiles with the virus of lymphocytic choriomeningitis. Amer. J. publ. Hlth. *29:* 1103–1108 (1939).

SHAUGHNESSY, H. J. and ZICHIS, J.: Infection of guinea pigs by application of virus of lymphocytic choriomeningitis to their normal skins. Proc. Soc. exp. Biol., N. Y. *42:* 755–757 (1939).

SHAUGHNESSY, H. J. and ZICHIS, J.: Infection of guinea pigs by application of virus of lymphocytic choriomeningitis to their normal skins. J. exp. Med. *72:* 331–343 (1940).

SHAVER, D. N.; BARRON, A. L., and KARZON, D. T.: Cytopathology of human enteric viruses in tissue culture. Amer. J. Path. *34:* 943–963 (1958).

SHVAREV, A. I. and REMEZOV, P. I.: A clinical and virological study of lymphocytic choriomeningitis. Probl. Virol. *4:* 67–69 (1959).

SCHWARTZMAN, G.: Association of the virus of lymphocytic choriomeningitis with erythrocytes of infected animals. J. Bact. *46:* 482–483 (1943).

SHWARTZMAN, G.: Recovery of the virus of lymphocytic choriomeningitis from the erythrocytes of infected animals. J. Immunol. *48:* 111–127 (1944).

SCHWARTZMAN, G.: Alterations in pathogenesis of experimental lymphocytic choriomeningitis caused by prepassage of the virus through heterologous host. J. Immunol. *54:* 293–304 (1946).

SIDWELL, R. W.; DIXON, G. J.; SELLERS, S. M., and SCHABEL, F. M., jr.: *In vivo* antiviral activity of 1,3-bis (2-chloroethyl)-1-nitrosourea. Appl. Microbiol. *13:* 579–589 (1965).

SIDWELL, R. W.; ARNET, T. G., and DIXON, G. J.: *In vitro* studies on the antiviral activity of 1,3-bis (2-chloroethyl)-1-nitrosourea. Appl. Microbiol. *14:* 405–410 (1966).

SIGURDARDÓTTIR, B. and THORMAR, H.: Isolation of a viral agent from the lungs of sheep affected with maedi. J. infect. Dis. *114:* 55–60 (1964).

SIGURDSSON, B.: Maedi, a slow progressive pneumonia of sheep: An epizoological and a pathological study. Brit. vet. J. *110:* 255–270 (1954a).

SIGURDSSON, B.: Rida, a chronic encephalitis of sheep with general remarks on infections which develop slowly and some of their special characteristics. Brit. vet. J. *110:* 341–354 (1954b).

SIGURDSSON, B.: Adenomatosis of sheep's lungs. Experimental transmission. Arch. ges. Virusforsch. *8:* 51–58 (1958).

SIGURDSSON, B. and PÁLSSON, P. A.: Visna of sheep. A slow, demyelinating infection. Brit. J. exp. Path. *39:* 519–528 (1958).

SIGURDSSON, B.; GRÍMSSON, H., and PÁLSSON, P. A.: Maedi, a chronic progressive infection of sheep's lungs. J. infect. Dis. *90:* 233–241 (1952).

SIGURDSSON, B.; PÁLSSON, P. A., and TRYGGVADÓTTIR, A.: Transmission experiments with maedi. J. infect. Dis. 93: 166–175 (1953).

SIGURDSSON, B.; PÁLSSON, P. A., and GRÍMSSON, H.: Visna, a demyelinating transmissible disease of sheep. J. Neuropath. exp. Neurol. *16:* 389–403 (1957).

SIGURDSSON, B.; THORMAR, H., and PÁLSSON, P. A.: Cultivation of visna virus in tissue culture. Arch. ges. Virusforsch. *10:* 368–381 (1960).

SIGURDSSON, B.; PÁLSSON, P. A., and VAN BOGAERT, L.: Pathology of visna. Transmissible demyelinating disease in sheep in Iceland. Acta neuropath. *1:* 343–362 (1962).

SIKORA, E.: Protective effect of neonatal thymectomy on lymphocytic choriomeningitis virus disease in mice. N. Y. State Dep. Health, Ann. Rep. Div. Lab. Res., pp. 43–44 (1963).

SIKORA, E. and HOTCHIN J.: Effect of amethopterin on the foot-pad response of mice to lymphocytic choriomeningitis virus. N. Y. State Dep. Health, Ann. Rep. Div. Lab. Res., pp. 40–41 (1962).

SILICOTT, W. L. and NEUBUERGER, K.: Acute lymphocytic choriomeningitis. Report of three cases with histopathologic findings. Amer. J. med. Sci. *200:* 253–259 (1940).

SIMONS, M. J. and FITZGERALD, M. G.: Rubella virus and human lymphocytes in culture. Lancet *ii:* 937–940 (1968).

SIMONS, M. J. and JACK, I.: Lymphocyte viraemia in congenital rubella. Lancet *ii:* 953–954 (1968).

SINGER, D. B.; RUDOLPH, A. J.; ROSENBERG, H. S.; RAWLS, W. E., and BONIUK, M.: Pathology of the congenital rubella syndrome. J. Pediat. *71:* 665–675 (1967).

SINGER, D. B.; SOUTH, M. A.; MONTGOMERY, J. R., and RAWLS, W. E.: Congenital rubella syndrome. Lymphoid tissue and immunologic status. Amer. J. Dis. Child *118:* 54–61 (1969).

SINSHEIMER, R. L.: A single-stranded deoxyribonucleic acid from bacteriophage ΦX174. J. molec. Biol. *1:* 43–53 (1959).

SKOGLAND, J. E. and BAKER, A. B.: An unusual form of lymphocytic choriomeningitis. Arch. Neurol., Chicago *42:* 507–512 (1939).

SLATER, J. S.: Nitrogenous constituents of serum and urine in normal and scrapie sheep. Res. Vet. Sci. *6:* 92–99 (1965a).

SLATER, J. S.: Succinic dehydrogenase, cytochrome oxidase and acid phosphatase activities in the brains of scrapie-infected goats and mice. Res. Vet. Sci. *6:* 155–161 (1965b).

SMADEL, J. E.: Common neurotropic virus diseases of man. Their diagnosis and mode of spread. U. S. Nav. Med. Bull. *40:* 1021–1036 (1942).

SMADEL, J. E. and WALL, M. J.: A soluble antigen of lymphocytic choriomeningitis. III. Independence of anti-soluble substance antibodies and neutralizing antibodies and the role of soluble antigen and inactive virus and immunity to infection. J. exp. Med. *72:* 389–405 (1940).

SMADEL, J. E. and WALL, M. J.: Identification of the virus of lymphocytic choriomeningitis. J. Bact. *41:* 421–430 (1941).

SMADEL, J. E. and WALL, M. J.: Lymphocytic choriomeningitis in the Syrian hamster. J. exp. Med. *75:* 581–591 (1942).

SMADEL J. E.; BAIRD, R. D., and WALL, M. J.: A soluble antigen of lymphocytic choriomeningitis. I. Separation of soluble antigen from virus. J. exp. Med. *70:* 53–66 (1939a).

SMADEL, J. E.; BAIRD, R. D., and WALL, M. J.: Complement-fixation in infections with the virus of lymphocytic choriomeningitis. Proc. Soc. exp. Biol., N. Y. *40:* 71–73 (1939b).

SMADEL, J. E.; WALL, M. J., and BAIRD, R. D.: A soluble antigen of lymphocytic choriomeningitis. II. Characteristics of the antigen and its use in precipitin reactions. J. exp. Med. *71:* 43–53 (1940).

SMADEL, J. E.; GREEN, R. H.; PALTAUF, R. M., and GONZALES, T. A.: Lymphocytic choriomeningitis: Two human fatalities following an unusual febrile illness. Proc. Soc. exp. Biol., N. Y. *49:* 683–686 (1942).

SMITH, M. G.: The salivary gland viruses of man and animals (cytomegalic inclusion disease); in: Progr. med. Virol. vol. 2, pp. 171–202 (Karger, Basel/New York 1959).

SMITH, M. G. and VELIOS, F.: Inclusion disease or generalized salivary gland virus infection. Arch. Path. *50:* 862–884 (1950).

SMITHARD, E. H. R. and MACRAE, A. D.: Lymphocytic choriomeningitis. Associated human and mouse infections. Brit. med. J. *1:* 1298–1300 (1951).

SOITUZ, V.; TAM, D., and NICOLESCU, H.: Attempted infection of pigs with the virus of equine infectious anemia. Ann. Inst. Pat. Igien. Anim. *4:* 103 (1953).

SOOTHILL, J. F.; HAYES, K., and DUDGEON, J. A.: The immunoglobulins in congenital rubella. Lancet *i:* 1385–1388 (1966).

SPENDLOVE, R. S.; LENNETTE, E. H., and JOHN, A. C.: The role of the mitotic apparatus in the intracellular location of reovirus antigen. J. Immunol. *90:* 554–560 (1963).

SQUIRE, R. A.; MONTALI, R. J., and BUSH, M.: Pathogenetic aspects of equine infectious anemia. J. amer. vet. med. Ass. *155:* 355–358 (1969).

STAMP, J. T.: Scrapie disease of sheep. A review of the contradictory evidence as to the nature of the disease. Vet. Rec. *70:* 50–55 (1958).

STAMP, J. T.: Scrapie: A transmissible disease of sheep. Vet. Rec. *74:* 357–362 (1962).

STAMP, J. T.: Scrapie and its wider implications. Brit. med. Bull. *23:* 133–137 (1967).

STAMP, J. T.; BROTHERSTON, J. G.; ZLOTNIK, I.; MACKAY, J. M. K., and SMITH, W.: Further studies on scrapie. J. comp. Path. *69:* 268–280 (1959).

STANLEY N. F.: Reovirus – a ubiquitous orphan. Med. J. Austr. *2:* 815–818 (1961a).

STANLEY, N. F.: Relationship of hepatoencephalomyelitis virus and reoviruses. Nature, Lond. *1:* 687 (1961b).

STANLEY, N. F.: Reoviruses. Presb. St. Luke's Hosp. med. Bull. Chicago, 3 (4), 146 (1964).

STANLEY, N. F.: The aetiology and pathogenesis of Burkitt's African lymphoma. Lancet *i:* 961–962 (1966).

STANLEY, N. F.: Reoviruses. Brit. med. Bull. *23:* 150–155 (1967).

STANLEY, N. F. and KEAST, D.: A reovirus-specific antigen in murine lymphoma 2731/L and in cultured Burkitt's lymphoma cells. Austr. J. exp. Biol. med. Sci. *45:* 517–525 (1967).

STANLEY, N. F. and LEAK, P. J.: Murine infection with reovirus type 3 and the runting syndrome. Nature, Lond. *199:* 1309–1310 (1963).

STANLEY, N. F. and PAPADIMITRIOU, J. M.: Burkitt's lymphoma and reovirus. Brit. med. J. *2:* 767 (1966).

STANLEY, N. F.; DORMAN, D. C., and PONSFORD, J.: Studies on the pathogenesis of a hitherto undescribed virus (hepatoencephalomyelitis) producing unusual symptoms in suckling mice. Austr. J. exp. Biol. med. Sci. *31:* 147–159 (1953).

STANLEY, N. F.; LEAK, P. J.; WALTERS, M. N. I., and JOSKE, R. A.: Murine infection with reovirus. II. The chronic disease following reovirus type 3 infection. Brit. J. exp. Path. *45:* 142–149 (1964).

STANLEY, N. F.; WALTERS, M. N. I.; LEAK, P. J., and KEAST, D.: The association of murine lymphoma with reovirus type 3 infection. Proc. Soc. exp. Biol., N. Y. *121:* 90–93 (1966).

STEIN, C. D. and GATES, D. W.: The neutralizing effect of antiserum from recovered carriers of equine infectious anemia on the virus of the disease. Vet. Med. *45:* 152–156 (1950).

STEIN, C. D. and MOTT, L. O.: Studies on congenital transmission of equine infectious anemia. Vet. Med. *37:* 370–377 (1942).

STEIN, C. D. and MOTT, L. O.: Equine infectious anemia in brood mares and their offspring. Vet. Med. *41:* 274–278 (1946).

STEIN, C. D. and OSTEEN, O. L.: Studies on immunization in equine infectious anemia. Amer. J. vet. Res. *2:* 344–348 (1941).

STEIN, C. D. and SONGER, J. R.: Some observations on further attempts to transmit equine infectious anemia to lambs and pigs. J. amer. vet. med. Ass. *128:* 604–608 (1956).

STEIN, C. D.; OSTEEN, O. L.; MOTT, L. O., and SHAHAN, M. S.: Experimental transmission of equine infectious anemia by contact and body secretions and excretions. Vet. med. *39:* 46–52 (1944).

STEIN, C. D.; MOTT, L. O., and GATES, D. W.: Some observations on carriers of equine infectious anemia. J. amer. vet. med. Ass. *126:* 277–287 (1955).

STERN, H.: Isolation of cytomegalovirus and clinical manifestations of infections at different ages. Brit. med. J. *1:* 665–669 (1968).

STERN, H. and TUCKER, S. M.: Cytomegalovirus infection in the newborn and in early childhood. Three atypical cases. Lancet *ii:* 1268–1271 (1965).

STETSON, C. A., jr.: Endotoxins and bacterial allergy; in: Cellular and humoral aspects of the hypersensitive states, pp. 442–450 (Hoeber-Harper, New York 1959).

STEWART, S. E. and HAAS, V. H.: Lymphocytic choriomeningitis virus in mouse neoplasms. J. nat. Cancer. Inst. *17:* 233–245 (1956).

STEWART, S. E.; EDDY, B. E.; HAAS, V. H., and BORGESE, N. G.: Lymphocytic choriomeningitis virus as related to chemotherapy studies and to tumor induction in mice. Ann. N. Y. Acad. Sci. *68:* 419–429 (1957).

STEYN, D. G.: East African virus disease in pigs. 18th Rept. Director vet. serv. Animal Ind. Onderstepoort (South Africa) *1:* 99–109 (1932).

STOCK C. C. and FRANCIS, T., jr.: The inactivation of the virus of lymphocytic choriomeningitis by soaps. J. exp. Med. *77:* 323–336 (1943).

STOCKMAN, S.: Scrapie: An obscure disease of sheep. J. comp. Path. *26:* 317–327 (1913).

STOCKMAN, S.: Contribution to the study of the disease known as scrapie. J. comp. Path. *39:* 42–71 (1926).

STOLLER, A. and COLLMANN, R. D.: Incidence of infective hepatitis followed by Down's syndrome nine months later. Lancet *ii:* 1221–1223 (1965).

STONE, S. S. and HESS, W. R.: Antibody response to inactivated preparations of African swine fever virus in pigs. Amer. J. vet. Res. *28:* 475–481 (1967).

STONE, S. S.; DELAY, P. D., and SHARMAN, E. C.: The antibody response in pigs inoculated with attenuated African swine fever virus. Canad. J. comp. Med. *32:* 455–460 (1968).

STORER, J. B.: Nonspecific life shortening in male mice exposed to the mammary tumor agent. J. nat. Cancer Inst. *37:* 211–215 (1966).

STRAUSS, L. and BERNSTEIN, J.: Neonatal hepatitis in congenital rubella. A histopathological study. Arch. Path. *86:* 317–327 (1968).

STREISSLE, G. and MARAMOROSCH, K.: Reovirus and wound-tumor virus: Serological cross reactivity. Science *140:* 996–997 (1963).

STULBERG, C. S.; BERMAN, L., and PAGE, R. H.: Comparative viral susceptibilities of eight culture strains (Detroit) of human epithelial-like cells. Virology *2:* 844–845 (1956).

STULBERG, C. S.; ZUELZER, W. W.; PAGE, R. H.; TAYLOR, P. E., and BROUGH, A. J.: Cytomegalovirus infections with reference to isolations from lymph nodes and blood. Proc. Soc. exp. Biol., N. Y. *123:* 976–982 (1966).

SUTER, E. and KIRSANOW, E. M.: Hyperreactivity to endotoxin in mice infected with mycobacteria. Induction and elicitation of the reactions. Immunology, Lond. *4:* 354–365 (1961).

SUTNICK, A. I.; LONDON, W. T.; GERSTLEY, B. J. S.; CRONLUND, M. M., and BLUMBERG, B. S.: Anicteric hepatitis associated with Australia antigen. J. amer. med. Ass. *205:* 670–674 (1968).

SYVERTON, J. T.; McCOY, O. R., and KOOMEN, J. R.: The transmission of the virus of lymphocytic choriomeningitis by *Trichinella spiralis.* J. exp. Med. *85:* 759–769 (1947).

SZERI, I.; BÁNOS, Z.; ANDERLIK, P.; BÁLAZS, M., and FÖLDES, P.: Pathogenesis of the wasting syndrome following neonatal thymectomy. Acta microbiol. hung. *13:* 255–262 (1966).

TABUCHI, E.; ISHII, S., and SONODA, A.: Studies on the immunity of equine infectious anemia by the inoculation of larger volume of formolized virus. Hokkaido Prefect. Gov. Rept. of EIA *2:* 71–80 (1955).

TANOOKA, H. and HUTCHINSON, F.: Modifications of the inactivation by ionizing radiations of the transforming activity of DNA in spores and dry cells. Radiat. Res. *24:* 43–56 (1965).

TAYLOR, M. J. and MACDOWELL, E. C.: Mouse leukemia XIV. Freeing transplanted line I from a contaminating virus. Cancer Res. *9:* 144–149 (1949).

TELLEZ-NAGEL, I. and HARTER, D. H.: Subacute sclerosing leukoencephalitis: Ultrastructure of intranuclear and intracytoplasmic inclusions. Science *154:* 899–901 (1966a).

Tellez-Nagel, I. and Harter, D. H.: Subacute sclerosing leukoencephalitis. I. Clinico-pathological, electron microscopic and virological observations. J. Neuropath. exp. Neurol. *25:* 560–581 (1966b).

Temin, H. M.: The effects of actinomycin D on growth of Rous sarcoma virus *in vitro*. Virology *20:* 577–582 (1963).

Temin, H. M.: The participation of DNA in Rous sarcoma virus production. Virology *23:* 486–494 (1964).

Ten Bensel, R. W. and St. Geme, J. W., jr.: A search for the reservoir of cytomegalovirus in salivary gland tissue. J. Pediat. *72:* 479–482 (1968).

Thiede, W. H.: Cardiac involvement in lymphocytic choriomeningitis. Arch. intern. Med. *109:* 50–54 (1962).

Thompson, G. R. and Aliferis, P. A.: A clinical-pathological study of Aleutian mink disease; an experimental model for study of the connective-tissue disease. Arthritis Rheum. *7:* 521–533 (1964).

Thormar, H.: Stability of visna virus in infectious tissue culture fluid. Arch. ges. Virusforsch. *10:* 501–509 (1960).

Thormar, H.: An electron microscope study of tissue cultures infected with visna virus. Virology *14:* 463–475 (1961).

Thormar, H.: Neutralization of visna virus by antisera from sheep. J. Immunol. *90:* 185–192 (1963a).

Thormar, H.: The growth cycle of visna virus in monolayer cultures of sheep cells. Virology *19:* 273–278 (1963b).

Thormar, H.: Physical, chemical and biological properties of visna virus and its relationship to other animal viruses. NINDB Monograph No. 2. Slow, latent and temperate virus infections, pp. 335–340. (US Dept. of Health, Education and Welfare, Washington, D. C. 1965a).

Thormar, H.: A comparison of visna and maedi viruses. 1. Physical, chemical and biological properties. Res. Vet. Sci. *6:* 117–129 (1965b).

Thormar, H.: Effect of 5-bromodeoxyuridine and actinomycin D on the growth of visna virus in cell cultures. Virology *26:* 36–43 (1965c).

Thormar, H.: A study of maedi virus; in Severi Proc. inter. conf. Lung tumours in animals, Perugia, Italy, 1965, pp. 393–402 (1966a).

Thormar, H.: A study of visna and maedi viruses and their relationship to other viruses of animals, pp. 1–29 (Dansk Videnskabs Forlag, Copenhagen 1966b).

Thormar, H.: Observations on visna virus-infected cell cultures stained with acridine orange. Acta path. microbiol. scand. *68:* 54–58 (1966c).

Thormar, H.: Cell-virus interactions in tissue cultures infected with visna and maedi viruses; in: Current topics in microbiology and immunology, pp. 22–32 (Springer, New York 1967).

Thormar, H.: Visna and maedi virus antigen in infected cell cultures studied by the fluorescent antibody technique. Acta path. microbiol. scand. *75:* 296–302 (1969).

Thormar, H. and Cruickshank, J. G.: The structure of visna virus studied by the negative staining technique. Virology *25:* 145–148 (1965).

Thormar, H. and Helgadóttir, H.: A comparison of visna and maedi viruses. II. Serological relationship. Res. Vet. Sci. *6:* 456–465 (1965).

THORMAR, H. and PÁLSSON, P. A.: Visna and maedi – two slow infections of sheep and their etiological agents; in: Perspectives in virology, vol. 5, pp. 291–308 (Academic Press, New York 1967).

THORMAR, H. and PETERSEN, I.: Photoinactivation of visna virus. Acta path. microbiol. scand. *62:* 461–462 (1964).

THORMAR, H. and SIGURDARDÓTTIR, B.: Growth of visna virus in primary tissue cultures from various animal species. Acta path. microbiol. scand. *55:* 180–186 (1962).

THORMAR, H. and VON MAGNUS, H.: Attempts to isolate virus from the cerebrospinal fluid of patients with multiple sclerosis. Acta neurol. scand. *39:* 209–212 (1963a).

THORMAR, H. and VON MAGNUS, H.: Neutralization of visna virus by human sera. Acta path. microbiol. scand. *57:* 261–267 (1963b).

THORMAR, H.; GÍSLASON, G., and HELGADÓTTIR, H.: A survey of neutralizing antibodies against maedi virus in sera from flocks of sheep affected with maedi and from healthy flocks. J. infect. Dis. *116:* 41–47 (1966).

THORP, F., jr.; JUDD, A. W.; GREY, M. L., and SCHOLL, L. B.: Scrapie in sheep. Michigan State Coll. Vet. *13:* 36–37 (1952).

TIERKEL, E. S.: Rabies, in Advances in veterinary science, vol. 5, pp. 183–226 (Academic Press, New York 1959).

TOBIN, J. O. H.: The growth of lymphocytic choriomeningitis virus in the developing chick embryo. Brit. J. exp. Path. *35:* 358–364 (1954).

TODD, F. A.: Equine infectious anemia: A research problem. J. amer. vet. med. Ass. *148:* 1051–1052 (1966).

TONDURY, G. and SMITH, D. W.: Fetal rubella pathology. J. Pediat. *68:* 867–879 (1966).

TONGEREN, H. A. E. VAN: A familial infection with hepatoencephalomyelitis virus in the Netherlands. Study on some properties of the infective agent. Arch. ges. Virusforsch. *7:* 429–448 (1957).

TOOLAN, H. W.: Experimental production of mongoloid hamsters. Science *131:* 1446–1448 (1960).

TOOLAN, H. W.: Studies on the H viruses. Proc. amer. Ass. Cancer Res. *5:* 64 (1964).

TOOLAN, H. W.: H-1 virus viremia in the adult hamster. Proc. Soc. exp. Biol., N. Y. *119:* 715–717 (1965).

TOOLAN, H. W.: The picodna virus: H, RV, and AAV; in: International review of experimental pathology, vol. 6, pp. 135–180 (Academic Press, New York 1968).

TOOLAN, H. W.; DALLDORF, G.; BARCLAY, M.; CHANDRA, S., and MOORE, A. E.: An unidentified filterable agent isolated from transplanted human tumors. Proc. nat. Acad. Sci., Wash. *46:* 1256–1258 (1960).

TRAUB, E.: A filterable virus from white mice. Immunology, Lond. *29:* 69 (1935a).

TRAUB, E.: A filterable virus recovered from white mice. Science *81:* 298–299 (1935b).

TRAUB, E.: The epidemiology of lymphocytic choriomeningitis in white mice. J. exp. Med. *64:* 183–200 (1936a).

TRAUB, E.: Persistence of lymphocytic choriomeningitis virus in immune animals and its relation to immunity. J. exp. Med. *63:* 847–861 (1936b).

TRAUB, E.: An epidemic in a mouse colony due to the virus of acute lymphocytic choriomeningitis. J. exp. Med. *63:* 533–546 (1936c).

TRAUB, E.: Immunization of guinea pigs with a modified strain of lymphocytic choriomeningitis virus. J. exp. Med. *66:* 317–324 (1937).

TRAUB, E.: Factors influencing the persistence of choriomeningitis virus in the blood of mice after clinical recovery. J. exp. Med. *68:* 229–250 (1938a).

TRAUB, E.: Immunization of guinea pigs against lymphocytic choriomeningitis with formolized tissue vaccines. J. exp. Med. *68:* 95–110 (1938b).

TRAUB, E.: Epidemiology of lymphocytic choriomeningitis in a mouse stock observed for four years. J. exp. Med. *69:* 801–817 (1939).

TRAUB, E.: Über den Einfluss der latenten Choriomeningitis-Infektion auf die Entstehung der Lymphomatose bei weissen Mäusen. Zbl. Bakt. *147:* 16–25 (1941).

TRAUB, E.: Specific immunity as a factor in the ecology of animal viruses; in: Perspectives in virology, vol. 1, pp. 160–183 (John Wiley & Sons, New York 1959).

TRAUB, E.: Über die immunologische Toleranz bei der lymphozytären Choriomeningitis der Mäuse. Zbl. Bakt. *177:* 472–487 (1960a).

TRAUB, E.: Observations on immunological tolerance and 'immunity' in mice infected congenitally with the virus of lymphocytic choriomeningitis (LCM). Arch. ges. Virusforsch. *10:* 303–314 (1960b).

TRAUB, E.: Über die natürliche Übertragungsweise des Virus der lymphozytären Choriomeningitis (LCM) bei Mäusen und ihre Parallelen zum Übertragungsmodus gewisser muriner Krebsviren. Zbl. Bakt. *177:* 453–471 (1960c).

TRAUB, E.: Demonstration, properties and significance of neutralizing antibodies in mature mice immune to lymphocytic choriomeningitis (LCM). Arch. ges. Virusforsch. *10:* 289–302 (1960d).

TRAUB, E.: Multiplication of LCM virus in lymph node and embryo cells from nontolerant and tolerant mice. Arch. ges. Virusforsch. *11:* 473–486 (1961a).

TRAUB, E.: Interference with Eastern equine encephalomyelitis (EEE) virus in the brains of mice immune to lymphocytic choriomeningitis (LCM). Arch. ges. Virusforsch. *11:* 419–427 (1961b).

TRAUB, E.: Can LCM virus cause lymphomatosis in mice? Arch. ges. Virusforsch. *11:* 667–682 (1962).

TRAUB, E.: Studies on the mechanism of immunity in murine LCM. Arch. ges. Virusforsch. *14:* 65–86 (1963).

TRAUB, E. and KESTING, F.: Further observations on the behavior of the cells in murine LCM. Arch. ges. Virusforsch. *13:* 452–469 (1963a).

TRAUB, E. and KESTING, F.: Experiments on heterologous and homologous interference in LCM-infected cultures of murine lymph node cells. Arch. ges. Virusforsch. *14:* 55–64 (1963b).

TRAUB, E. und SCHÄFER, W.: Serologische Untersuchungen über die Immunität der Mäuse gegen die lymphozytische Choriomeningitis. Zbl. Bakt. *144:* 331–345 (1939).

TRAUTWEIN, G.: Experimental study of Aleutian disease. Arch. exp. Vet. Med. *18:* 287–395 (1964).

TRAUTWEIN, G. W. and HELMBOLDT, C. F.: Aleutian disease of mink. I. Experimental transmission of the disease. Amer. J. vet. Res. *23:* 1280–1288 (1962).

TREUSCH, J. V.; MILZER, A., and LEVINSON, S. O.: Recurrent lymphocytic choriomeningitis. Report of a case in which treatment was with pooled normal adult serum. Arch. intern. Med. *72:* 709–714 (1943).

TRIANDAPHILLI, I.; BARLOW, J. L., and COHEN, S. M.: Immunofluorescence in the serodiagnosis of lymphocytic choriomeningitis. N. Y. State Dep. Health, Ann. Rep. Div. Lab. Res., pp. 52–53 (1964).

TSAI, K. S.; GRINYER, I.; PAN, I. C., and KARSTAD, L.: Electron microscopic observation of crystalline arrays of virus-like particles in tissues of mink with Aleutian disease. Canad. J. Microbiol. *15:* 138–140 (1969).

ULE, G.: Kleinhirnrindenatrophie vom Körnertyp. Dtsch. Z. Nervenheilk. *168:* 195–226 (1952).

UPHOFF, D. E. and HAAS, V. H.: Immunologic response to lymphocytic choriomeningitis virus in lethally irradiated mice treated with bone marrow. J. nat. Cancer Inst. *25:* 779–786 (1960).

UTZ, J. P.: Viruria in man; in: Progr. med. virol., vol. 6, pp. 71–81 (Karger, Basel/New York 1964).

VEERARAGHAVEN, N.; GAJANNA, A.; RANGASAMI, R.; SARASWATHI, K. C.; DEVARAJ, R., and HALLAN, K. M.: Studies on the salivary excretion of rabies virus by the dog from Surandai. Pasteur Inst. of Southern India, Coonoor; Ann. Rept. of the Director, 1965 und Scientific Rept. 1966, pp. 91–97 (Diocesan Press, Madras 1967).

VELHO, E.: La peste porcine africaine. Bull. Off int. Epizoot. *48:* 395–402 (1957).

VERMEIL, C.: Limites de l'association symbiotique Toxoplasma gondii ultra virus de la chorio-méningite lymphocytaire. Arch. Inst. Pasteur *33:* 55–59 (1956).

VESIKARI, T. and VAHERI, A.: Rubella: a method for rapid diagnosis of a recent infection by demonstration of the IgM antibodies. Brit. med. J. *i:* 221–223 (1968).

VIETS, H. R. and WATTS, J. W.: Acute aseptic meningitis. J. nerv. ment. Dis. *80:* 253–273 (1934).

VIGOVSKII, A. I. and GUTSEVICH, A. V.: Preliminary results of investigation of natural foci of lymphocytic choriomeningitis in West Ukraine. Parasitology, Cambr., pp. 889–891 (1961).

VOGT, H.: Chronische Verlaufsform der benignen lymphozytären Meningitis. Dtsch. Arch. klin. Med. *183:* 501–514 (1939).

VOLKERT, M.: Studies on immunological tolerance to LCM virus. Preliminary report on adoptive immunization of virus carrier mice. Acta path. microbiol. scand. *56:* 305–310 (1962).

VOLKERT, M.: Studies on immunological tolerance to LCM virus. 2. Treatment of mice by adoptive immunization. Acta path. microbiol. scand. *57:* 465–487 (1963).

VOLKERT, M.: Studies on immunologic tolerance to LCM virus; in: Perspectives in virology, vol. IV, chapt. 16, pp. 269–282 (Harper & Row, New York 1965).

VOLKERT, M. and LARSEN, J. H.: Studies on immunological tolerance to LCM virus. 3. Duration and maximal effect of adoptive immunization of virus carriers. Acta path. microbiol. scand. *60:* 577–587 (1964).

VOLKERT, M. and LARSEN, J. H.: Studies on immunological tolerance to LCM virus. 5. The induction of tolerance to the virus. Acta path. microbiol. scand. *63*:161–171(1965a).

VOLKERT, M. and LARSEN, J. H.: Studies on immunological tolerance to LCM virus. 6. Immunity conferred on tolerant mice by immune serum and by grafts of homologous lymphoid cells. Acta path. microbiol. scand. *63:* 172–180 (1965b).

VOLKERT, M. and LARSEN, J. H.: Immunological tolerance to viruses; in: Progr. med. virol., vol. 7, pp. 160–207 (Karger, Basel/New York 1965c).

VOLKERT, M.; LARSEN, J. H., and PFAU, C. J.: Studies on immunological tolerance to LCM virus. 4. The question of immunity in adoptively immunized virus carriers. Acta path. microbiol. scand. *61:* 268–282 (1964).

VOLKERT, M. and LUNDSTEDT, C.: The provocation of latent lymphocytic chorio-meningitis virus infections in mice by treatment with anti-lymphocytic serum. J. exp. Med. *127:* 327–339 (1968).

WAGNER, R. R. and SNYDER, R. M.: Viral interference induced in mice by acute or persistent infection with the virus of lymphocytic choriomeningitis. Nature, Lond. *196:* 393–394 (1962).

WAINWRIGHT, S. and MIMS, C. A.: Plaque assay for lymphocytic choriomeningitis virus based on hemadsorption interference. J. Virology *1:* 1091–1092 (1967).

WALTERS, M. N. I.; JOSKE, R. A.; LEAK, P. J., and STANLEY, N. F.: Murine infection with reovirus. I. Pathology of the acute phase. Brit. J. exp. Path. *44:* 427–436 (1963).

WALTERS, M. N. I.; LEAK, P. J.; JOSKE, R. A.; STANLEY, N. F., and PERRET, D. H.: Murine infection with reovirus. III. Pathology of infections with types 1 and 2. Brit. J. exp. Path. *46:* 200–212 (1965).

WALTON, J. N.: Myopathy in sheep. Lancet *ii:* 841–842 (1956).

WATANABE, S.: Studies on equine infectious anemia virus in tissue culture. II. Serial cultivation of equine infectious anemia virus in the tissue culture derived from the horse and its reversion test to the horse. Jap. J. vet. Sci. *22:* 79–88 (1960).

WAY, R. C.: Cardiovascular defects and the rubella syndrome. Canad. med. Ass. J. *97:* 1329–1334 (1967).

WEBB, H. E.: Viruses and the neuroglia with special reference to scrapie, kuru and disseminated sclerosis. Proc. roy. Soc. Med. *60:* 698–702 (1967).

WEBB, H. E. and SMITH, C. E. G.: Relation of immune response to development of central and nervous system lesions in virus infections of man. Brit. med. J. *2:* 1179–1181 (1966).

WEBB, P.A.; JOHNSON, K. M.; MACKENZIE, R. B., and KUNS, M. L.: Some characteristics of Machupo virus, causative agent of Bolivian hemorrhagic fever. Amer. J. trop. Med. Hyg. *16:* 531–538 (1967).

WEBB, H. E.; WIGHT, D. G. D.; PLATT, G. S., and SMITH, C. E. G.: Langat virus encephalitis in mice. I. The effect of the administration of specific antiserum. J. Hyg. *66:* 343–354 (1968a).

WEBB, H. E.; WIGHT, D. G. D.; WIERNIK, G.; PLATT, G. S., and SMITH, C. E. G.: Langat virus encephalitis in mice. II. The effect of irradiation. J. Hyg. *66:* 355–364 (1968b).

WEBB, H. E.; WETHERLEY-MEIN, G.; MOLOMUT, N., and PADNOS, M.: First cautious trial of MP virus in human cancer cases reported. Antibiotic News, July-Aug., p. 5 (1968c).

WEIGAND, H. and HOTCHIN, J.: Studies of lymphocytic choriomeningitis in mice. II. A comparison of the immune status of newborn and adult mice surviving inoculation. J. Immunol. *86:* 401–406 (1961).

WEILAND, M. H. and HOTCHIN, J. E.: A cytotoxic effect of antiserum on virus-infected cells. N. Y. State Dep. Health Ann. Rep. Div. Lab. Res., pp. 26–27 (1959).

WEISSENBACHER, M. C.; SCHMUÑIS, G. A., and PARODI, A. S.: Junin virus multiplication in thymectomized mice. Effect of thymus and immunocompetent cells grafting. Arch. ges. Virusforsch. *26:* 63–73 (1969).

WELLER, T. H. and HANSHAW, J. B.: Virologic and clinical observations on cytomegalic inclusion disease. New Engl. J. Med. *266:* 1233–1244 (1962).

WELLER, T. H. and ROWE, W. P.: The human cytomegalovirus; in: Diagnostic procedures for viral and Rickettsial diseases, 3rd. ed., p. 707 (Amer. Pub. Hlth. Ass. Inc., New York 1964).

WELLER, T. H.; ALFORD, C. A., jr., and NEVA, F. A.: Retrospective diagnosis by serologic means of congenitally acquired rubella infections. New Engl. J. Med. *270:* 1039–1041 (1964).

WELLER, T. H.; ALFORD, C. A., jr., and NEVA, F. A.: Changing epidemiologic concepts of rubella, with particular reference to unique characteristics of the congenital infection. Yale J. biol. Med. *37:* 455–472 (1965).

WENNER, H. A.: Isolation of LCM virus in an effort to adapt poliomyelitis virus to rodents. J. infect. Dis. *83:* 155–163 (1948).

WHITE, L. R.; LEIKIN, S.; VILLAVICENCIO, O.; ABERNATHY, W.; AVERY, G., and SEVER, J. L.: Immune competence in congenital rubella: Lymphocyte transformation, delayed hypersensitivity, and response to vaccination. J. Pediat. *73:* 229–234 (1968).

WHITNEY, E.: Response of infant and adult mice to lymphocytic choriomeningitis virus infection. Proc. Soc. exp. Biol. N. Y. *78:* 247–250 (1951).

WHITNEY, E.; KRAFT, L. M.; LAWSON, W. B., and GORDON, I.: Noninfectious complement-fixing antigen from embryonated hens' eggs infected with lymphocytic choriomeningitis virus. Abstract Bact. Proc., p. 50 (1953).

WIGHT, P. A. L.: The histopathology of the spinal cord in scrapie disease of sheep. J. comp. Path. *70:* 70–83 (1960).

WIGHT, P. A. L.: The histology of the spinal and sympathetic ganglia and the adrenal glands in scrapie disease of sheep. J. comp. Path. *71:* 53–59 (1961).

WIKTOR, T. J.; FERNANDES, M. V., and KOPROWSKI, H.: Cultivation of rabies virus in human diploid cell strain, WI-38. J. Immunol. *93:* 353–366 (1964).

WIKTOR, T. J.; FERNANDES, M. V., and KOPROWSKI, H.: Detection of a lymphocytic choriomeningitis component in rabies virus preparations. J. Bact. *90:* 1494–1495 (1965).

WIKTOR, T. J.; KAPLAN, M. M., and KOPROWSKI, H.: Rabies and lymphocytic choriomeningitis virus (LCMV). Infection of tissue culture; enhancing effect of LCMV. Ann. med. exp. Fenn. *44:* 290–296 (1966).

WIKTOR, T. J.; KUWERT, E., and KOPROWSKI, H.: Immune lysis of rabies virus-infected cells. J. Immunol. *101:* 1271–1282 (1968).

WILCOX, J. H. and MUSSBAUM, R. E.: Observations on the chromosomes of spleen cells of mice affected with scrapie. Vet. Rec. *82:* 171–172 (1968).

WILLIAMS, R. C., jr.: Anti-γ-globulin factors and immunofluorescent studies in Aleutian disease of mink. NINDB Monograph No. 2. Slow, latent and temperate virus infections, pp. 329–332 (US Dept of Health, Education and Welfare, Washington, D. C. 1965).

WILLIAMS, R. C., jr.; WILLIAMS, L. P., and WOLHEIM, F. A.: Immunoglobulins in mink ranchers associated with Aleutian disease. J. amer. med. Ass. *194:* 135–138 (1965).

WILLIAMS, R. C., jr.; RUSSELL, J. D., and KENYON, A. J.: Anti-gamma-globulin factors and immunofluorescent studies in normal mink and mink with Aleutian disease. Amer. J. vet. Res. *27:* 1455–1460 (1966).

WILSNACK, R. E. and ROWE, W. P.: Immunofluorescent studies of the histopathogenesis of lymphocytic choriomeningitis virus infection. J. exp. Med. *120:* 829–841 (1964).

WILSON, D. R.: Unpublished work 1954 (cit. STAMP *et al.*, J. comp. Path. *69:* 268–280 [1959]).

WILSON, D. R.; ANDERSON, R. D., and SMITH, W.: Studies in scrapie. J. comp. Path. *60:* 267–282 (1950).

WINKLER, U.: Über die fehlende Photo- und Wirtszellreaktivierbarkeit des UV-inaktivierten RNS-Phagen Fr. Photochem. Photobiol. *3:* 37–43 (1964).

WOODS, W. A.; JOHNSON, R. T.; HOSTETLER, D. D.; LEPOW, M. L., and ROBBINS, F. C.: Immunofluorescent studies on rubella-infected tissue cultures and human tissues. J. Immunol. *96:* 253–260 (1966).

WOOLEY, J. G.; ARMSTRONG, C., and ONSTOTT, R. H.: The occurrence in the sera of man and monkeys of protective antibodies against the virus of lymphocytic choriomeningitis as determined by the serum-virus protection test in mice. Publ. Hlth Rep., Wash. *52:* 1105–1114 (1937).

WOOLEY, J. G.; STIMPERT, F. D.; KESSEL, J. F., and ARMSTRONG, C.: A study of human sera antibodies capable of neutralizing the virus of lymphocytic choriomeningitis. Publ. Hlth Rep., Wash. *34:* 938–944 (1939).

WRIGHT, H. T.: Congenital anomalies and viral infections in infants. Calif. Med. *105:* 345–351 (1966).

WYATT, J. P.; SAXTON, J.; LEE, B. S., and PINKERTON, H.: Generalized cytomegalic inclusion disease. J. Pediat. *36:* 271–294 (1950).

YAFFE, D.: The distribution and *in vitro* propagation of an agent causing high plasma lactic dehydrogenase activity. Cancer Res. *22:* 573–580 (1962).

YAOI, H.; NAGATA, A.; GOTO, N., and SAITO, K.: Experimental studies on equine infectious anemia (swamp fever). Report 1. Re-transmission of Arakawa's virus to horse. Arch. ges. Virusforsch. *8:* 621–631 (1958).

YAOI, H.; NAGATA, A.; GOTO, N. et SAITO, K.: Etude expérimentale de l'anémia infectieuse des équidés. 1. Essai de retransmission a des chevaux du virus d'Arakawa. Bull. off. int. Epizoot. *51:* 76–81 (1959a).

YAOI, H.; GOTO, N.; SANO, H., and YAMASAWA, R.: Studies on the virus of equine infectious anemia. Report 2. Neutralization and protection tests with Arakawa's virus. Yokohama med. Bull. *10:* 125–130 (1959b).

YAOI, H.; GOTO, N., and NAGATA, A.: Studies on the virus of equine infectious anemia. Report 5. An attempt of isolating the virus by serial passage in mice by intracerebral route. Yokohama med. Bull. *10:* 265–279 (1959c).

YAOI, H.; NAGATA, A., and SAITO, K.: Studies on the virus of equine infectious anemia. Report 6. Isolation of the virus by serial transmission in rabbits. Yokohama med. Bull. *11:* 1–20 (1960).

YOUN, J. K. and BARSKI, G.: Interference between lymphocytic choriomeningitis and Rauscher leukemia in mice. J. nat. Cancer Inst. *37:* 381–388 (1966).

ZIEGLER, M.: Vergleichende histologische Untersuchungen über die infektiöse, perniziöse und chronische progressive Anämie des Pferdes. Zugleich ein Beitrag zur Frage ihrer einheitlichen Ätiologie und ihrer Pathogenese. Z. Infekt. Krankh. parasit. Krankh. Hyg. Haustiere *25:* 1–8 (1924).

ZIEGLER, M.: Zur Histologie der ansteckenden Blutarmut. Berl. Münch. tierärztl. Wschr. *41:* 751–752 (1925).

ZINDER, N. D.: RNA phages; in: Ann. rev. microbiol., vol. 19, pp. 455–472 (Annual Reviews, Palo Alto 1965).

ZLOTNIK, I.: Vacuolated neurones in sheep affected with scrapie. Nature, Lond. *179:* 737 (1957a).

ZLOTNIK, I.: Significance of vacuolated neurones in the medulla of sheep affected with scrapie. Nature, Lond. *180:* 393–394 (1957b).

ZLOTNIK, I.: The histopathology of the brain stem of sheep affected with natural scrapie. J. comp. Path. *68:* 148–166 (1958).

ZLOTNIK, I.: Cerebellar and midbrain lesions in scrapie. Nature, Lond. *185:* 785 (1960).

ZLOTNIK, I.: The histopathology of the brain of goats affected with scrapie. J. comp. Path. *71:* 440–448 (1961).

ZLOTNIK, I.: The pathology of scrapie: A comparative study of lesions in the brain of sheep and goats. Acta neuropath., suppl. *1:* 61–70 (1962a).

ZLOTNIK, I: A comparative study of early brain lesions of goats inoculated with scrapie goat brain by the intracerebral and the subcutaneous routes. J. comp. Path. *72:* 366–373 (1962b).

ZLOTNIK, I.: The pathology of scrapie. Report of Scrapie Seminar, Washington, D. C., 1964, pp. 213–224 (US Dept. of Agriculture, ARS 91–53, Washington, D. C. 1966a).

ZLOTNIK, I.: The transmission of scrapie to mice and hamsters. Report of Scrapie Seminar, Washington, D. C., 1964, pp. 263–269 (US Dept. of Agriculture, ARS 91–53, Washington, D. C. 1966b).

ZLOTNIK, I.: Spread of scrapie by contact in mice. J. comp. Path. *78:* 19–22 (1968).

ZLOTNIK, I. and BARLOW, R. M.: The transmission of a specific encephalopathy of mink to the goat. Vet. Rec. *81:* 55–56 (1967).

ZLOTNIK, I. and KATIYAR, R. D.: The occurrence of scrapie disease in sheep of the remote Himalayan foothills. Vet. Rec. *73:* 543–544 (1961).

ZLOTNIK, I. and RENNIE, J. C.: The occurrence of vacuolated neurones and vascular lesions in the medullas of apparently healthy sheep. J. comp. Path. *67:* 30–36 (1957).

ZLOTNIK, I. and RENNIE, J. C.: The pathology of the brain of mice inoculated with tissues from scrapie sheep. J. comp. Path. *72:* 360–365 (1962).

ZLOTNIK, I. and RENNIE, J. C.: Further observations on the experimental transmission of scrapie from sheep and goats to laboratory mice. J. comp. Path. *73:* 150–162 (1963).

ZLOTNIK, I. and RENNIE, J. C.: Experimental transmission of mouse passaged scrapie to goats, sheep, rats and hamsters. J. comp. Path. *75:* 147–157 (1965).

ZLOTNIK, I. and RENNIE, J. C.: The effect of heat on the scrapie agent in mouse brain. Brit. J. exp. Path. *48:* 171–179 (1967).

ZLOTNIK, I. and STAMP, J. T.: Scrapie disease of sheep. Wld Neurology *2:* 895–907 (1961).

ZUCKERMAN, A. J.: Viral hepatitis and the Australia/SH antigen. Nature, Lond. *223:* 569–572 (1969).

ZUCKERMAN, A. J. and TAYLOR, P. E.: Persistence of the serum hepatitis (SH-Australia) antigen for many years. Nature, Lond. *223:* 81–82 (1969).